KU-262-487

An Introduction to Complementary Medicine

Edited by Terry Robson BA, DipEd, ND

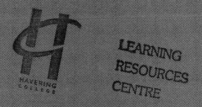

LEARNING
RESOURCES
CENTRE

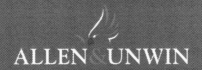

ALLEN & UNWIN

First published in 2003
© this collection Terry Robson 2003
© individual chapters remains with their authors 2003

All rights reserved. No part of this book may be reproduced
or transmitted in any form or by any means, electronic or
mechanical, including photocopying, recording or by any
information storage and retrieval system, without prior permission
in writing from the publisher. The *Australian Copyright Act 1968*
(the Act) allows a maximum of one chapter or 10 per cent of this
book, whichever is the greater, to be photocopied by any educational
institution for its educational purposes provided that the educational
institution (or body that administers it) has given a remuneration
notice to Copyright Agency Limited (CAL) under the Act.

83 Alexander Street,
Crows Nest NSW 2065 Australia
Phone: (61 2) 8425 0100
Fax: (61 2) 9906 2218
E-mail: info@allenandunwin.com
Web: www.allenandunwin.com

National Library of Australia
Cataloguing-in-Publication entry:

Robson, Terry.
  An introduction to complementary medicine.
  Includes index.

ISBN 174114 0544.

1. Alternative medicine. I. Title.

615.5

Set in 11/13 pt Janson Text by Midland Typesetters, Maryborough, Victoria
Printed in Australia by Griffin Press, South Australia

10 9 8 7 6 5 4 3

CONTENTS

PREFACE

A book such as this covers a considerable breadth of territory. It spans Vedic texts, the work of Hippocrates and the latest scientific and medical journals. It journeys through China, India, Australia, Europe, New Zealand, Papua New Guinea, Latin America and the USA. Inevitably its expansive wingspan is dictated by its topic.

Complementary medicine is often defined by the modalities that it encompasses. Additionally it may be seen as denoting a group of theories that share certain central philosophical tenets that fall broadly into the category of holism. However it is delineated, complementary medicine is a broad and inclusive church. Indeed, complementary medicine is such a diverse field that even naming it presents challenges.

The phrase 'complementary and alternative medicine' and the consequent acronym 'CAM' are frequently used to describe the field of medicine covered in this book. Unfortunately, 'alternative' has come to connote 'fringe'. As the reader will discern, however, there is no longer anything marginal about the therapies discussed here. Additionally the 'alternative' must have an initial reference point. This implies that it only has an existence in relation to that predetermining reference point. In this instance the implication would be that the therapeutic modalities covered are but an 'alternative' to the central pillar of medicine, the orthodox approach that bases itself on biomedical principles. Far from this, the approaches to health and illness outlined in this text stand independently of orthodox medicine. Accordingly, it has been decided not to use the word 'alternative' but rather employ the phrase 'complementary medicine' as the descriptor for the content of this text. Additionally, as the Conclusion states and as the whole of the book attests, the future of medicine resides in combining the orthodox medical approach with the philosophies and practices detailed here. Hence the modalities dealt with in this book are truly complementary to orthodox medicine.

While matters of terminology are being addressed it is worth pointing out that the chosen convention for dating in this book is BCE and CE rather than BC and AD. BCE denotes Before Common Era and CE indicates Common Era. They refer to the same time periods as BC and AD respectively. The 'common era' convention is one that is gaining academic currency and, given the broad cultural base of this book, it seemed eminently appropriate.

It is not expected that the contents of this book will be exhaustive of all the fields that fall under the complementary medicine umbrella. Rather, what has been chosen is a representative sample of the core modalities that constitute the practice of complementary medicine in the western world. The omission of a modality does not therefore in any way impugn the efficacy of that modality but simply reflects the limitations of publishing and the fact that lines must be drawn somewhere.

What does exist in this book is the passion and expertise that each of the authors has for their field. In becoming acquainted with this book the reader will also come abreast of the dynamic forces that are contributing to the shape of future medicine. It is not intended as a text that will form the basis of practice in any one modality, but it is a broad guide to each of these therapeutic approaches and how each relates to the broader medical community. It is to be hoped that the wisdom and passion that the reader encounters in these pages will spark their own desire for further exploration of the healing potential that these pages illuminate.

Terry Robson

ACKNOWLEDGEMENTS

Many thanks must go to each of the authors who gave their time, diligence and good humour to the process of bringing this book together. Their chapters represent but the tip of a skilled and passionate dedication to their field. It is with gratitude and admiration that their gift of sharing is recognised.

Thanks are also due to Emma Cant who oversaw the whole process and brought a calm surety to it all.

Finally, I must thank my lovely wife, Davina. Without her enduring love and gentle support an endeavour such as this would be utterly impossible.

T J R
Sydney 2003

CONTRIBUTORS

Stephen Andrew BA, BEd(Counselling)
Stephen Andrew is based in Melbourne, Australia, and teaches counselling theory and
practice at La Trobe University and Swinburne University. He runs a private practice
and counsels clients who access the Gambler's Help organisation. Stephen holds a
Bachelor of Arts majoring in psychology and philosophy and a Bachelor of Education
specialising in counselling. He is registered as a psychologist in Victoria, Australia.

Alan Bensoussan PhD
Alan Bensoussan is the Director of the Centre for Complementary Medicine
Research and Head of the Chinese Medicine Unit at the University of Western
Sydney. Dr Bensoussan has been in clinical practice in Chinese medicine for twenty
years and is an active researcher. He has published two books and works in an
advisory capacity for both government and industry and frequently serves as a
short-term consultant to the World Health Organization.

Simon Borg-Olivier MSc, BAppSc(Physiotherapy), MAPA
Simon Borg-Olivier has been teaching yoga for twenty years and is co-director of
'Yoga Synergy'. Simon graduated from the University of Sydney with a Bachelor
of Science in human biology and mathematics, a Master of Science in molecular
biology and Bachelor of Applied Science in physiotherapy. As well as conducting
yoga classes Simon regularly travels throughout Australasia teaching the applied
anatomy and physiology of hatha yoga.

Karen Bridgman MAppSc(Social Ecology), MSc(Hons), PhD, ND, BDM, DipHom
Karen Bridgman lectures at the University of Western Sydney, is a consultant to
the manufacturing industry and runs an organic herb business. She holds a
Master of Applied Science in social ecology, a Master of Science (Honours) and
a Doctor of Philosophy, with a doctorate entitled '"Her-story" and mythology
of women in medicine'. Karen has practised as a naturopath and herbalist for
22 years and is currently working in a medical practice and in a private
pathology laboratory.

Phillip S. Ebrall BAppSc(Chiropractic), PhD, FICC
Phillip Ebrall is a senior lecturer in Chiropractic with RMIT University Melbourne. Dr Ebrall is a member of the editorial board of the *Chiropractic Journal of Australia, Journal of Manipulative and Physiological Therapeutics* and *Clinical Chiropractic*, and an advisor/consultant to Chiropractic Education Australia. He has published a number of chapters in chiropractic texts, almost 50 papers in the indexed, peer-reviewed chiropractic literature and is the author of the textbook *Assessment of the Spine*. Dr Ebrall gained his PhD in 2000 and is a Fellow of the International College of Chiropractors.

Nicole Heneka ND, DBM, DipNut, DipHom, DRM
Nicole Heneka is a naturopath, health consultant and lecturer. She currently lectures at Nature Care College, Sydney, Australia, and has previously lectured at other natural therapy colleges in Sydney. Nicole has been in private practice since 1994 and is the author of several in-house textbooks and research papers covering areas such as nutritional biochemistry, the Bach Flowers and botanical medicine.

Ian Howden BCom, ARoH
Ian has been in private practice as a homœopath for over 25 years. Since 1996 he has been foundation lecturer in homœopathy in the Bachelor of Naturopathy degree at Southern Cross University in New South Wales. In the 1970s Ian taught sociology at the University of New South Wales and the University of Wollongong and he has published in the areas of sociology, flower essences and homœopathy. He is active in research and has a particular interest in anthroposophical medicine. Thanks are due to Dr Tom Jagtenberg for his invaluable contribution to Chapter 11.

Assunta Hunter BA(Hons), ND, MWH
Assunta Hunter is a lecturer in complementary medicine at the Australian Centre for Complementary Medicine Education and Research (ACCMER), a joint venture of the University of Queensland and Southern Cross University. She has a Masters degree from Melbourne University in women's health and has an active research interest in the role of herbal medicine in this area. She is a practising herbalist and has been involved in naturopathic education for eighteen years.

Nicholas Lucas BSc, MHSc(Osteopathy)
Nicholas Lucas is a lecturer in osteopathic medicine in the School of Exercise and Health Sciences at the University of Western Sydney, Sydney, Australia. He is a registered osteopath and a director of Sydney Musculoskeletal Medicine, a clinic in Sydney specialising in the diagnosis and management of syndromes associated with musculoskeletal pain and dysfunction. He is also an editor of the *Journal of Osteopathic Medicine*.

Bianca Machliss BSc, BAppSc(Physiotherapy), MAPA
Bianca Machliss is co-director of 'Yoga Synergy' and has been teaching yoga since 1990. Bianca has a Bachelor of Science in human biology and psychology and a Bachelor of Applied Science in physiotherapy from the University of Sydney. Bianca teaches to hundreds of yoga students each week and is actively engaged in training yoga teachers to become safe and effective complementary health practitioners.

Martha Macintyre BA(Hons), CertSocAnth, PhD
Martha Macintyre is senior lecturer in medical anthropology at the Centre for the Study of Health and Society at the University of Melbourne. She has conducted research into economic development, social change and health in Papua New Guinea and on immigrant women's health in Australia.

Shaun Matthews MB, BCh, CertAyuMed, Cert. Yoga Teacher Training
Dr Shaun Matthews lectures at the School of Public Health and Community Medicine at the University of New South Wales and coordinates the faculty of Ayurvedic Studies at Nature Care College in Sydney. Shaun studied medicine in Ireland and Australia and has been a general practitioner since 1992. He has trained in Ayurveda at Gujarat Ayurveda University and Yoga Teacher Training at the Bihar School of Yoga in India. He is in private practice at the Bondi Whole Health Centre in Sydney.

Robert Moran BSc, BSc, MHSc(Osteopathy)
Robert Moran is a research fellow and lecturer in osteopathy in the School of Health Science, at UNITEC Institute of Technology, Auckland, New Zealand. He is a qualified osteopath and director of PhysiqueCare, a clinic in Auckland specialising in osteopathy and Pilates rehabilitation. He is also an editor of the *Journal of Osteopathic Medicine*.

Stephen P. Myers PhD, BMed, ND
Stephen Myers is the Director of the Australian Centre for Complementary Medicine Education and Research (ACCMER), a joint venture of the University of Queensland and Southern Cross University. Until 2001 he was the Foundation Head of the School of Natural and Complementary Medicine at Southern Cross University, Lismore, Australia, where he still plays an active role. He initially qualified as a naturopathic practitioner and later in western medicine. He has a PhD in basic and clinical pharmacology. His current passion is to play a role in building an active research culture in complementary medicine.

Kylie A. O'Brien BAppSc(Chinese Medicine), BSc(Optometry), MPH
Kylie O'Brien holds a Bachelor of Applied Science in Chinese medicine, Bachelor of Science in Optometry and Masters of Public Health and is a registered Chinese medicine practitioner in Victoria. She works in the Department of Medicine, Monash Medical School, conducting research into complementary medicine and Chinese medicine, and has also worked in the Department of Human Services on the implementation of the *Chinese Medicine Registration Act 2000*. She is actively involved in the development of Chinese medicine education.

Corinne G. Patching van der Sluijs BHlthSc(Chinese Herbal Medicine), BSc(Biology), DipEd
After completing a Bachelor of Science in biology and a Diploma of Secondary Education at Murdoch University, Perth, Corinne Patching van der Sluijs spent several years teaching at a large international school in Hong Kong. She then completed a Bachelor of Health Sciences in Chinese Herbal Medicine at the University of Technology, Sydney, being awarded the University Medal. She is currently conducting postgraduate research on menopause at the University of Western Sydney.

Terry Robson BA, DipEd, ND
Terry Robson works as a health journalist and is a health reporter for radio and television networks around Australia. Terry is a fully qualified naturopath (Nature Care College) who has worked in private practice, the manufacture of complementary medicines and as deputy editor of *International WellBeing* magazine. He holds a Bachelor of Arts (Australian National University) majoring in psychology and ancient history/archaeology and a Diploma of Education (University of Sydney).

Pamela Snider ND
Pamela Snider is a naturopathic physician and professor of Naturopathic Clinical Theory at Bastyr University, Seattle. From 1994 to 2003 she was Associate Dean for the Naturopathic Medicine Program and Public and Professional Affairs at Bastyr. She was appointed to the federal Medicare Coverage Advisory Committee in February 2003. Pamela is a leading North American spokesperson in integrative healthcare and naturopathic medicine with an emphasis on interdisciplinary collaboration and public health.

Vicki M. Tuchtan BAppSc(PhysEd), AdDip(Myotherapy), GradDipAroma
Vicki Tuchtan is currently the National Head of Teaching and Learning at the Australian College of Natural Medicine, and is undertaking a doctoral thesis at the Queensland University of Technology researching massage and pain management. A physical educator with clinical experience in massage and myotherapy, Vicki has lectured extensively in bioscience and manual therapies and is also undertaking a Masters in education. Vicki writes a regular column, titled 'Acting Naturally', for the *Courier-Mail* newspaper.

Mark A. Webb BSc, DipAroma, DRM
Mark Webb has a Bachelor of Science degree in biochemistry and plant biology and diplomas in Aromatherapy and Remedial Massage. Mark is currently continuing with additional studies in aromatic and botanical medicine. His career in aromatherapy includes researching, teaching, clinical practice and writing. He is the author of *Bush Sense—Australian Essential Oils and Aromatic Compounds*.

Ian White BSc, ND, DBM
Ian White is the founder of the Australian Bush Flower Essences and a fifth-generation Australian herbalist. After obtaining his Bachelor of Science from the University of New South Wales and graduating from the New South Wales College of Natural Therapies, Ian has practised as a naturopath for 25 years. Ian continues to develop the bush essence range and is the author of three major books. He runs regular seminars and workshops on the bush essences in over 30 countries.

Hans Wohlmuth BSc, ND, MNHAA
Hans Wohlmuth is a lecturer in pharmacognosy and phytotherapy in the School of Natural and Complementary Medicine at Southern Cross University, Lismore, Australia. He trained in natural medicine in Denmark and has a degree in biological science from Macquarie University. Hans is a former herbal practitioner and executive member of the National Herbalists Association of Australia and the author of an introductory botany text. He acts as a consultant to government and the medicinal plant industry and is actively engaged in medicinal plant research.

Charlie Changli Xue BMed, PhD, FAACMA, RCMP
Charlie Changli Xue holds a Bachelor of Medicine in Chinese medicine and a PhD. He is the Head of the Chinese Medicine Unit and Director of the Chinese Medicine Research Group at RMIT University. He serves as a short-term consultant to the World Health Organization on a regular basis and has been a member of the Chinese Medicine Registration Board of Victoria since 2000. He has been leading the development of Chinese medicine education and research at RMIT since 1995. Since 1987 Dr Xue has had teaching, research, clinical practice and academic administration experience in mainland China, Hong Kong and Australia.

Jared L. Zeff ND, LAc
Jared Zeff is a member of the faculty at Bastyr University, Seattle, and teaches in the naturopathic medicine program. He holds degrees in science and naturopathic medicine and maintains a private practice in Vancouver, Washington. He has been in private practice since 1979, but has maintained a dual career, teaching in naturopathic medical colleges, where he earned a full professorship in 1988. From 1988 to 1993 he served as Academic Dean at National College.

FOREWORD
By Joseph E. Pizzorno, ND

One of the challenges of naming our medicine as 'complementary' or 'alternative' is that, right at the start, it defines us by what we are not rather than by what we are. The problem is magnified by defining us by the therapies we use rather than the philosophies that inform the care we provide. Not only does this approach define us inaccurately, it lumps in practices, practitioners and interventions that have little or no relationship to our systems of healing, other than being non-conventional, and often are a public risk. In a perfect world, how would we be named, how would we be defined?

I would use the term 'natural medicine', not because Nature is the source of our therapies, but rather because Nature is the source of our healing philosophies. What makes our medicine special and appealing to the public is our profound belief in the powerful healing ability within each unique individual. When appropriately applied, our therapies support and enhance each individual's unique ability to heal. While all have this innate healing ability, each manifests it in utterly unique ways. This requires a high level of personalisation of therapy to effectively provide natural health care, another of the reasons patients are attracted to us.

An Introduction to Complementary Medicine does an admirable job of describing the philosophies of the natural medicine professions, their historic origins and the appropriate use of their healing modalities.

If the past defined us as alternative and the present defines us by our philosophies, how might we be defined in the future? I think this will be primarily determined by the choices each of the natural healing professions makes in the areas of research and education. Our practice protocols and clinical efficacy have until now been driven by our philosophical precepts and historic therapies. The past two decades have seen a dramatic, and welcome, increase in research establishing the efficacy (or, in some cases, lack of efficacy) of the natural healing therapies and advancing our understanding of their mechanisms of action. With this improved understanding of our therapies should come an increased ability to more accurately and effectively apply them to our patients. How might we achieve this improvement in quality of care?

I believe that the major advances in our understanding of genomics and functional testing will provide, for the first time, a sound scientific basis for the therapy personalisation that is so welcomed by our patients, but so difficult to achieve with the tools available to us in the past. The Ayurvedic doshas, the Traditional Chinese Medicine five elements, the Naturopathic Medicine body types and the Homœopathic constitutions, all share the common characteristic of attempting to categorise and define individual physiological uniqueness. As better tools become available to enable us better understand not only how our therapies work, but the unique physiology of each patient, we can more accurately personalise the care we provide.

Achieving this will require research that looks at the integration of philosophy, therapies and patient uniqueness. Once we have better elicited and documented how these interact, we then need to inform our educational systems to ensure that both new and existing practitioners are able to practise an ever improving quality of care.

An Introduction to Complementary Medicine is a good textbook on what *is*. Many of those who read this book will the architects of what *will be*. I believe strongly that just as the tools of rigorous, objective scientific inquiry dramatically improved the safety and efficacy of conventional medicine, so too will application of those tools to natural medicine dramatically advance our safety and efficacy. However, we must be very thoughtful in what we research. Frankly, I see very limited value in comparing the efficacy of St John's wort to Prozac. Yes, we do want to know which works best, is safest and costs least. But is natural medicine really about substituting a green drug for a synthetic one? I think not.

Of far greater importance is subjecting our philosophies and precepts to scientific rigour. Some may fear this, in the belief that western biomedical understanding and tools are not suitable for such an investigation. Perhaps this is true in some instances. Clearly, randomised clinical trials of therapies isolated from the context in which they are normally used are not a valid study of healing systems or the personalisation of care they provide. Nonetheless, investigation of clinical outcomes can be accomplished regardless of philosophy or therapy. If we choose, for example, to detoxify a patient, then regardless of the method used we should be able to document an objective change in the patient's health, independent of practitioner effects.

I believe the future of the natural healing professions to be very bright. Accompanying the growing public and professional acceptance and understanding of our therapies is a growing body of research documenting their efficacy. The profound wisdom of natural medicine, combined with the remarkable physiological understanding of modern medical science, provides the foundation for a much needed revolution in healthcare.

INTRODUCTION

The evolving medical paradigm
Terry Robson

The notion of the 'status quo' in a living system is a myth. Stasis does not occur in any living entity or network. Medicine deals with life and hence is alive itself. Naturally, then, it is no surprise that the philosophical model of medicine under which the western world has operated for the better part of the twentieth century is changing fundamentally. While change in life is always confronting it is equally inevitable. The true question lies not in whether the current dominant medical paradigm will change but rather how it will change.

The particular phase of evolution facing twenty-first century medicine is unique but not entirely new. Global mythology reveals that the quest for a world-view that yields health and wellbeing is timeless. In Central African mythology there is a dangerous one-legged, one-armed half man known as the 'Chiruwi', or 'mysterious thing'. This creature challenges anyone he encounters to a fight with the promise that if vanquished he will reveal many medicines and the lucky victor will become skilled in the healing arts (Campbell 1993). Perhaps western medicine is currently in the process of dealing with a cultural Chiruwi.

Another mythical figure relevant to the medical situation of the third millennium comes in the form of the Greek God of the mountainside, Pan. This playful and energetic god could be fearsome and he instilled in humans who ventured carelessly into his domain a sudden and groundless fright, or 'pan-ic'. On the other hand Pan offered bounty to those who honoured him. To these worshippers he would offer health and the wisdom to reach the universal source (Campbell 1993).

In an unconscious homage to Pan and the Chiruwi there is a distinct global movement to embrace something beyond the biomedical model of medicine that has been the beloved child of science. Global organisations, governments, science and individuals are turning in ever greater numbers to the complementary paradigm of medicine. In a sense, there is a metaphoric move toward honouring the nature god Pan in the hope that perhaps he will offer the wisdom that will lead to truly fundamental healing. This is not to say that there is a mood to discard totally the advances of biomedical medicine. A Luddite yearning for simpler days past will not move medicine forward. Rather what is occurring is the shaping of a post-modern medical paradigm.

Terms of engagement

To begin a discussion of the changes that are taking place in medicine it is necessary to define terms. For much of the twentieth century the biomedical model was the dominant medical paradigm and we will refer to it as 'orthodox medicine'. It features a drug and surgical approach to disease management. Underpinning these curative tools is a scientific and reductionist attitude toward the human body that tracks disease to its biochemical roots.

Essentially the orthodox philosophy sees medical science as applied biology and its practitioners as diagnostic biochemists. It is based on the principle of Cartesian Dualism which implies that, even if there were no mind in it, the nerves, muscles and blood vessels of the body would have the same functions. This separation of mind and body was espoused by Rene Descartes in the seventeenth century and has served as the underpinning of the orthodox approach since that time.

The separation of mind and body paved the way for the development of a medical approach based on measurable quantities. This was what allowed medicine to become a science and possess directly predictive properties. The dualist notion was born just as the scientific revolution of the seventeenth century was under way. Isaac Newton's mechanistic theories were emerging and it was only natural that the orthodox science of medicine came to view the human body as a machine (Foss 2002). Orthodox medicine has been incredibly successful. It has prolonged lives and, along with improvements in hygiene, been part of a social and medical milieu that has seen many diseases eradicated. Yet the latter part of the twentieth century and now the twenty-first century has seen a widespread movement toward another medical model.

'Complementary medicine' is a term that encompasses a range of practices and philosophies. Some are ancient and some are relatively new but what they have in common is that they are based on theories or explanatory mechanisms that are not in keeping with the orthodox biomedical model (Bensoussan 1999). Some of the leading medical modalities that come under the heading of 'complementary medicine' are featured in Part 2 of this book including among their number herbal medicine, homœopathy, acupuncture, nutrition, massage and counselling. These modalities are diverse but they hold common central attitudes. Complementary medicine rejects the dualism of orthodox philosophy while accepting the science of medicine. Fundamentally, complementary modalities embrace 'a concept of medicine as a science of the human person and insist on an understanding of disease as something that involves a systemic dislocation of the whole person, not just of the body' (Foss 2002: 126).

Within complementary medical modalities there are variations on this philosophy (see Part 2) yet the holistic view that health is a dynamic interplay between mind, body and spirit is common to all. Certainly the premises of complementary medicine are finding increasing support with scientists, governments and people the world over.

The people

On a global scale there is substantial and justifiable acceptance of the many benefits that orthodox medicine brings. Simultaneously, however, the western world, birthplace of orthodox medicine, is embracing complementary medicine in an emphatic way. The World Health Organization (WHO) estimates that the global market for complementary therapies stands at 60 billion US dollars a year and is growing steadily. This represents a worldwide trend that is reflected in individual countries in significant ways.

Data from the British parliament support the idea that complementary medicine use in Britain is high and is increasing. In 1999 in Britain 93 million pounds was spent on complementary medicine and five million Britons visited the 50 000 complementary practitioners who operate there. By 2002 the amount that Britons spent on complementary medicines had risen to 126 million pounds (Reuters 2002). Australia is also experiencing an exponential increase in the use of complementary medicine. It is estimated that Australians spent 2.3 billion Australian dollars on complementary therapies and medicine in the year 2000, which is a 120 per cent increase on what they spent in 1993 (MacLennan *et al.* 2002). Overall in 2000 Australian people spent four times more money from their pockets on complementary medicine than they spent on prescription drugs.

The same report (MacLennan 2002) indicated that in the USA expenditure on complementary medicines in 2000 was 34 billion US dollars. The popularity of complementary medicine with the American people is widely attested. Nearly 68 per cent of all American adults have used at least one complementary therapy at some time in their lives and of these 50 per cent continue to use complementary medicine twenty years later (Eisenberg *et al.* 2001). High retention rates such as this reflect the fact that complementary medicine and its philosophy can become a way of life for those who use it. A more recent study (Rivera *et al.* 2002) based in El Paso, Texas, suggests that the number of people using complementary medicine may be still increasing. This study found that 77 per cent of those surveyed were using complementary medicine.

In France 75 per cent of the population has used complementary medicine at least once and in Germany 77 per cent of pain clinics provide acupuncture (WHO 2002a). In Germany as well, a study of adults with hayfever, asthma, eczema and food allergies found that more than one in four of these people used complementary medicine to treat their allergic condition (Schafer *et al.* 2002). Of these people 78 per cent used the complementary treatments because they assumed there would be fewer side effects. Although the assumption that 'natural is safe' is a fallacious one, the perceived relative safety of complementary medicine is proving a significant factor in driving people to embrace it as part of their health regime. Equally, however, people clearly perceive that complementary medicine is efficacious.

A study from a New York City pain clinic (von Peter *et al.* 2002) found that 85 per cent of patients had used complementary medicine to relieve their pain. Further, 60 per cent believed that their complementary medicines had worked. This points to the fact that the ground swell of support for complementary medicine is not arising out of some misguided search for absent nurturing or 'feel-good' treatments. When it comes to choosing health options individuals are pragmatic enough to insist that their treatments are efficacious. Often, people will turn to complementary medicine if they perceive that orthodox medicine is not delivering the health outcomes they desire (Bensoussan 1999). The surging tide of pragmatism that is seeing people across the world turn to a combination of orthodox and complementary medicine is leading science to address the wisdom that lies in these complementary therapies.

The science

In the face of immense public interest science is turning its attention to the question of health and health management. As this process occurs what is unfolding is that, both on a philosophical and fundamental level, science can embrace and learn from a 'complementary' approach to healing.

Bodies of intelligence

As has been suggested above, complementary medicine treats the body as a holistic organism with dynamic processes that operate to keep that body in balance. Implicit to this paradigm is the acceptance that all parts of a human being are connected and that disease in one area can result from imbalance in another area. This conflicts with the traditional approach of orthodox medicine that targets symptoms in discrete body areas. Evolving scientific theory, however, is finding ways to encompass the holistic philosophy.

One of the newer scientific world-views is complexity theory. This theory is applied to a variety of fields including ecology, physics, economics and computing where complex structures exist. In essence, complexity theory holds that once the rules governing these systems are found, it is possible to make effective predictions and even to control apparently complex entities. One salient point that is also emerging from complexity theory is that the properties of the system cannot necessarily be tracked to individual components but arise from the whole system. The implications of this notion for medicine are clear.

If complexity theory holds true then disease arises from the whole body, not its discrete parts. Effectively, pathology arises 'when the body self-organises in response to some disturbance but becomes confused and ends up worse at self-regulation than before' (Hyland 2001: 33). In this light the mechanistic notions of orthodox medicine cannot hope to achieve cure but can only patch holes in the network that is the human body. Under complexity theory, genes, lifestyle and environment all interact to impact on the network that is the human body and the result is either disease or health. This paradigm is coincident with theories of holistic healing and reflects that at the true sharp end of science, the underpinnings of holistic medicine are being reinforced. The complete coalescence of science and complementary theory will not happen immediately. Nevertheless the signs and symptoms that science is actively considering complementary medicine are manifold.

Everything old . . .

Deliberate investigation of complementary medicines is taking place within the orthodox scientific establishment in many ways. As the bibliography for this book attests, there is a plethora of studies in the medical and scientific journals examining the components of complementary medicine from acupuncture to herbal medicine to yoga. A striking illustration of modern science meeting traditional methods is research in Wales that may result in a 600-year-old book yielding new drugs.

In a village called Myddfai in Wales in the early thirteenth century a physician called Rhiwallon founded a line of healers that spread throughout the Welsh land. This line of physicians persisted for hundreds of years but around the year 1400 the Myddfai healers penned their most important text, the *Red Book of Hergest*. Contained in this book were over 500 remedies using more than 200 different plants. Modern pharmacists are engaged in examining the Myddfai cures to see what chemicals they may yield that can be turned into pharmaceutical drugs (Whitfield 2002). Similar pursuits are occurring in the southern hemisphere.

In Australia the Commonwealth Scientific and Industrial Research Organisation (CSIRO) has announced that it will be turning considerable attention to the investigation of the healing properties of herbs. In addition to examining traditional western herbs such as garlic, the CSIRO also intends to examine native plants for their economic and medicinal potential. The dilemma facing scientific inquiry into herbs is that isolating so-called 'active ingredients' from herbs violates holistic principles and is likely to have a negative effect on efficacy. Still, interest is the first step toward understanding.

Herbs, however, are not the only ancient medicines that are experiencing a rising tide of scientific interest. If ever there was a symbol through which the orthodox medical establishment has expressed its disdain for the healing wisdom that had passed before, it was the leech. The image of patients festooned with leeches has been emblematic of the supposed naivety of historical healing. Indeed, the leech was a popular medical tool throughout much of history. Babylonian writings suggest that the leech was being used medicinally as long as 3500 years ago. The Egyptians also embraced leeches as healing tools and the Europeans took up the annelids with equal verve. So popular was leech therapy with medieval European healers that physicians of this time were actually known as 'leeches' (Fields 1991). It is estimated that by 1850 French physicians were using 100 million leeches per year so it is not surprising that in the nineteenth century the European leech was dancing along the edge of extinction.

Medicinal leeches were used over the centuries for bloodletting and were applied to congested or inflamed parts of the human body. Many ailments were subjected to the application of leeches. In America in the nineteenth century, leeches were used as a common home remedy to treat gum disorders and haemorrhoids, and to relieve the pain of large bruises (Fields 1991). The advent of improved understanding of bacteriology and infection in the latter nineteenth century led to a significant focus on hygiene and a drop in popularity for the leech. Thus in the twentieth century, orthodox medicine scoffed at the apparently farcical adherence to the leech therapy of earlier centuries. In the last decade of the second millennium CE, however, leeches have made a medical comeback.

It has been found that in cases of venous congestion, where re-establishing the flow of blood is essential, leeches have great therapeutic value. As they consume their meal of blood, leeches promote blood flow through the tissue. Even after a leech is full of blood and detaches from the body, the anticoagulants it secretes into the tissue allow the wound to ooze blood for hours afterwards. These effects cannot be replicated by application to the site of anticoagulants such as heparin. Evidence is also growing to support the pain-relieving effects of leeches for conditions such as arthritis.

One study has evaluated the effectiveness of leeches in relieving arthritis of the knee (Michaelsen *et al.* 2002). This study took place at the University of Essen, Germany, and involved sixteen patients with confirmed osteoarthritis of the knee. Ten of the patients were treated with leeches and six were controls. For those in the leech group, four leeches were applied around the knee joint for a period of 80 minutes each day. Both the control and the leech group were given conventional treatment for pain excluding non-steroidal anti-inflammatories. Those in the leech group experienced a rapid relief of pain which was faster than those in the control group, with sustained improvement after four weeks and no major complications. This is just one of many studies reporting that leech therapy can reduce pain and improve joint mobility in arthritis. To testify that orthodox medicine is genuinely interested in leeches, there are moves afoot to develop mechanical leeches that secrete chemicals similar to real leeches but which are also insatiable. Time will tell whether a mechanical leech can provide all of the subtle benefits that the living creature can yield. This is not to particularly advocate leech therapy, but to illustrate that science is increasingly validating ancient medical wisdom.

Nutrients or nutraceuticals

At the most basic level food is the root of health and, perforce, disease. The axiom that food should be synonymous with medicine has now passed into popular consciousness and parlance. Perhaps the most tangible manifestation of the acceptance by orthodox science and medicine of the curative power of nutrition is the development of what are known as 'functional foods' or 'nutraceuticals'.

Since the British navy realised that limes could ward off scurvy, three centuries of investigation has revealed that food contains substances that are vital to health. In that time many vitamins and minerals have been discovered. In the early part of the twenty-first century, however, another revolution is taking place in the foods available to human beings. The modern diet is based on a few central plants that have been domesticated and bred to be increasingly bland. This narrowing and blanching of the human food chain has resulted in a relative deficiency of health-promoting substances in the average western diet. The missing substances are neither nutrients nor toxins but lie somewhere in between and their lack is resulting in modern humans being 'pharmacologically impoverished' (Tudge 2001). To make up for this deficit, modern science has turned its attention to the development of 'nutraceuticals'.

These nutraceuticals are foods that richly supply the consumer with substances that are generally missing from modern food but which are health promoting. Leading among these are yoghurts containing *Lactobacillus* bacteria and margarines fortified with plant sterols. It is estimated that by the year 2006 the market in nutraceuticals will be worth 35.4 billion US dollars annually (Datamonitor 2002). This is not to advocate nutraceuticals, as the option of consuming a greater diversity of fruit and vegetables would be a premium, and far preferable, strategy in establishing health. Nevertheless this immensely popular sector of health management reflects clearly that orthodox science and the medicine that it inspires has embraced one of the premises of complementary medicine, which is the simple notion that lifestyle, including diet, has real and significant impacts on health.

Thus on many levels orthodox medicine and complementary medicine are already moving together. At government and bureaucratic levels, this move is happening at an even more rapid pace.

The bureaucracy

Simon Mills, respected British medical herbalist, has put the situation succinctly: 'Public demand for complementary medicine has grown to a level where communication and co-operation with orthodox health services is necessary' (Mills 2001: 160). Perhaps the most significant recognition of this fact has come from the World Health Organization (WHO).

In light of the sweeping interest in complementary medicine the WHO has released a detailed policy paper on this topic (WHO 2002b). As a starting point the WHO defines 'traditional medicine' as including diverse medical practices incorporating plant, animal and mineral-based medicines, spiritual therapies, manual techniques and exercises. In areas such as Africa, Asia and Latin America traditional medicine is often used to meet primary healthcare needs and is also part of a wider belief system and is considered a part of everyday life and wellbeing. The WHO observes that in the western world where orthodox medicine has been the dominant paradigm, complementary medicine is the manifestation of traditional medicine. Going further, the WHO indicates that the reason for the western world's turn toward complementary medicine is 'concern about the adverse effects of chemical medicines, a desire for more personalised health care and greater public access to health information' (WHO 2002b: 1). In light of these trends the WHO has made several significant recommendations.

First, the WHO has observed that as of the year 2000, 25 countries reported having a national traditional medicine policy. These policies are recommended to other countries with recommendations to create legal mechanisms that will promote equity in access to traditional/complementary medicines and to ensure sound practice and efficacy of the therapies provided. In saying this the WHO acknowledges that for complementary therapies:

> . . . their common basis is a holistic approach to life, equilibrium between the mind, body and the environment and an emphasis on health rather than disease. Generally, the provider focuses on the overall condition of the individual patient rather than on the particular ailment or disease from which the patient may be suffering. This more complex approach to health care makes traditional/complementary medicine very attractive to many. But it also makes scientific evaluation highly difficult since so many factors must be taken into account (WHO 2002b: 2).

Broadly the WHO has four major objectives regarding complementary medicine:

- **To integrate complementary/traditional medicine with national health-care systems.**
- **To promote the safety and quality of complementary medicines.**
- **To increase affordability and access to complementary medicines.**
- **To promote therapeutically sound use of complementary medicine by both users and providers.**

It is encouraging that such a high-level bureaucracy recognises that complementary medicine is an integral component of a future medical paradigm. Such recognition, however, can be a two-edged sword. Around the world the orthodox medical establishment is staking its claim to evaluate complementary medicine. In the USA the Congress has created the National Centre for Complementary and Alternative Medicine (NCCAM) at the National Institute of Health. The centre's mission is to explore complementary healing practices in the context of science (Nahin & Straus 2001). In New Zealand the government has decided that orthodox medical bodies are not qualified to evaluate complementary remedies. Similarly in Australia the Complementary Medicines Evaluation Committee includes complementary medicine practitioners, suppliers and scientists. By contrast, however, in the European Union a series of directives threaten to curtail complementary medicine availability, particularly in Britain. All this is an inevitable consequence of the nexus of change in which society, and medicine, finds itself.

Notwithstanding such pitfalls there is certainly a mood abroad to see medicine step to a new level that incorporates orthodox and complementary medicine. The twenty-first century is a post-modern era and medicine is evolving to meet the needs of its time.

Post-modern medicine

There was a time when the term 'modern' was synonymous with 'good' or 'best'. Possibly as a result of the Darwinian revolution in thought, the 'modern' was conceived to be at the apex and what had passed before was, by definition, lesser. Such a view is increasingly holding less credence. There is a rising perception that the philosophical milieu must itself evolve to a new level if the planet and the individuals on it are to survive. In essence, a yearning for something beyond the modern is emerging. Hence in many spheres post-modern schools of thought are arising.

'Modernity' could be said to correspond to the changes of the Industrial Age and perhaps to have begun in the mid-eighteenth century. Under the 'modern' paradigm science provides the ultimate model for understanding. Science is theoretically neutral and objective and scientists are ideally supposed to operate through their unbiased, rational capacities. Of course, whether such a 'disembodied scholar' can ever exist is problematic and a debate unto itself. The post-modern world by contrast coincides roughly with the Information Age and its parameters are fundamentally different from that which has passed before. In the post-modern reality, knowledge cannot be divorced from ethical considerations. The mechanical dictums of the Industrial Revolution are no longer enough and methodologies that encompass more than the strictly measurable are in demand. In medicine this is manifesting as the turn away from reductionist biochemistry toward the holistic notions of complementary healing. The exact shape of post-modern medicine remains to be elucidated, yet a few elements of it are already clear.

The health paradigm of the twentieth century treated the human body as if it were a car that could simply be repaired with a quick trip to the garage, otherwise known as the doctor's surgery. The post-modern view is that visible symptoms both mask and arise from deeper problems that might not be physical, or tangible, at all (Theobald 1999). Implicit to this model is that the patient must look within themselves, rather than only to a doctor or practitioner, when a disease occurs. In the Information Age, every person has the right, and the access, to information about their health and illness. Physicians are no longer the repositories of exclusive knowledge but are expert partners to the individual in their healing process. Thus an individual operating under the post-modern medical model has far greater responsibility for their health and commensurate control over their own healing process. This humanising and individuation of the medical process is a significant driver of the need for a more subjective notion of healing as opposed to the objectivism of the scientific biomedical model. People have an innate sense that they are more than a collection of chemicals. This innate sense of a greater synthesising force has been evidenced throughout history by the diverse manifestations of religion across time and geography. Hence, post-modern medicine approaches health from the perspective of the whole person.

New models for medicine are evolving in response to the post-modern ethos. They go by such names as psychobiology, somatic psychotherapy, psychosomatic medicine and biopsychosocial medicine. In some senses they are new in that they incorporate the elements of the biomedical model and then expand upon it. Yet they are also old in that the principles they espouse have been abroad for millennia and enunciated by philosophies like Ayurveda and Traditional Chinese Medicine. Fundamentally, the post-modern medical paradigm accepts that mind and body are not discrete but are inextricably bound. Beyond this, where biomedicine conceived matter as being divisible into atomic fundamentals, the post-modern paradigm recognises that matter is composed of systems of energy and information transfer. Information can be transferred at any level. Within any one person the nervous, endocrine and immune systems are in constant communication (Conlan 1999). Externally the individual communicates through both verbal and physical language. Disruptions in the energetic and informational state of the individual can lead to illness. Thus under the post-modern view, all levels of the individual must be addressed to achieve healing. The biopsychosocial model is a useful illustration of this approach.

Biopsychosocial medicine was developed by Dr George Engel and was first clearly enunciated by him in 1977. Engel began as a devoted student of the biomedical model of medicine but soon came to an appreciation of the role of the psyche in illness. His understanding of ulcerative colitis is illustrative of his philosophy. Through his own work Engel observed that ulcerative colitis was a disease of the bowel mucosa with implication of the vascular system. In addition, however, Engel examined 700 cases of ulcerative colitis and found personality traits that predisposed to the disease. He found that ulcerative colitis patients tended to be compulsive, dependent and had problems with relationships that stemmed from a retention of the mother–child relationship dynamic (Brown 2000). Engel found that this type of personality predisposed the bowel tissue to changes that occur in ulcerative colitis. Thus he was elucidating the inseparability of mind and body as well as the relationship of that mind and body unit to the environment in which it exists. Engel embellished this model over the decades until he enunciated the 'bio-psychosocial model', which is an approach to the management of disease that factors in the biological, psychological and sociological aspects of the individual.

Whatever the name given to the discipline, the uniting factor of post-modern medicine is that it recognises the importance of relationship: both the relationship of the mind and body and of the whole person to the environment. The name gaining popularity as the descriptor for this post-modern paradigm is 'integrated medicine'.

An integrated model

The newly installed President of the American Medical Association, Dr Wendell C. Phillips, made a bold statement. He said: 'The chief role of the physician of the future will be to keep his patients well rather than treat them when they are sick'. These commendable sentiments were somewhat before their time as they were expressed in 1926 (Science Newsletter 1926). Dr Phillips' utopian vision has not come to pass and orthodox medicine wavers perilously on the precipice of being simply the technical management of disease (Prince Charles 2001). Orthodox medicine has focused on specific disease intervention and has ignored concepts of self-healing and holism. Complementary healing has blossomed into this vacuum, yet the way forward is not simply to tack elements of complementary healing onto the orthodox edifice. Similarly, to discard all that orthodox medicine and science has achieved would be farcical. Advocates of orthodox and complementary medicine alike are acknowledging that an integrated model is the future of medicine.

Integrated medicine will have as its premise a search for health and healing rather than disease and treatment. Patients will be viewed as whole beings with minds and spirits as well as bodies and not just as a biochemical puzzle to be solved. Technology will sit alongside lifestyle factors as primary instruments of healing (Rees 2001). Most importantly, integrated medicine will encourage greater involvement of the patient in the healing process. It will recognise that information is an individual's right and that health is an individual's responsibility. 'Integration' in this context can be seen to have a broad application to the medical future.

Future medicine will not only be an integration of the orthodox and complementary paradigms but will depend on an integration at the individual level. This will involve an integration of the mind, spirit and body as well as an integration of the individual into their larger environment. Individuals will be more informed about and responsible for their own health. The medical community will treat people as unique and individuals will embrace a notion of health that goes beyond the absence of disease. Health will be acknowledged as a dynamic process that arises from the internal balanced integration of the individual and that person's interactions with their community. The challenge of the integrated model is dealt with in the Conclusion to this volume but suffice it to say that the integrated medical future is one of individual empowerment and immense potential. The philosophies and methods outlined in the rest of this book are contributing forces that shape the present and future of medicine. They are diverse yet unified and their blend is a significant part of the rich mixture that is the future of healing and, therefore, of the human race.

Recommended reading

Conlan, R. 1999, *States of Mind*, John Wiley and Sons, New York.

Foss, L. 2002, *The End of Modern Medicine*, State University of New York Press, Albany.

Nuland, S.B. 2000, *The Mysteries Within*, Touchstone, New York.

Theobald, R. 1999, *Visions and Pathways for the 21st Century*, Southern Cross University Press, Lismore, Australia.

World Health Organization 2002, 'Traditional medicine—growing needs and potential', *WHO Policy Perspectives On Medicine* No. 2, May.

PART 1
Philosophies of healing

1

Ayurveda
Shaun Matthews

Ayurveda, the traditional system of medicine that arose out of the Indian subcontinent, has been practised for well over 6000 years. The word Ayurveda is derived from two words in Sanskrit, the language of ancient India: *Ayus*, meaning life, and *veda*, meaning knowledge or science. Ayurveda is thus the science of life, or, more aptly, the art of living. It looks to understand all of life, from birth to death, including the physical, emotional, mental and spiritual aspects of human existence.

As such Ayurveda is a truly holistic paradigm of healing, helping people to live their lives in harmony with nature, nature here being both without, and within, one's relationship with the outside world as well as with one's own body. It examines the individual's relationship with food and herbs, the weather and the seasons, their relationship with fellow human beings and, ultimately, their relationship with themselves.

In India it is known as 'the mother of all healing' as it is said to care for all creatures as a mother does for her children. Ayurveda also describes approaches to improving the health of animals and even plants. As well as drawing from a long history of clinical experience, Ayurveda honours the role of intuition in the healing process. Intuition is seen as a god-given gift that can be utilised by physician and patient alike. Thus, unlike western medicine, it has a place for knowledge that comes from subjective as well as objective experience.

Ayurveda presents a model of health and disease that understands living systems in essentially energetic terms, and in this way it neatly brings together interactions between the mind, body and spirit. The term 'bodymind' better reflects the orientation of Ayurveda, which tends to view the human organism as a whole.

The term Asthanga Ayurveda refers to the fact that Ayurveda is traditionally described as having eight limbs, which are:

1. **Kaya Chikitsa—medical therapeutics**
2. **Shalakya Tantra—treatment of diseases of the head and neck**
3. **Shalya Tantra—surgery**
4. **Kaumarabhritya—paediatrics**
5. **Agada Tantra—toxicology**

6. **Bhutavidya—psychology and psychiatry**
7. **Rasayana—the science of rejuvenation**
8. **Vajikarana—the science of aphrodisiacs**

Ayurveda as a healing science does not exist in isolation; indeed it is part of a tradition of Vedic sciences. Its sister sciences include Jyotish (Vedic astrology), Yoga and Vaastu (Vedic architecture and space harmonisation). Yoga therapy is becoming increasingly well known in western countries, in which various yogic practices are used to treat a range of diseases. In this tradition patients are given instruction in yoga postures (*asanas*), breathing exercises (*pranayama*) and meditation to help restore the flow of vital energy (*prana*) around the body. Various saltwater cleansing practices are also utilised in yoga therapy to purify the 'bodymind'.

The history of Ayurveda

Ayurveda is held to have been originally propounded by Brahma, the creative intelligence behind the universe. Its teachings were written down during the Vedic period in India from 4000 to 2000 BCE. The four Vedas, or books of sacred knowledge, are some of humanity's oldest literature and contain many references to the essential principles of Ayurveda.

Since the Vedic period, Ayurveda has had a chequered history and, as Table 1.1 shows, a lot of Ayurvedic knowledge has been lost over the years, particularly during the Muslim and European invasions of India. In Kerala state in the south of India, generally acknowledged as the home of Ayurveda, the oral tradition of Ayurvedic learning has been spared. Thus it is not uncommon to find families in Kerala that have been practising Ayurveda in a father to son tradition for over 400 years. In India

Table 1.1   Ayurveda through the ages

4000–2000 BCE—the Vedic period in India
1500 BCE—appearance of *Charaka Samhita*, Ayurveda's foremost medical text
600 BCE—Ayurvedic teaching institution at Takshashila established
300 BCE—Emperor Ashoka converts to Buddhism, Ayurveda enjoying state patronage
300 CE—Nalanda Buddhist University, housing 10 000 students, teaching Ayurveda
800 CE—spread of Indian culture, including Ayurveda, to Tibet, Sri Lanka and Southeast Asia
1000–1200 CE—Muslim invasions of India and destruction of centres of learning and Ayurvedic texts
1600–1700 CE—the opening of European trade routes to the East
1750–1950 CE—British occupation of India
1835 CE—active suppression of indigenous systems of healing by the British
1947 CE—Indian independence and renaissance of Ayurveda
1990s—emerging interest in western countries in Ayurveda as a holistic healing science

today there are over 50 universities with faculties of Ayurveda and many new private colleges of Ayurveda are being founded. However, only a small percentage of the national health budget goes to Ayurveda, so facilities in public hospitals are often limited. In the south of India many new Ayurvedic spas and health resorts have opened in recent years and are becoming popular with foreign tourists and students.

The aims of Ayurveda

Ayurveda, as well as being a medical system that seeks to relieve the suffering of humanity through different treatment strategies, is also focused on preserving the health of healthy people and helping people in general to attain the four principal aims of life in Ayurveda: *dharma, artha, kama* and *moksha.*

Dharma is a complex concept which has been interpreted in different ways through the ages. When used at the level of the individual, it refers to that path through life that allows for a person to achieve their full potential and to fulfil their own unique destiny. A person's dharma is a calling to honour and actualise their uniqueness as a human being. It is not a selfish endeavour but rather something that will 'carry' them through their life. Honouring their dharma may involve doing things that are boring, inconvenient and even painful; however, living in accordance with their dharma is innately satisfying at a deep level. Their dharma not only contributes to their own personal wellbeing but it is also beneficial for their families and communities. Dharma has a protective function in a person's journey through life, and enables them to find out where their own individual thread fits into the overall tapestry of life.

The second Vedic aim, artha, relates to the pursuit of security, which may be through gathering wealth, power and/or fame. It is also the means by which a person is able to support themselves in their journey through life. Kama, the third Vedic aim, relates to the pursuit of pleasure, in the form of simple mundane desires such as the desire to enjoy one's children, a beautiful piece of music or the warmth of the sun's rays on one's back. The fourth aim of life is moksha, which means 'liberation'. It relates to the spiritual domain of our lives and is concerned with such questions as 'Who am I?' and 'What will happen to me when I die?'. It involves coming to terms in a meaningful way with the transitory nature of our lives on this planet.

The philosophical basis of Ayurveda

Ayurveda draws from a rich mix of philosophical systems that have their origins in ancient India. Those systems that accept the authority of the Vedas are referred to

Table 1.2 Ayurvedic classification of philosophical systems

Astika philosophical systems	*Nastika philosophical systems*
Samkhya	Buddhism
Yoga	Jainism
Nyaya	Charvaka
Vaisheshika	
Purva Mimamsa	
Vedanta	

as *astika* and those that do not accept the authority of the Vedas are called *nastika* (see Table 1.2). Ayurveda's approach is essentially synthetic, maintaining that truth can be seen from many different points of view, all equally valid.

Of these systems, Samkhya provides Ayurveda with its theory of creation and outlines the workings of the mind. It is the oldest school of Indian philosophy and is generally seen as the first attempt to harmonise the philosophy of the Vedas through reason. It is a systematic account of the process of evolution and attempts to comprehend the universe as the sum total of 25 categories.

According to Samkhya the misery of the soul comes about because of its intimate association with the physical body. Bondage is said to be an illusion caused by incorrect knowledge of the true nature of reality. It is held that discriminative knowledge will release the soul from misery. Samkhya is concerned with the empirical world and is governed by the rules of reason and what can be known. It postulates two ultimate realities, *Purusa* and *Prakruti*. Purusa is cosmic spirit, the animating principle of nature; by virtue of Purusa we become aware of the existence of the physical world. Prakruti is cosmic substance, the primary source of all things. All objects of the world, including the body, the mind, the senses and the intellect are derived from Prakruti.

Mahat is the first product of the evolution of Prakruti and is often translated as cosmic intelligence. *Ahamkara*, the second product of Prakruti, is the 'I'-forming principle, which gives us the feeling of 'I' and mine. It causes the disparate parts of a being to relate to each other as part of a separate but unified organism. On account of the ahamkara, or ego, we wrongly consider ourselves to be the agent or cause of our actions. Ahamkara manifests into the five sense faculties, the five motor organs and the mind, or *manas*. The five motor organs, or organs of actions, are the mouth, the hands, the feet, the reproductive organs and the excretory organs. It also further manifests into the five senses with their corresponding elements or *bhutas* (see Figure 1.1).

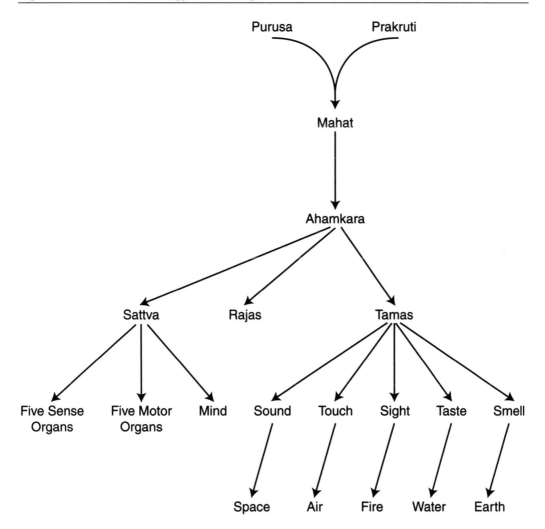

Figure 1.1   The cosmology of Samkhya

Purusa   Prakruti

Mahat

Ahamkara

Sattva   Rajas   Tamas

Five Sense   Five Motor   Mind   Sound   Touch   Sight   Taste   Smell
Organs   Organs

Space   Air   Fire   Water   Earth

The Triguna

Samkhya teaches that Prakruti has three *gunas*, or primary attributes, *Sattva*, *Rajas* and *Tamas*. These principles are said to exist behind all substances in the universe and account for the diverse range of objects in experience. Sattva is the principle of harmony and brings lasting happiness. Rajas is the principle of dynamism and brings pain in the long run. Tamas is the principle of inertia and brings dullness or lack of feeling.

The three gunas are particularly important in how Ayurveda understands the functioning of the mind. As Sattva starts to predominate, the mind becomes clearer and is better able to avoid harmful activities. If Rajas or Tamas predominate, the mind becomes more agitated or dull, respectively, and is therefore more likely to make wrong decisions, to become forgetful or fearful. Rajas and Tamas cause psychological disease, which can contribute to physical disease.

The Five Great Elements

The ancient *rishis*, or enlightened seers, are said to have asked the question, 'How can we know the universe?'. Ultimately they realised that we experience the universe through our five senses; accordingly Ayurveda describes five elements, one for each of the sense organs. These are earth, water, fire, air and space, which correspond to the solid state, the liquid state, the power to transform the state of a substance, the gaseous state and the space in which everything exists.

It is held that every substance in the universe is made up of these five elements and can be classified according to its predominant element. For example, an object which is solid at room temperature is said to be mainly composed of the earth element.

The Three Doshas

Within living systems, such as the human 'bodymind', Ayurveda describes three energetic forces known as *doshas*. They are derived from the Five Great Elements and are known as *Vata*, *Pitta* and *Kapha* dosha. Vata arises from the elements of space and air, Pitta arises from fire and water, and Kapha arises from earth and water. The doshas are the inherent motivating principles of life and, being invisible forces, can only be demonstrated by inference. They permit embodied life to exist.

Vata is responsible for movement, Pitta is responsible for transformation and Kapha is the cohesive principle in living organisms. At a physiological level Vata governs nervous system functioning, Pitta governs digestion and Kapha lubricates, maintains and contains the other two doshas.

The doshas are known by their gunas, or qualities. Vata dosha is light, dry, cool, rough, mobile, subtle and astringent in taste. It carries out a diverse range of functions in the body including the conduction of nerve impulses and the expulsion from the body of faeces, sweat, urine, menstrual fluid, semen and the foetus. Additionally, Vata dosha regulates the circulation of the blood, breathing and movement along the digestive tract and governs the movement of the mind.

Pitta dosha is hot, moist, intense, sharp, fleshy smelling and sour in taste. It is responsible for the formation of tissues and waste products and controls the metabolism of the body. It governs the flow and secretion of bile and enzymes into the gastrointestinal tract and the flow of hormones into the bloodstream. Pitta dosha regulates hunger, thirst, body temperature and sexual desire.

Kapha dosha is cold, heavy, moist, oily, stable, smooth, slow, firm and sweet in taste. It enables the growth and sustenance of the body and provides an appropriate watery medium in which cellular activities can flourish. Kapha dosha is responsible for nurturing and rejuvenating the body and preventing wear and tear. It also maintains the strength and the immunity of the body.

The doshas are found throughout the body, but are more prominent in certain parts of the body. Vata is located below the navel, especially in the bladder, large bowel, the pelvis, the bones and the legs. Pitta is located between the navel and the chest, especially the small intestine, liver, stomach, blood and the lymph. Kapha is located above the diaphragm, especially the thorax, head and neck, the upper part of the stomach and in the fat tissues of the body.

The Law of Like and Unlike

Ayurveda understands the relationship between the microcosm of the human 'bodymind' and the macrocosm of the external world through the Law of Like and Unlike. A substance is seen as a carrier of a number of qualities, called *gunas*. The law looks at the gunas of a thing in order to see how it will influence the microcosm of the human 'bodymind'. These qualities can influence a human being in different ways and may be nourishing, balancing or disturbing. Things with like qualities will cause an increase in those qualities, for example lying in the sunlight on a warm day causes an increase of warmth in the body. Things with unlike qualities will cause a decrease in those qualities, for example drinking a glass of ice-cold water will cause our innately warm bodies to cool down. In this way the food we eat, the herbs we ingest, the weather and the people we associate with have an effect on the qualities of our 'bodyminds'.

The constitutional approach of Ayurveda

Ayurveda places great importance on understanding the innate constitution of a person, which is known as one's *prakruti*, or nature. Prakruti refers to a person's physical and mental constitution, which is fixed at the moment of conception and is determined by conditions in the parents' 'bodyminds' at the time of sexual union. Accordingly, the constitution is influenced by four principal factors: the genes of the father, the genes of the mother, the mother's diet and habits during pregnancy and the state of the womb, and the season at the time of conception. The constitution does not change during one's lifespan. The combination of basic elements present at birth, as expressed in the three doshas, remains constant.

Ayurveda describes seven basic constitutional types:

1. **Vata-dominated prakruti**
2. **Pitta-dominated prakruti**
3. **Kapha–dominated prakruti**
4. **Vata–Pitta prakruti (bidoshic)**
5. **Pitta–Kapha prakruti (bidoshic)**
6. **Kapha–Vata prakruti (bidoshic)**
7. **Vata–Pitta–Kapha prakruti (equal amounts of the three doshas are present)—this is rare**

The Vata, Pitta and Kapha constitutional types

The Vata constitutional type tends to have a light build, often suffers from cold extremities and is prone to dry skin and constipation. They are temperamentally more sensitive and more 'highly strung', are naturally creative though prone to anxiety and insecurity when out of balance. The Pitta constitutional type tends to have a medium build and are warm to touch. They are fiery by nature and are prone to overheating and hyperacidity of the digestive tract. Generally Pitta types enjoy being productive though are susceptible to anger and frustration when out of balance. The Kapha constitutional type tends to have a heavy build and oily skin and is prone to mucus and gaining excess weight. They are naturally calm and easygoing, and perform tasks in a slow and thorough manner. However, Kapha types are more likely to suffer from lethargy and melancholy when out of balance. (See Table 1.3.)

The doshas in health and disease

The concept of balance is a key principle in Ayurveda. When the doshas are in balance we experience good physical health and mental wellbeing. Digestion is powerful, there is abundant energy, easy elimination, a calm mind and clear senses. The doshas in balance function together; however, when they are out of balance they create disharmony and can produce disease if corrective measures are not taken.

Aggravation or increase in Vata dosha causes dryness and agitation in the 'bodymind' and may manifest as constipation, dry skin, anxiety, ungroundedness and insecurity. Aggravation or an increase in Pitta dosha causes excessive heat and inflammation in the 'bodymind' and may manifest as fever, red skin rashes, hyperacidity, ulcers, anger, frustration and self-criticisim. Aggravation or an increase in Kapha dosha causes problems with excessive mucus and swelling in the 'bodymind' and may manifest as excessive weight gain, colds, bronchitis, fluid retention and lethargy and possessiveness.

Table 1.3   Ayurvedic constitutional assessment

Vata	Pitta	Kapha
Frame		
• thin	• medium	• thick
Hair		
• dry, kinky	• soft, oily, early grey	• thick, oily, wavy
Teeth		
• big, crooked	• moderate, yellowy	• strong, white
Eyes		
• small, dry, dull	• sharp, penetrating	• big, attractive
Skin		
• dry, rough	• fair, sunburn easily	• thick, oily
Appetite		
• variable	• strong, excessive	• slow, steady
Speech		
• fast	• sharp, cutting	• slow, monotonous
Elimination		
• constipated easily	• soft, loose	• slow, heavy bowel habit
Physical activity		
• very active	• moderate	• lethargic
Mind		
• restless, 'spacy' at times	• analytical, sharp	• methodical
Emotional temperament		
• fearful, anxious	• irritable, fiery	• calm, easygoing
Memory		
• forgetful	• sharp	• slow but prolonged
Dreams		
• fearful, lots of movement	• violent, energetic	• watery, romantic
Sleep		
• light, difficulty falling asleep	• sound	• heavy, prolonged
Finances		
• spend quickly	• moderate	• good money saver

Agni—the digestive fire

Ayurveda places great emphasis on the maintenance and restoration of one's digestive capacity in the prevention and treatment of disease. The word *agni* in Sanskrit means 'fire'—the biological fire that governs metabolism. It refers not only to our digestive fire but also to the transforming force within all of us. Agni is present in the body in three main areas, known as the *jatharagni*, the five *bhutagnis* and the seven *dhatu-agnis*. The jatharagni is located in the stomach and gastrointestinal tract and is responsible for 'cooking' the food through the action of saliva, hydrochloric acid, different enzymes, bile and pancreatic juice. It also separates the nutrient portion of food from the wastes and makes possible the absorption of nutrients in the intestines and their further transformation into plasma, the nutrient fluid portion of blood. The five bhutagnis are mainly housed in the liver. They adapt the broken-down food into a substance which can be assimilated by the tissues of the body. The seven dhatuagnis are located in the tissues of the body. They are responsible for the synthesis of the basic tissue elements in the body and exist as seven groups of enzymes. They synthesise the seven *dhatus*, or body tissues, from the 'cooked' food.

The agni of the gastrointestinal tract is directly linked to the agni of the tissues and contributes to it and gives it strength. In this way the strength of tissue metabolic processes is fundamentally dependent on the strength of the agni in the gastrointestinal tract. As well as maintaining the nutrition of the tissues agni is also responsible for the proper functioning of the immune system. It destroys unwanted toxins, bacteria and parasites along the length of the gastrointestinal tract and also is involved in the production of antibodies that circulate in the blood.

If a person's agni is unable to digest food properly, food components accumulate in the large intestine and turn into a foul-smelling and sticky substance, termed *ama*. It has the qualities of being unripe, uncooked, immature or undigested and clogs the intestines, where it undergoes chemical changes creating toxins. When ama is absorbed from the intestines it finds its way into the bloodstream, causing blockage of the channels of the body's tissues. This process tends to take place in an individual's weakest organs. As the blockage leads to stagnation, ama accumulates more and more, reducing the immune mechanisms in the particular organ. The end result of this process is the manifestation of disease in the affected organ.

The cause of disease

Ayurveda recognises that the cause of disease lies in our daily diet, lifestyle and behaviour. The immediate cause of disease is imbalance of the three doshas Vata, Pitta and Kapha, and this may or may not be accompanied by the presence of ama or toxins resulting from impairment of the agni, or digestive fire. Imbalances of the doshas can be triggered by external factors such as the weather or by internal factors such as suppressed emotions.

There are three main causes of disease described in Ayurveda which are said to underlie the process of disease formation. The first and ultimate cause of disease is *prajnaparadha*, which literally means 'crimes against wisdom'. This refers to doing things that you know will not be beneficial for you, such as staying out in the sun in midsummer when you know it will cause sunburn or eating that bar of chocolate when you know it will make you feel sick afterwards. This wilfulness on the part of the individuals causes them to ignore the inherent rhythms of nature, that is, their own nature as well as the nature that is outside of them.

The second main cause of disease according to Ayurveda is *asatmyendriyartha samyoga*, which literally means 'unwholesome contact of the senses with their objects'. This relates to exposing your sense organs to things that are essentially detrimental to your organism, such as the watching of pornography or gratuitous violence on television, listening to loud rock music or eating excessive amounts of chilli. These exposures have an adverse impact on the mind, which will in turn affect the tissues of the body and vice versa.

The third significant cause of disease is *kala parinama*, which denotes the effects of seasonal changes which take place naturally and which have an effect on the mind, the doshas and the strength of the body. For example, the cold winds of autumn are said to aggravate Vata dosha which acts as a trigger for diseases such as influenza and bronchitis.

Ayurvedic diagnostic approaches

The assessment of a patient coming for treatment proceeds through three steps: questioning, visual examination and palpation. The classical eightfold Ayurvedic examination generally includes examination of a person's physical features, nails,

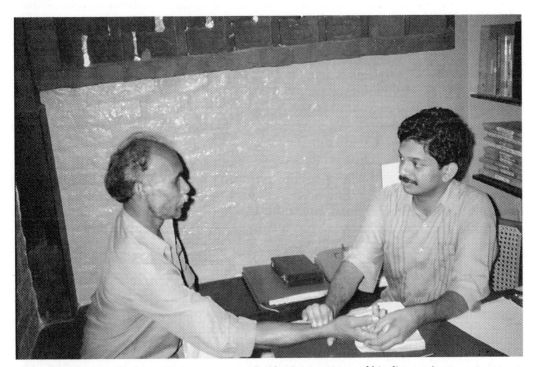

A South Indian Ayurvedic practitioner using pulse diagnosis as part of his diagnostic assessment. (Shaun Matthews)

skin, eyes, tongue, stools, urine and pulse. Some practitioners are particularly skilled in the art of pulse diagnosis which is utilised in identifying dysfunction in specific organs in the body and in diagnosing constitutional type.

Prior to instigating treatment an evaluation of the strength of the patient is also carried out. This takes into account the patient's constitutional type, any current doshic imbalance, the vitality of their tissues, their body build and measure, what food and herbs they are habituated to taking, their willpower, the state of their digestive fire, or agni, their capacity for exercise and their age.

Ayurveda teaches that there are three pillars of good health. These are proper diet, adequate rest and appropriate use of sexual vitality. Ayurveda has a strong focus on self-healing, empowering the individual to take responsibility for their health and wellbeing. By learning to use their energies in the right way, the individual can play an important role in the prevention of disease and rejuvenation of the 'bodymind'. This aspect of Ayurveda is known as *swasthavrtta*, which literally means 'establishing oneself in healthy habits'. To achieve this, daily and seasonal routines are recommended in order to prevent disturbances of the digestive fire and aggravation of the three doshas.

Ayurvedic treatment modalities

Ayurvedic treatment is based around the removal of the cause of doshic imbalance or disease. To facilitate this process the Ayurvedic physician is required to be different things at different times. They may need to act as a teacher, a priest, a counsellor, a motivator, an initiator of change and even as a cook. The physician works to support nature, which is seen as fundamentally intelligent. As nature's innate healing power is respected, the burden of treatment rests on the physician's shoulders, but not the burden of cure.

The Ayurvedic practitioner uses a multitude of treatment methods in their approach to the treatment of disease. These approaches can broadly be categorised under the headings of physical, psychological and spiritual therapies, though there is considerable overlap between these approaches to healing the 'bodymind'.

Physical therapies

Physical therapies include the use of food as medicine and the prescription of both kitchen and medicinal herbs as well as various mineral preparations. Ayurvedic treatments also incorporate aromatherapy using specific essential oils, colour therapy and various forms of massage. Ayurvedic massage makes use of oils medicated with herbs according to time-honoured traditions and can involve the manual stimulation of vital energy points in the body called *marma* points.

Ayurveda incorporates specific strategies to rejuvenate the 'bodymind', using special herbs and behavioural regimens to prevent ageing, strengthen immunity and improve mental functioning. These approaches are known as *Rasayana*, or the science of rejuvenation. There are also specific herbs used to promote virility in men and to enhance fertility in women. This aspect of Ayurveda is known as *Vajikarana*, or the science of aphrodisiacs.

In order to purify the 'bodymind' of long-standing toxins and to expel disease- producing doshas from the body, Ayurveda has developed *Panchakarma*, or the five deep-cleansing therapies. These therapies require special dietary preparation, 'oleation' of the body with oils and ghee and induced sweating. This is followed by vomiting, purgation or enema treatment, after which the patient must rest. Other forms of Panchakarma include bloodletting, sometimes using leeches, and the application of medicated oil drops or powder to the nasopharynx as a means of treating diseases of the

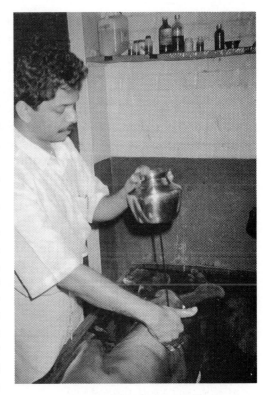

Dhara—a form of Ayurvedic massage using special oils which have been medicated with herbs. (Shaun Matthews)

head and neck. Panchakarma is especially effective in the treatment of chronic diseases such as rheumatoid arthritis, hyperacidity and nervous paralysis.

Psychological therapies

The aim of this group of treatment approaches is to give the patient greater peace of mind and to help them in working with debilitating, negative emotions. Traditionally, in an Indian context, the treatments might involve music therapy, to induce an uplifting mood, and various meditation practices. Also prescribed is *mantra*, which involves the silent repetition of sacred sounds by the patient and which can be very beneficial in stabilising the mind, and chanting aloud. In order to cultivate Sattva or mental harmony, *satsang* or association with wise teachers is recommended. In a contemporary western context, psychological support from counsellors and psychotherapists can be invaluable in helping people deal with difficult life situations and internal dilemmas. Group psychotherapy in the form of personal development seminars, religious groups and twelve-step programs can also be very helpful to individuals at this level.

Spiritual therapies

Spiritual therapies are prescribed when there is no obvious physical or psychological cause for a disease. Various religious and occult methods are used to harmonise negative energy. These methods include the chanting of mantras, fire ceremonies, pilgrimages and the offering of oblations.

Ayurvedic nutrition

Ayurveda aims to help the individual get the most nourishment from the food they consume. To achieve this end it brings a number of recommendations to bear on how we grow, store, process and prepare the food. By becoming more aware of these distinctions (see Table 1.4 for questions to ask), people are then better able to discriminate about the nutritional content of food items.

Table 1.4   Expanding one's awareness of food

1. What is the basic nature of the food?
2. How is it grown (i.e. organic, hydroponic, biodynamic, mono-agriculture, natural forest)?
3. How is it harvested and stored?
4. Has it been grown locally? Has it been grown in an area suited to its cultivation?
5. How has it been processed?
6. How has it been prepared?
7. Has it been mixed with other foods?
8. Is the food in season?
9. Is it appropriate for one's constitutional type?
10. Is it appropriate for one's current health imbalance?
11. Is it in the appropriate amount?
12. Is it being taken at the appropriate time?
13. Is the person eating the food used to having it in their diet?
14. What sequence is the food being taken in?

Ayurvedic herbology

Ayurvedic herbology is known as *dravyaguna*, where *dravya* means 'substance' and *guna* means 'quality'. A herb is seen as a substance with a particular set of qualities (see Table 1.5) which is prescribed by an Ayurvedic physician in order to produce a specific effect on the 'bodymind' of the patient.

Table 1.5   The energetics of herbs

Guna	—the qualities of a herb (i.e. moist, dry, light, heavy)
Rasa	—the taste of the herb. The six tastes are sweet, sour, salty, pungent, bitter and astringent. Each taste has a different range of effects on the body
Virya	—the potency of the herb (i.e. whether it has a cooling or heating effect on the body)
Vipaka	—the post-digestive effect of the herb on the body
Prabhava	—the specific power of the herb, used to explain the occult properties of herbs. It also refers to the power of rituals, mantras and gemstones in the preparation of herbal medicines

Although Ayurvedic physicians sometimes prescribe single herbs, herbal medicines are often prescribed in the form of herbal compounds containing several different herbs. This has the effect of:

1. **increasing the healing powers of the medicine prescribed;**
2. **expanding the field of activity of the medicine; and**
3. **compensating for potential side effects of particular herbs.**

In combining herbs the Ayurvedic physician must select a herb appropriate for the individual person and their particular condition.

There are five main methods of herbal preparation, designed for different therapeutic effects or to help preserve their potencies. They are as follows:

1. *Svarasa*, **or fresh juice of the herb, is obtained by crushing or pounding the fresh plant and then straining the liquid through a cloth. For dry herbs a weaker preparation can be made by adding water to the dry herb or powder, letting it sit for 24 hours and then straining the liquid to make a juice substitute.**
2. *Kalka*, **or herbal paste, is obtained by crushing the fresh plant to the point where it becomes a soft mass. Dry herbs with some water added can also be used to create a workable paste.**
3. *Kvatha*, **or decoction, involves boiling the herbs over a low flame. One part of fresh herb is added to sixteen parts by weight of water and the mixture boiled down to one-fourth. Clay pots are used for cooking decoctions.**
4. **In a hot infusion, or** *phant*, **the herbs are added to boiling water and allowed to steep for at least half an hour. The ratio of herbs to water is one to eight. The herbs are strained and the liquid used.**
5. **In a cold infusion, or** *hima*, **herbs are let stand in cold water for up to twelve hours. This method is preferred for delicate herbs and those with a cooling energy.**

Beyond these five major methods, other preparations of herbs are also used. *Churna* refers to a powder traditionally prepared with a mortar and pestle and filtered through linen, or ground mechanically with a herb grinder. These are often easier to make when there are many ingredients and require a lower dosage than raw herbs as they allow more of the herb to be ingested directly. Powders are usually taken with an *anupana*, a substance such as honey, ghee or milk, which acts as a vehicle for the herb and helps to facilitate absorption.

Medicated wines including *arishtas* made from decoctions and *asavas* made from expressed juices are often used as vehicles for other medicines and to kindle the agni of digestive fire. A yeast culture is added to the juice or decoction and allowed to ferment for a period of days to months. Medicated jellies called *avalehas* are used as tonics and rejuvenatives, such as the famous general tonic in India, Chyavan Prash. Pills and tablets known as *guti* and *vati* are popular and are made from decoctions.

Medicated ghee, or *ghrita*, help to increase agni and are especially useful as rasayana or rejuvenatives for the brain and nervous system. Medicated oils, or *taila*, are used externally in massage and are also taken internally. Sesame oil is generally favoured. Milk decoctions are made using one part of herbs, eight parts of milk and 32 parts of water. The mixture is boiled on a low heat until all the water has evaporated.

Ayurveda and spiritual life

Ayurveda is concerned with providing a strong physical basis for our spiritual practice. It can be described as the therapeutic arm of the spiritual sciences of India such as Yoga, Vedanta, Buddhism and Tantra. As such Ayurveda draws from these traditions in its approach to spiritual life. The human being is seen as a body–mind–spirit complex, our physical body being a crystallisation of deeply rooted mental tendencies passed on from previous lifetimes. In this view our true nature is seen as eternal and unchanging, sometimes referred to as consciousness, or *atman*. Each human being is eventually drawn to that spiritual path best suited to their individual makeup.

Various paths, or *margas*, have been distinguished over the millennia to meet the needs of different human beings in their search to realise their true nature. Some of the main margas described include Raja Yoga (the path of the mystic), Bhakti Yoga (the path of devotion), Jnana Yoga (the path of wisdom) and Karma Yoga (the path of social service). Vedanta can be said to fall under the heading of Jnana Yoga for practical purposes and Tantra involves various meditation practices including mantra, visualisation, pranayama and both external and internal rituals.

Research in Ayurveda

In the last 25 years the effectiveness of Ayurvedic herbal preparations has gained increasing recognition as modern research methods are applied to Ayurvedic herbs. However, to date, the number of trials performed on Ayurvedic herbs is still relatively small when compared to the number of trials performed each year on modern pharmaceutical preparations.

Modern western medicine tends to want to isolate the active principle of a herb and then measure the therapeutic effect, whereas Ayurveda uses naturally occurring plant substances, taken in their entirety. As mentioned above, Ayurveda also tends to use compound herbal preparations often with ten or more different herbs in them and this can cause difficulties when using western scientific research methods.

Some Ayurvedic herbs that have been researched in modern times include *Curcuma longa* (haridra) for its anti-inflammatory properties, *Rauwolfia serpentina* (sarpagandha) for its anti-hypertensive effects, *Bacopa monnieri* (brahmi) for enhancing cognitive functioning in the elderly and *Zingiber officinale* (sunthi) for the treatment of morning sickness. As the wealth of the Ayurvedic pharmacopoeia gets more acknowledgement from western researchers, and the side effects of modern drugs become more unacceptable, it is likely that more researchers in the West will be drawn to study Ayurvedic herbs and herbal compounds.

Contemporary Ayurveda

Ayurveda is a living science that has renewed itself through the ages. Thus it recognises the need for integrating its approaches to healing into the particular culture and place in which it is being practised. At the level of physical therapies this means the utilisation of locally grown food and herbs and resources available in that country. At the level of psychological and spiritual therapies this means using approaches to working with the mind that are best suited to the psyche and temperament of the people of that country. As Ayurveda develops in western countries it will be the task of practitioners and teachers of Ayurveda to modify treatment strategies to better suit local conditions.

Conclusion

Ayurveda draws from a rich philosophical tradition which views the human being as a mind–body–spirit complex and recognises the innate connections between the physical, emotional, mental and spiritual aspects of human life. The 'bodymind' is understood in energetic terms, through the functioning of the three doshas—Vata, Pitta and Kapha. Vata being the principle of movement, Pitta the principle of transformation and Kapha the principle of cohesion in living systems. Every human being is seen as having a unique 'bodymind' constitution, created at the moment of conception. This is understood in terms of the three doshas and their relative strengths in the constitution. The aim of Ayurveda is to create a condition of balance in the bodymind through the manipulation of the internal and external environment of the person coming for treatment.

Ayurveda utilises physical, psychological and spiritual therapies to facilitate better health. An Ayurvedic physician will prescribe dietary changes, along with kitchen and medicinal herbs to help balance the bodymind. A consultation will also involve an assessment of the person's lifestyle and exercise patterns and may include the prescription of yoga postures, breathing practices and meditation. Psychological support in the form of referral to a counsellor may sometimes be required, particularly in a contemporary western setting. Traditionally spiritual support in the form of the prescription of mantras, fire ceremonies and pilgrimages is also utilised.

In more recent times Ayurvedic treatment methods are being researched in both India and western countries. The effectiveness of Ayurvedic herbs in the management of chronic conditions such as dementia is starting to gain recognition as more trials are being funded and performed.

Thus as a holistic and comprehensive paradigm of healing Ayurveda has much to offer the practice of medicine in western countries in the twenty-first century. Indeed it is already starting to find its place, as healthcare practitioners the world over look beyond the confines of those models of health focused largely on the physical plane of existence.

Further reading

Dash, Bhagwan and Junius, Manfred 1983, *A Handbook of Ayurveda*, Concept Publishing Company, New Delhi.

Frawley, David and Ranade, Subhash 2001, *Ayurveda: Nature's Medicine*, Lotus Press, Wisconsin.

Frawley, David 1997, *Ayurveda and the Mind*, Lotus Press, Wisconsin.

Lad, Vasant 1985, *Ayurveda: The Science of Self-healing*, Lotus Press, Wisconsin.

Svoboda, Robert 1992, *Ayurveda: Life Health and Longevity*, Arkana, London.

2

Indigenous healing
Martha Macintyre

The term 'indigenous' means simply that the people, animals or plants referred to are native to a particular place, region or zone. In recent years it has been used to designate those peoples who constitute the original population in a nation. Thus in Australia, the Americas and Canada the indigenous or Aboriginal people are the descendants of those who inhabited the country prior to colonisation. Often the effects of invasion, conquest, land appropriation and depopulation by introduced diseases are such that the indigenous peoples become minorities within modern nations. In other parts of the world, such as Africa and the Pacific, the indigenous populations have continued as the dominant groups and their cultural systems have not been subjected to the same dramatic disruptions and changes associated with Western colonisation.

However, throughout the past century imperial expansion, foreign aid, economic development and processes of globalisation have ensured that these people too have encountered, been subjected to and in various ways embraced or incorporated Western medical systems into their understandings of health and illness.

In this chapter the emphasis is on the systems of healing in contemporary indigenous and tribal societies. The ideas of health and illness that operate in small-scale communities are as numerous and diverse as the cultures that persist. While they are often referred to as 'traditional' and most derive from ancient knowledge and practices, the healing systems of indigenous and tribal people in the twenty-first century are often dynamic reflections of their capacity to adapt and change while sustaining core elements of their cultures. Almost all of these systems evolved in non-literate cultures, where knowledge is transmitted orally and techniques learned by observation. While these methods ensure that the ideas and practices remain integral to the culture that generated them, it also means that most information is accessible to outsiders only through the work of anthropologists (see the recommended texts at the end of the chapter).

Given the range and variation in cultural constructions of health and illness across indigenous and tribal societies, this chapter will present brief descriptions of some of the traditional knowledge systems relating to healing that persist among the indigenous peoples of Australia, Canada, Indonesia and Latin America, as well as those of tribal people in Papua New Guinea. These are offered as illustrative rather than representative examples of the ways that indigenous understandings of healing continue to operate in the context of a globalised world.

Conceptualisations of health and illness in traditional societies

The experiences of being ill or healthy are always culturally mediated. The cosmologies or world-views of people provide the terms in which they experience health or illness and represent these experiences to others. Medical anthropologists distinguish between the medical concept of 'disease', which is a specifically defined biological dysfunction, and 'illness', the condition of feeling unwell within distinctive cultural parameters. This enables anthropologists to emphasise the ways that a materialist, allopathic medical system of knowledge fails to encompass the holistic view of health as a complex condition involving the person, the social group, the environment, spiritual or supernatural forces and morality. In most traditional systems, health and illness are thought of in ways that are very different from the approach of Western medical science.

Traditional systems often draw on wider perspectives of wellbeing in order to express their notions of health. The Cree of the Great Whale area in eastern Canada have a term that describes health which is best translated as 'being alive well' (Adelson 2000: 59), thus encapsulating ideas of endurance, vitality and health. Adelson's study of contemporary Cree health begins with a quote from an elder who declared 'If the land is not healthy then how can we be?'(2000: 3). This hypothetical question might be posed in any culture, but for Canadian and Australian Aboriginal peoples it has been identified as the crux of their views of health (Franklin & White 1991). For most indigenous people whose cultures have developed through complex patterns of custodianship, care and exploitation of land and sea resources, health is grounded in social relationships that structure their use of the land and its bounty. A flourishing cultural identity and consistent identification with specific places are in many respects as crucial to a vital, healthy existence as a strong sense of self and physical wellbeing.

In this sense then, holism is a very broad concept when applied to indigenous health, as it incorporates ideas about the person as a physical and spiritual entity into a landscape that encompasses land, food resources, sacred places and the social group or tribe who inhabit that space. Whereas Western and some ancient Asian healing traditions are holistic in the sense of integrating mental, physical and spiritual facets of the individual person, indigenous holism is more socially expansive. Aboriginal Australians and Canadians especially stress the integration of the person into a world that is simultaneously geographical, social, material and spiritual. Western medical systems that see physiological wellbeing of an individual as the definition of health often are seen therefore as inadequate to the needs of indigenous people (Das 1990; Reid 1983).

Ideas of the body and the person

While it is impossible to generalise about indigenous concepts of personhood, it is important to keep in mind that other cultures have quite different ideas about the attributes of human bodies. In particular, the distinction between mind and body that characterises much Western medical thought is rare in tribal philosophies. For example, in Misima Island in Papua New Guinea an individual is perceived as being composed of elements that are unique and intrinsic but include such things as shadow or reflected image, aspects that Western thought would locate as extraneous properties dependent on light and external factors. Thus the Misiman person consists of flesh, bone and blood, energy or 'life force', breath, spirit or soul, and shadow or image (Macintyre 1990). In this community then, 'seeing a ghost' might mean that a sleeping person's image has separated from its source and is wandering around independently. Alternatively it could be the shade or soul of a person whose body, life force and breath have departed, leaving the deceased as a visible but intangible 'person' who still wants to communicate with relatives.

In considering the different ideas of personhood, it is instructive to appreciate that understandings of procreation, of the coming into being of a person, often encapsulate indigenous ideas about humanity and individuality. Two examples of alleged 'ignorance of paternity' by tribal people illustrate the ways that cultural differences, rather than lack of knowledge, determine the variations in ideas about persons, bodies and human reproduction.

Bronislaw Malinowski published a study of the sexual lives of people in the Trobriand Islands of Papua New Guinea (Malinowski 1932). He described their explanations of reproduction as displaying ignorance of the physiological processes of procreation. Trobrianders attributed human pregnancy to the actions of spirits, who ensured that a reincarnated 'spirit baby' would be transported from the spirit world of the dead and into the body of a clanswoman. Physical symptoms of pregnancy, such as the cessation of menstruation and morning sickness, were attributed to the actions of the spirit baby within the woman's body. Similar views of the spiritual means of procreation have been attributed to Australian Aboriginal cultures, where a woman perceives herself to be impregnated by a spirit that inhabits a particular place, which henceforth becomes a way of identifying the person in life.

Rather than being instances of tribal ignorance, these representations of procreation processes are examples of anthropological misunderstanding and ethnocentric interpretation. The assumption is that Western science has the correct explanation and Trobrianders and Aboriginals have faulty or misconstrued views of the ways that humans conceive. In fact, both indigenous groups recognised that sexual intercourse was necessary if a woman was to become pregnant. Beyond this, however, they are privileging the social identity of a new member of a clan over the biological entity of a 'baby' and so emphasise those processes which are crucial in connecting the infant to its forebears, its parents and kin, its territory and the spirits that ensure the continuity of humans within their environment. In effect it is an insistence on the social identity of a new baby rather than identification of it as simply a biological product.

These cases also reveal another fundamental difference between indigenous and Western scientific ideas of the forces that shape, determine and ensure human life. In many traditional knowledge systems there is no distinction between 'supernatural' and 'natural' elements that accords with Western materialist explanations. While many tribal people would acknowledge that the ways of spirits are mysterious, this does not make them sceptical about the impact of spirits and other unseen forces (that Western people call 'supernatural') on their daily lives, and especially on their health. Moreover, the link between people, spiritual forces and land or territory reinforces conceptualisations of what it is to be human in a tribal society. The categories that Westerners use to distinguish mind and body, natural and supernatural, or spirit and matter mean that they demarcate entities and their properties. In many indigenous knowledge systems the boundaries are permeable and flexible. So, for instance, the insistence that a person might sicken and die away from their territory or that food from elsewhere will not sustain good health derives from ideas about the necessity of connectedness between spirits, land, food resources and people. The Cree man's question 'If the land is not healthy then how can we be?' expresses the centrality of 'relatedness' or cosmological integration in indigenous ideas of health.

What causes illness?

Contrary to the common misconception that tribal people are 'prisoners of belief' or irrational adherents of superstition, most anthropologists who have studied indigenous health and illness have noted that people are curious about the causes of any misfortune and draw on complex notions of cause and effect to account for its manifestations. One of the most famous studies, *Witchcraft, Oracles and Magic among the Azande* (Evans-Pritchard 1937), explored the explanatory theories that these African people drew on to account for injury and illness. He discussed the ways that so-called 'superstitious' belief in oracles and the attribution of all misfortune to witchcraft are fundamentally rational, based in a knowledge system that incorporates the supernatural into the natural domain. Yet he also noted that people adapted their beliefs, expressed doubts and made allowances for different circumstances (Evans-Pritchard 1937: 195).

In many indigenous systems we find that people offer different levels of explanation, separating immediate (physical) cause from underlying social or 'supernatural' causation. Thus a person who falls from a tree and has a broken leg will be diagnosed as having broken bone because of the impact and being in need of treatment to help mend the bone. At the same time, however, the healer might attribute the misfortune itself to malevolent sorcery that ensured that the injured person would behave in particular ways. The treatment therefore has to deal with misfortune at both levels, the physical injury and the sorcery that brought it about.

Sorcery

In her study of sorcery and healing among the Yolngu people of northern Australia, Janice Reid wrote:

> Yolngu ideas about the cause and treatment of serious sickness rest on one assumption: that humans have the capacity to mobilise and to control the power which exists in the universe and are themselves vulnerable to attacks by others using that power (Reid 1983: 34).

In many indigenous societies, people attribute injury and illness to sorcery. As Reid observes for the Yolngu, the sorcerer is able to inflict harm on his (sorcerers are usually male) victims by drawing on supernatural powers and esoteric knowledge about dangerous forces and substances in his universe. The affliction by sorcery might be recognised as the immediate cause, but the underlying cause is usually social. In considering their affliction, the victim asks not only 'Who made me ill?' but 'What is wrong that someone wants to harm me?' and so delves into the social origin of the disorder. Jealousy, greed and other malevolent or anti-social impulses are often considered to be the root cause of sorcery activities.

Among the Tubetube people of Papua New Guinea, sorcery was consciously directed towards people who had offended the sorcerer in some way. Most clan leaders were considered to be powerful sorcerers, so sorcery could thus be a political sanction against rivals or enemies (Macintyre 1987). There were numerous types of sorcery and knowledge or techniques could be acquired from an adept (skilled person) by giving gifts of valuables. Some sorcery involved magical spells; other sorcery included the use of potent substances such as poisonous fish or plants. The sorcerer would put the poison in food or sometimes on a sliver of hard wood placed where a person would injure themselves.

The medical anthropologist Gilbert Lewis carried out research among the Gnau in Papua New Guinea and documented the numerous types of sorcery that people of the West Sepik region understand as the causes of disease and death (Lewis

2000). Gnau people identify numerous varieties of sorcery, some of which operate without human agency and others that use substances to cause harm. Elaborate divination rituals invoking spirits that will reveal and expel the sorcery are enacted as the means of comprehending causes of illness and healing the afflicted person.

In many tribal cultures there are forms of sorcery that involve taking something that has been part of a person (such as hair, nail parings, urine or faeces) and performing some magic on it that makes the person ill. One important aspect of the sorcerer's powers is that he usually has the capacity to reverse the effects of a curse or spell and thus his magical potency can be used to counteract ill-effects as well as generate them.

Witchcraft

Witches do not usually have the dual capacity to inflict or alleviate harm and their activities are often seen as purely destructive in intent. It is important to note that the distinction between sorcery and witchcraft is not always clear and the use of these English words as translations from indigenous terms makes definitions even more problematic. In some cultures witches are female and sorcerers male, but this might be an artefact of anthropological translation. Usually witches are identified as thoroughly negative, socially disruptive people whose activities are vindictive or irrational in that they do not use their destructive magical powers in the interest of anyone but themselves. However, many anthropologists have concluded that witchcraft accusations often serve as a form of social control, especially in societies where all deaths are attributed to magic influence. In an overview of social pressures to conformity in small-scale societies, Roger Keesing concluded:

> Witchcraft accusations . . . give a splendid means to get rid of those who cheat, deviate, or succeed too much—and a splendid incentive to be an upstanding citizen. Fear that witchcraft will be directed against one makes conformity to the norms of social life strategically wise (Keesing 1981: 319).

Witchcraft usually refers to forms of evil magical power that are derived entirely from the supernatural domain. In the islands of the Louisiades in southeast Papua New Guinea, witchcraft is transmitted from mother to daughter (Macintyre 1987) and is construed as a physical substance that is present in their bodies. Witchcraft activities are often perceived as involuntary. Witches are thought to kill their victims in order to consume them and to be indiscriminate in their activities, often causing the deaths of close relatives. These connotations have unfortunately meant that recently people suffering from HIV/AIDS have on occasions been identified as witches and heavily stigmatised in some Papua New Guinea communities.

Spirits

'Spirits' is a very loose term that is applied to supernatural beings or entities who direct or influence the lives of the social group or community. Traditionally, most tribal societies, including Aboriginal peoples in Australia and North America, held animistic beliefs about their environment. Plants, animals and natural features such as waterfalls and mountains have spirits that are regarded as powerful agents in respect of human activities and prosperity. Sometimes mythical spirits that have a crucial role in ensuring fertility, food supply and social wellbeing are identified with specific natural features such as waterholes, reefs, mountains or places in the familiar landscape.

The term 'spirits' can also be applied to the souls or ghosts of deceased ancestors, beings who maintain their interest in the social life of their community. In some indigenous cosmologies, such as that of the Misimans mentioned above, 'spirits' might also be the immaterial element of a living person that has detached from the physical body and is able to move around, visit and communicate with people, warning them of danger, reminding them of obligations or inflicting harm because of offences they have committed. Many illnesses are attributed to the actions of spirits in respect of trespass or sacrilege of their sacred places. Illness is thus a consequence of a breach of a law, with the spirits as agents. Given the wide range of supernatural beings that can be called spirits, a few examples give some indication of the ways that spirits are considered to cause harm, illness or death.

Janice Reid, in discussing Australian Aboriginal understandings of illness causation, describes instances among the Yolngu where illness was attributed to 'wangarr', the creator spirits of the Dreamtime (Reid 1983: 52). Wangarr are central to the traditional belief system and take a variety of forms—some are natural species or landforms, others are individuated beings with human-like qualities. The spirits inflict harm on humans who in some way offend them—either by failing to respect laws or obligations, such as entering or defiling a sacred place, or by misusing a sacred object associated with the spirit.

Among the Cree of the Great Whale River, human survival depended on successful hunting and this in turn required appropriate deference to the spirits of animals, places and elemental forces. Adelson sets down some of the Cree stories that demonstrate the ways that a hunter had to observe rituals that honoured their 'spirit guides', such as building 'shaking tents' in order to ensure that their food supply continued (Adelson 2000: 27–9).

On Tubetube island in Papua New Guinea, the spirits of recently deceased people are thought to inflict illness on those living relatives who have not observed mourning rituals or taboos (Macintyre 1987). Sometimes the spirit is angry with a particular person and so makes them the victim of a dramatic accident, such a being struck by a falling tree or stung by a poisonous fish. On other occasions a child of the offender will be stricken with malaria. Spirits who are guardians of places or crucial subsistence activities such as gardening or fishing can choose to punish by withdrawing their interest in a person's success (thereby threatening them with starvation) or by visiting them in the form of a poisonous snake or fish. Thus 'natural' occurrences, such as snake bite or fish poisoning and even crop failure due to drought, are thought to be the work of spirits.

Moral failure and breaches of taboos

In some indigenous societies, moral failure or breaches of traditional laws are believed to carry their own punishments, often taking the form of illness. Among the Yolngu, for example, strict food taboos accompany ceremonies and Reid reports of men from Yirrkala who attended a ceremony where they were unfamiliar with the rules: 'Although they were told to eat only lean animals and fish, some ate fatty animals and, as a result were stricken with leprosy' (Reid 1983: 53). While human agents sometimes inflict harm on people who trespass on or desecrate sacred places, breaches of restrictions relating to sacred sites often carry immediate supernatural punishments. Similarly, food taboos associated with special states such as menstruation or pregnancy carry with them their own consequences when breached, so a mother who eats a forbidden food is viewed as causing congenital deformity or stunting her baby's growth.

On Tubetube, the breaking of taboos such as incest or killing of a close family member are thought to be abominable crimes that cause the perpetrator's blood to putrefy. The symptoms of this disease include high fevers and eruptions of boils all over the body but, as with Aboriginal beliefs about the consequences of moral failure (Reid 1983: 52–3), the mechanisms whereby the illness develops are not scrutinised. The absence of a detailed analysis of the ways in which an illness or injury are caused by supernatural agents is a further indication of the ways that indigenous people tend not to separate the immaterial, supernatural elements from the material, physical dimensions of their universe. It is so obvious to people that the breach of a taboo or the desecration of a sacred place will have negative impacts on the person that asking 'How does the person get sick?' is commensurate with asking someone in a Western culture who has been hit by a bus 'How did you get hurt?'. Just as Westerners accept that the natural laws of physics will mean that a human body is unable to withstand the impact of a moving vehicle without injury, so breaking a tribal taboo or sacred law will have its inevitable effects.

Culture-bound syndromes

Some medical anthropologists have identified 'culture-bound syndromes' (Kleinman 1980), meaning specific illnesses that are not recognised as diseases by Western medicine. Aboriginal bone-pointing, or 'singing' a person to death, would be a classic instance. This is a disputed concept as often the symptoms are consonant with medical diagnoses but the cultural causal explanation is not. For example, on Lihir in Papua New Guinea people sometimes experience a mild illness, involving lethargy and headache, when a visitor departs from their village. They call this *piot* and explain it as a quality of the person who visits which is manifest in the capacity to make people feel tired and unwell. Thus a person who has strong *piot* will leave some of it in the village where it will affect the hosts. To avoid this, Lihirians will place a receptacle of water at the door of the visitor's house. They believe that the *piot* will go into the water and so can be disposed of somewhere where it can do no harm. (**Note:** references to practices on Tubetube and Lihir in Papua New Guinea where no citation is given are drawn from the author's research on those two islands.)

Healing systems in tribal and indigenous societies

Healing in most societies entails different sorts of knowledge. Some is available to everyone; some is esoteric or secret and can involve long apprenticeships as the skills and secrets are transmitted from one generation to the next. The healing treatments vary in respect of the ways that people conceptualise the functions of the human body and the causes of illness. In most cultures there is a body of common knowledge about traditional treatments for common ailments. Very often this takes the form of teaching people the names and habitats of specific plants or substances that alleviate symptoms or effect cures. Catherine Berndt (1982: 128) describes the ways that knowledge about causes and treatments of a range of illnesses are trans-mitted in the context of Aboriginal myths, but a great deal of information is imparted to people in the context of everyday life as adults tend to the sick, or as people move around in their environment and are instructed about the dangers, uses and healing powers of specific plants.

Herbal treatments

Herbal treatments are common in many tribal communities (Cambie & Ash 1994) and the most useful plants are commonly domesticated or grown in places close to settlements so that people have easy access to them. Throughout the Pacific, for example, it is common to see specific varieties of hibiscus (*Hibiscus tiliaceus* and *Hibiscus rosa-sinensis*) grown near houses. These plants have numerous uses. The pounded leaves are mixed with cold water to relieve stomach aches or to induce labour in pregnant women; steeped in hot water the mixture has laxative effects. The outer bark is used for eye infections and a decoction made from the sap cures scabies; in some places the leaves are used to cover sores or wounds as they are thought to inhibit infection. Knowledge and use of these treatments are not secret and most adults self-medicate. Awareness of herbal treatments for common ailments tends to be general, although some people take more interest than others and so become more knowledgeable.

In egalitarian tribal societies, healing is usually a domestic, family affair and so older, more experienced members of a group, 'wise men and women', tend to be the first consulted. Only when the common, accessible interventions fail do people consult experts.

Massage, bone-setting and physical interventions

In many tribal societies specific people are known to be skilled in culturally specific treatments of the body. While not universal, bloodletting is found as a treatment for illness in many societies. On Lihir in Papua New Guinea, fevers, headaches and some forms of mental illness continue to be treated by a female ritual specialist who uses small sharp shells (or, more commonly nowadays, shards of glass) to make small incisions across the brow of the sufferer, thereby releasing the 'bad

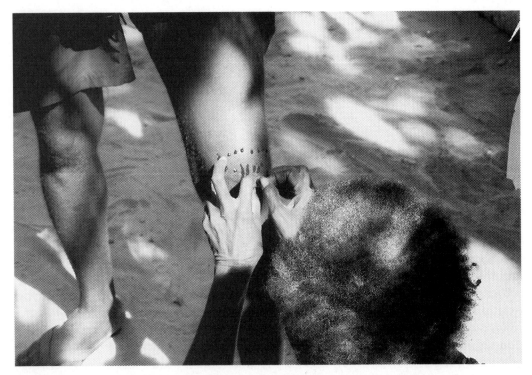

Bloodletting a swollen knee by making small incisions with a shard of glass. (Martha Macintyre)

blood' that Lihirians believe causes the symptoms. If the headache is persistent, or if the person has had a fall that appears to have resulted in pressure on the brain, the healer cuts deep into the flesh and scrapes away part of the bone, thereby relieving the pressure. This form of surgery, called in English 'cranial trepanation', is very ancient and has been practised in many societies.

Given the fact that tribal peoples were traditionally subsistence producers, injuries involving broken bones could be serious handicaps, for a person might be unable to participate fully in activities such as hunting, fishing or gardening if lamed by a fracture. Bone-setters were therefore highly regarded healers, often transmitting their knowledge through specific familial lines. Sometimes the techniques were purely manipulative, sometimes they included magical and herbal treatments.

Massage techniques have been observed as indigenous treatments in many cultures (Connor *et al.* 1996: 157–97) for muscle pain and swelling as well as a method of administering herbal medication. In many Pacific societies sweet-smelling herbs are steeped in coconut oil which is then smoothed into the skin. Coconut oil itself has healing properties as it contains both antibiotic and anti-fungal agents and the plants are thought to enhance its effects. Less pleasant, but equally common, is the use of nettles or other stinging plants which are massaged into the skin to cure a range of ailments. The technique is often used by groups whose ideas of health are humoral, that is, where there is attention paid to 'hot and cold' aspects of the body. When a pain is considered to be 'cold' in origin, nettles are rubbed on the affected area in order to heat it and so restore an ideal balance.

Esoteric and magical knowledge

Often medical interventions involve a combination of traditional herbal treatments and the use of magical spells that people believe are the major source of efficacy. Knowledge of magic is often private and spells are only passed on to people who are trusted or through various exchange mechanisms whereby the 'apprentice' offers a valuable gift in exchange for the spell. The owners of healing spells are often the same sorcerers who are deemed able to inflict harm and sometimes the form of cure is simply a magical spell that reverses the effect of the one that initially made the person ill. Payment of some form is customary when a sorcerer or magical healer is consulted.

Magical healers who know how to counter the effects of sorcery often work by magically extracting objects or harmful substances from the sorcery-victim's body, often by sucking it out or stroking the part of the body where it is allegedly lodged. For example, the Aboriginal healers of the Kimberley region in Australia, who are called *mabarn*, suck the patient's chest or abdomen and draw out blood which is then placed in a receptacle and examined for sorcery objects. Water may be added

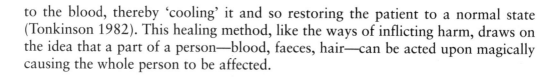

to the blood, thereby 'cooling' it and so restoring the patient to a normal state (Tonkinson 1982). This healing method, like the ways of inflicting harm, draws on the idea that a part of a person—blood, faeces, hair—can be acted upon magically causing the whole person to be affected.

Spirit healers and shamans

In many indigenous and tribal societies there are specific people who have special powers that enable them to heal illnesses that are caused by spirits or supernatural means. Such people are believed to have the capacity to communicate with spirits in dreams, visions or trances. Spirit mediums work in a variety of ways. Some simply call on spirits to assist them in interpreting an affliction. Sometimes the medium goes into a trance and speaks with spirits who offer an explanation of the cause of an illness and usually therefore the means of effecting a cure. In cultures where spirits of the dead are thought to inflict harm on people for wrongs perpetrated against them, in life or by not observing mourning obligations, the spirit medium will usually recommend a course of action that will appease the offended spirit and so alleviate the illness (Connor *et al.* 1996).

Shamanism is in some respects similar to spirit healing, but it often entails complex religious beliefs and the induction of ecstatic states as part of the healing rites. Shamans can be either male or female and their roles are conceptualised as enacting sacred knowledge and experience rather than simply practical expertise. Among Inuit peoples of North America and many of the indigenous tribal groups of the Brazilian rainforest area, shamans are people who, having experienced a major crisis (physical, psychological or spiritual), have gained extraordinary powers. It is thought that having been close to death they are thus endowed with the gift of moving through the domains of suffering and death into the world of the afterlife and so are able to comprehend all aspects of human experience. Shamanic healing among Australian Aboriginal groups often involved an apprenticeship or initiation, during which time a young boy was taken on a supernatural journey and became familiar with the beings of the Dreamtime. From that time they were able to see and communicate with the incorporeal element of all people, living and dead. Shamanic healing has much in common with other forms of religious healing carried out by priests and ritual specialists but shamans can heal in a variety of ways, including the use of plant medications.

Priests, religious healing and communal rituals

In many traditions there are communal rituals that are directed both towards maintaining the health of the group and healing specific people. In these rituals, often priests or religious leaders play special roles to ensure that the ceremonies are performed correctly while taking on the role of mediator between the worlds of spirits and living humans. The diversity of tribal cultures is reflected in the range of rituals, some involving large numbers of people coming together from a wide region, others being simpler, more domestic ceremonies. In some respects all major sacred rituals in tribal societies constitute the health of participants. They do this by ensuring continued fertility of the land and the people; by initiating young men and women into appropriate adult roles; by showing respect for the resources available for healthy survival; and by dealing with the deaths of individuals with due honour. Traditionally, rites at death were crucial in restoring social order, re-establishing propitious relations and maintaining social harmony after a death or calamity. In most indigenous communities failure in the proper performance of rituals is considered a reason for affliction, illness, death or failure of food supply.

The participation of community members in rituals affirms cultural unity as they involve the enactment of complex beliefs about the nature of human relations within an integrated universe. Gilbert Lewis's study, *A Failure of Treatment* (2000), illustrates the way that, even when rituals are not efficacious, the sequential performance of rituals aimed at determining the cause and eliminating the effects of illness serve to confirm people's cultural beliefs in the nature of health and illness. Similarly, Diane Bell comments about the Kaititj people of Central Australia: 'In the past, many women's ceremonies centred on the crises of life—birth, death, menarche—and the health of the small, intimately related band in which people lived most of the year' (Bell 1983: 197). The disruptions to tradition in Australian Aboriginal societies has meant that many groups have modified their ceremonial life, but as Bell's study of Kaititj women, *Daughters of the Dreaming* (1983), demonstrates, women's ceremonies continue to be seen as vital components in the maintenance of wellbeing in communities.

Syncretism and the uses of orthodox medicine

There are now very few tribal societies in the world where the only forms of medical treatment available to indigenous people are those traditionally used by their ancestors. In the Amazon region in South America, Papua New Guinea, Canada and Australia health services providing orthodox medical treatment have been established. Throughout the developing world, programs funded by the World Health Organization, foreign aid donors and national governments administer a wide range of primary healthcare treatments. There are international programs for immunisation against polio, diphtheria and whooping cough. Malaria, tuberculosis and HIV/AIDS are widespread in many developing countries where traditional systems of healing persist and public health campaigns are aimed at creating awareness to prevent epidemics, alleviating suffering, eliminating vectors and encouraging people to seek medical treatment. In most places in the world, maternal and child health programs are familiar to even the most remote communities.

In Canada and Australia, where social and cultural changes brought about by colonisation have had devastating effects on indigenous health, special programs have been established that aim at accommodating the cultural traditions of the minority populations. There are also specific campaigns directed at combating the diseases that have emerged in the context of forced settlement, dramatic changes in diet, the introduction of alcohol, high levels of violence and extreme poverty.

Sometimes the provision of orthodox medical services and treatments is sporadic and inadequate. As most tribal communities who continue to practise their traditions live in rural areas, their access to services is limited. Limited provision and restricted access are possibly the strongest factors in maintaining the use of traditional healing. While in some areas hostility towards governments makes people mistrustful of medical services, in most places where such treatment is available people use it. The reasons for this are not very complicated. The sorts of diseases that are common in poor, remote regions are often those that respond quickly to Western medical intervention. Pain relief, antibiotic treatments for respiratory and other infections or surgical interventions for traumatic injury are commonly the first resort when people become familiar with Western medicine. In the main, people are pragmatic and will try various treatments in the hope that one, or a combination of several, will relieve their suffering. Medical pluralism is common in most societies, including tribal and minority indigenous communities (Frankel & Lewis 1989; Mobbs 1991; Strathern & Stewart 2000).

Anthropological studies of medical pluralism (Reid & Trompf 1991) have shown that where access or availability is consistent people tend to use first the medical treatment they believe will work best at relieving pain and discomfort and then resort to alternatives if it has not been effective. In many tribal societies the hierarchy of resort with treatment is to use orthodox treatments if they are available as they deal with the symptoms very rapidly. Once relief has been effected, people will then use herbal or magical treatments to remove the cause of illness or to maintain their health. This reflects the fact that many indigenous people retain their ideas of illness causation even when they embrace other views of treatment. So, for example, a person who has developed pneumonia might first attend a clinic and take a course of antibiotics, but on returning to the village will approach a traditional healer to find out the (supernatural) cause of the affliction. If the disease is attributed to sorcery, then the same person will undertake the treatments proposed by the traditional expert, believing that unless the sorcery is dealt with the illness will recur or another will be manifest. Sometimes, too, the person might also use traditional herbal treatments to re-establish an idea of balance or to assist in the alleviation of symptoms.

The incorporation of beliefs, understandings and practices from other healing traditions is referred to as 'medical syncretism' and is an essential process in all cultures, including those in advanced industrial societies. Even in pre-colonial periods the exchange of magical knowledge, medicinal plants and healing techniques was an important communicative activity between tribal communities. Syncretism is thus the process whereby people adapt to changes and inflect the new knowledge they acquire with their distinct cultural perspective. While some people might feel that the blending and mixing of healing methods erodes traditional systems, these processes represent the dynamism and capacity for change that is the mark of all human societies.

Recommended reading

Frankel, Stephen and Lewis, Gilbert (eds) 1989, *A Continuing Trial of Treatment: Medical Pluralism in Papua New Guinea*, Kluwer Academic Publishers, Boston.

McElroy, Ann and Townsend, Pat 1996, *Medical Anthropology in Ecological Perspective*, 3rd edn, Westview Press, Boulder, Colorado.

Sargent, Carolyn F. and Johnson, Thomas M. 1996, *Medical Anthropology: Contemporary Theory and Method*, Praeger, Westport, Connecticut.

Strathern, Andrew and Stewart, Pamela J. 2000, *Curing and Healing: Medical Anthropology in Global Perspective*, Carolina Academic Press, Durham, North Carolina.

Reid, Janice (ed.) 1982, *Body, Land and Spirit: Health and Healing in Aboriginal Society*, University of Queensland Press, St Lucia.

3

Naturopathic medicine

Stephen P. Myers, Assunta Hunter, Pamela Snider, Jared L. Zeff

> Naturopathy, is the creation of conditions which enable the body to heal itself as far as it is capable of doing so (Roger Newman Turner 1984: 14).

Naturopathic medicine is an eclectic practice of healthcare united by core underlying principles. Central to these principles is the healing power of nature (*vis medicatrix naturae*), a concept ascribed to Hippocrates and one which is as old as the healing arts. The healing power of nature refers to the inherent self-organising and healing process of living systems that establish, maintain and restore health. In the words of Newman Turner (1984: 19), 'naturopathy is based on the recognition that the body possesses not only a natural ability to resist disease but inherent mechanisms of recovery and self-regulation'. Lewith (in Newman Turner 1984) suggests that the healing power of nature underpins nearly all the techniques in complementary medicine. The application of this concept gives rise to the use of natural methods to assist the healing process: the use of food, sunshine, water, rest and relaxation. Modern naturopathy has its basis in 'nature cure', an approach that originally focused on the application of these simple natural modalities but which now has been extended to include other therapeutic approaches such as herbal medicine, nutritional supplementation and tactile therapies.

Definition

Prior to 1989 naturopathic medicine was defined by its therapeutic modalities. There were several extant definitions but none acted as a unifier of the profession. In the United States, where naturopathy was recognised as an occupation by state licensing, it was defined by the US Department of Labor in its *Dictionary of Occupational Titles*. It defines a naturopath as one who:

> Diagnoses, treats and cares for patients using a system of practice that bases treatment of physiological function and abnormal conditions on natural laws governing the human body. Utilizes physiological, psychological and mechanical

methods such as air, water, light, heat, earth, phytotherapy, food and herbs therapy, psychotherapy, electrotherapy, physiotherapy, minor and orificial therapy, mechanotherapy, naturopathic corrections and manipulations, and natural methods or modalities together with natural medicines, natural processed food and herbs and natural remedies. Excludes major surgery, therapeutic use of X-ray and radium, and the use of drugs, except those assimilable substances containing elements or compounds which are components of body tissues and physiologically compatible to body processes for the maintenance of life (US Department of Labor 1991).

This emphasis on the modalities was in contrast to the philosophy-based approach defining the profession during the early part of the twentieth century. The principles and philosophy were well described at that time by the founders and leading authors in naturopathic medicine. With the rise of industrialised medicine and subsequent decline of traditional and alternative disciplines, the profession's ability to consistently voice its philosophy weakened. As naturopathic medicine re-emerged in the early 1970s, the profession's unique identity became a core issue.

In 1986 the American Association of Naturopathic Physicians (AANP), a newly revived professional association, under the presidency of Dr Cathy Rogers, commissioned Dr Pamela Snider and Dr Jared Zeff to create a unifying definition of naturopathic medicine. This project, which took over two years and was distinguished by an inclusive process, sought and received input from the entire US profession, its various agencies and many Canadian naturopathic physicians. The committee found a single element of agreement among the profession upon which it built its process. This element was the general agreement that the profession was unified by a philosophy, not by modalities. The committee sifted through input from the profession cataloguing six principles upon which the profession generally agreed. These six principles were placed before the House of Delegates of the AANP at its annual conference in September 1989 at Rippling River, Oregon, which unanimously approved them, reconfirming and articulating in modern terms its core principles as a professional consensus (see below).

Definition of Naturopathic Medicine
Naturopathic medicine is a distinct system of primary health care: an art, science, philosophy and practice of diagnosis, treatment and prevention of illness. Naturopathic medicine is distinguished by the principles which underlie and determine its practice. These principles are based upon the objective observation of the nature of health and disease, and are continually re-examined in the light of scientific advances. Methods used are consistent with these principles and are chosen upon the basis of patient individuality. Naturopathic physicians are primary health care practitioners, whose diverse techniques

include modern and traditional, scientific and empirical methods. The following principles are the foundation for the practice of naturopathic medicine:

Principles

The healing power of nature (vis medicatrix naturae)

The healing power of nature is the inherent self-organizing and healing process of living systems which establishes, maintains and restores health. Naturopathic medicine recognizes this healing process to be ordered and intelligent. It is the naturopathic physician's role to support, facilitate and augment this process by identifying and removing obstacles to health and recovery, and by supporting the creation of a healthy internal and external environment.

Identify and treat the causes (tolle causam)

Illness does not occur without cause. Causes may originate in many areas. Underlying causes of illness and disease must be identified and removed before complete recovery can occur. Symptoms can be expressions of the body's attempt to defend itself, to adapt and recover, to heal itself, or may be results of the causes of disease. The naturopathic physician seeks to treat the causes of disease, rather than to merely eliminate or suppress symptoms.

First do no harm (primum non nocere)

Naturopathic physicians follow three precepts to avoid harming the patient:

- **Naturopathic physicians utilize methods and medicinal substances which minimize the risk of harmful effects, and apply the least possible force or intervention necessary to diagnose illness and restore health.**
- **Whenever possible the suppression of symptoms is avoided as suppression generally interferes with the healing process.**
- **Naturopathic physicians respect and work with the *vis medicatrix naturae* in diagnosis, treatment and counselling, for if this self-healing process is not respected the patient may be harmed.**

Doctor as teacher (docere)

The original meaning of the root word for 'doctor', '*docere*', in Latin is teacher. A principal objective of naturopathic medicine is to educate the patient and emphasize self-responsibility for health. Naturopathic physicians also recognize and employ the therapeutic potential of the doctor-patient relationship.

Treat the whole person

Health and disease result from a complex of physical, mental, emotional, genetic, environmental, social and other factors. Since total health also includes spiritual health, naturopathic physicians encourage individuals to pursue their personal spiritual development. Naturopathic medicine recognizes the harmonious functioning of all aspects of the individual as being essential to health. The multifactorial nature of health and disease requires a personalized and comprehensive approach to diagnosis and treatment. Naturopathic physicians treat the whole person taking all of these factors into account.

Prevention

Naturopathic medical colleges emphasize the study of health as well as disease. The prevention of disease and the attainment of optimal health in patients are primary objectives of naturopathic medicine. In practice these objectives are accomplished through education and the promotion of healthy ways of living. Naturopathic physicians assess risk factors, heredity and susceptibility to disease, and make appropriate interventions in partnership with their patients to prevent illness. Naturopathic medicine asserts that one cannot be healthy in an unhealthy environment and is committed to the creation of a world in which humanity may thrive.

Practice
Naturopathic methods
Naturopathic medicine is defined primarily by its fundamental principles. Methods and modalities are selected and applied based upon these principles in the relationship to the individual needs of each patient. Diagnostic and therapeutic methods are selected from various sources and systems and will continue to evolve with the progress of knowledge.

Naturopathic practice
Naturopathic practice includes the following diagnostic and treatment modalities: utilization of all methods of clinical and laboratory diagnostic testing including diagnostic radiology and other imaging techniques; nutritional medicine, dietetics and therapeutic fasting; medicines of mineral, animal and botanical origin; hygiene and public health measures; naturopathic physical medicine including naturopathic manipulative therapies; the use of water, heat, cold, light, electricity, air, earth, electromagnetic and mechanical devices, ultrasound, and therapeutic exercise; homœopathy; acupuncture; psychotherapy and counselling; minor surgery and naturopathic obstetrics (natural childbirth). Naturopathic practice excludes major surgery and the use of most synthetic drugs.

Source: American Association of Naturopathic Physicians' definition of Naturopathic Medicine. Prepared for the Select Committee on The Definition of Naturopathic Medicine, Dr Pamela Snider and Dr Jared Zeff, Co-Chairs. Adopted 1 November 1989, Rippling River Convention, Oregon.

These six powerful concepts comprise both a unifying definition of naturopathic medicine and a theory of practice which follows from the defining principles. The definition and principles of practice provide a steady point of reference for all policy decision-making processes as a profession as well as assist an evolving understanding of health and disease (Snider & Zeff 1988).

History of naturopathic medicine

The constellation of practices that form naturopathic medicine today in Europe, Australia and the USA has its roots in the 'nature cure' movement of eighteenth- and nineteenth-century Europe. Some of these practices date back millennia and derive from the folk medicine of European cultures where the use of 'air, water and sunshine' as medicines was applied in the healing spas and health centres of Europe.

Nature cure as it was used in Europe incorporated a variety of techniques from adherence to a vegetarian diet to the use of water treatments and sunbathing as ways of treating specific conditions and promoting health. What united these therapies and provided the underpinning for the nature cure movement was a belief that this system of preventing and treating disease with natural agents was effective because it stimulated the body's self-curative processes and worked with the *vis medicatrix naturae* ('the healing power of nature').

The concept of the healing power of nature and the vitalistic philosophy that was its basis is attributed to Hippocrates (*c*.460–377 BCE). His treatise, *On Airs, Waters, and Places*, set forth his ideas on the importance of exploring every aspect of the patient's physical, social and emotional environment (Hippocrates 1987). The emphasis on the role of food, water and occupation as central to health and the development of disease is the beginning of a rational approach to medicine.

The person whose writings kept these ideas alive in the Arab world during the dark ages in Europe was Avicenna. His texts on medicine incorporated the works of the ancient Greeks, including Hippocrates, Galen and Dioscorides, and greatly extended and amplified the ideas which we now recognise as the foundations of naturopathy. In particular, his understanding of the elements, the humours and the constitution form the basis for individual prescribing and holistic treatment that is a central aspect of naturopathic medicine.

As it has developed in the course of the twentieth century, naturopathic medicine combined these ancient principles with the belief that the physician merely supports the active self-recuperative powers of the human body and applied this under-standing within the framework of modern scientific knowledge. In modern practice, then, naturopathy is an eclectic approach to practice that brings together techniques as diverse as hydrotherapy, dietary treatment, herbal medicine, massage, spinal manipulation and homœpathy.

The term 'naturopathy' was not coined until the late nineteenth century and is attributed to the German homœopath Scheel, who combined Latin and Greek root words to translate literally as 'nature disease' (Cody 1999). The term was utilised by Benedict Lust (1870–1945) to publicise his college in 1902. It was used as a way of describing both a style of healing and a way of life which he sought to introduce to America. Lust's experience of the nature cure movement derived directly from one of the major proponents of hydropathy, Father Sebastian Kneipp (1824–97).

The use of water as a therapy is a central form of treatment in many cultures. Hydrotherapy, a method of nature cure, combines therapeutic bathing with the specific use of mineral-rich waters internally. Throughout the nineteenth century hydropathy had a broad following in both Europe and the USA. In nineteenth-century Germany, hydropathy, as practised as part of nature cure, eventually combined the use of water and sunshine as treatments with herbal medicine and nutritional therapies (Kirchfeld & Boyle 1994). The hydrotherapy clinics of central Europe emphasised a vegetarian diet which avoided the use of all stimulants such as coffee, tea and tobacco and which encouraged healthy living in the form of adequate rest, relaxation and exercise as well as the cultivation of a positive mental outlook. Incorporating herbal medicine into this regime reinforced the therapeutic use of water as a treatment and the use of sunshine and relaxation as aspects of the healing process.

Lust combined the use of homœopathy, massage and manipulative techniques with the traditional nature cure practices of Kneipp. Lust was a great promoter of naturopathy in the USA through his colleges and the sanitaria he established around the country. He was a public figure, often persecuted by medical and religious groups that opposed natural medicine practitioners, particularly from the 1930s onward. From 1900 to 1920 there was a great interest in naturopathy in the USA and naturopaths were widely consulted (Wharton 1999).

Practitioners such as Priessnitz (1799–1852), Arnold Rikli (1823–1906) and Father Kneipp in Europe also promoted the practice of nature cure. Perhaps the best-known American practitioner and one of the earliest naturopaths in America was Henry Lindlahr (1862–1924). Lindlahr was himself treated by Father Kneipp and toured the nature cure establishments of Europe before studying medicine and osteopathy in America. On graduation he set up a sanitarium for nature cure and osteopathy in Chicago which integrated the use of manipulative therapy with nature cure techniques. Lindlahr went on to write two of the classic texts of early naturopathy, *The Practice of Nature Cure* and *Nature Cure: Philosophy and Practice Based on the Unity of Disease and Cure*. The traditional nature cure approach has sometimes been described as 'drugless medicine'.

Differences in practice around the world

Naturopathy developed in slightly different ways in Australia and Britain. In the nine-teenth century there were large numbers of nature cure practitioners in Australia. Many were trained in Europe or were self-trained. The use of hydrotherapy, herbal medicine and homœopathy was widespread, and techniques such as electrotherapy and medical clairvoyance were also combined with these naturopathic disciplines. Figures such as the homœopath Benjamin Fawcett lectured in Australia and published tracts about the practice of homœopathic medicine. John Broadbent published *The Australian Botanic Guide* and edited a professional journal for herbalists. The lack of medical practitioners in many areas was complemented by a range of non-orthodox practitioners who were well regarded in their local communities (Martyr 2002).

In Europe, nature cure maintained the popularity that had developed in the eighteenth and nineteenth centuries; however, the style of practice tended to be less eclectic than American practice. In the twentieth century natural medicine practitioners enjoyed varying degrees of popularity and legitimacy in different European countries. In Germany the practice of naturopathy was widespread and the popularity of natural medicine was boosted in the late 1930s by German nationalists, including Adolf Hitler. Currently, in Germany natural health practi-tioners are licensed as *Heilpraktikers* who train at accredited colleges and study for state licensing exams. *Heilpraktikers* work within the national health service, an unusual situation in Europe.

In England the practice of naturopathy was much less popular in the twentieth century than in the rest of Europe or the United States. Numbers of practitioners were smaller and there were few educational institutions. In England the practice of naturopathy is much closer to the tradition of 'drugless healing'. The eclectic approach to naturopathy, involving the use of therapies such as homœopathy, herbal medicine and dietary supplementation, was not popular in England. Osteopathy and naturopathy are combined in the teaching at the main college of naturopathy (the British College of Naturopathy and Osteopathy). This college has emphasised a fairly 'strict' nature cure approach to the training of naturopaths.

In much of the rest of western Europe naturopathic practice developed slowly from its antecedents in the traditional medical practices of those countries to its current form. Popularity waxed and waned in the nineteenth and twentieth centuries and this is reflected in very mixed legal, social and political positions in those countries today. In France, Belgium, Italy and Spain naturopathy is illegal while in the Netherlands the process of registration is underway (Fulder 1996).

Eclectic practice

Naturopathic physicians generally combine a range of therapeutic modalities within their treatments. In Britain and some European countries these therapies remain true to the nature cure paradigm. In Australia, New Zealand, Canada and the United States these therapies also include the use of natural medicines. The practice is truly eclectic with naturopaths choosing different sets of modalities that suit their style of practice. The core modalities which form the basis of naturopathic education in Australia are nutritional medicine, herbal medicine, physical medicine, homœopathic medicine and counselling. In North America many naturopathic programs also include Traditional Chinese Medicine, which has a different philosophical base and approach to practice. These modalities are outlined in their respective chapters.

The cornerstone of naturopathic medicine is sound nutrition (Zeff 1997). Diet is regarded as critical in stimulating the healing power of nature. Medical science has determined that malnourished individuals are susceptible to disease through multiple mechanisms. Equally, overnourished and significantly overweight individuals have higher rates of morbidity and mortality than those of average weight. Naturopaths firmly believe that the quality of food is an essential component of sound nutrition. An emphasis is placed on fresh fruits and vegetables and a decrease in artificial flavourings, colourings and preservatives. Naturopathic dietary practices include fasting, elimination diets and the addition of fruit and vegetable juices.

A basic holistic model

The concept of treating the whole person derives from an understanding that only treating the physical aspects of an individual is often inadequate to uncover the core of their illness. At its heart is the notion that an individual has many dimensions of which the physical is only one. Intrinsic to this concept is that these dimensions are unified to provide a whole individual who is greater then the simple sum of their parts. While the broad field of complementary medicine would agree with these statements, there is no real consensus as to what makes up these many dimensions. Different philosophies and world-views have models of the individual that differ significantly.

In order to teach this concept and to share a common language of holism the staff at Southern Cross University's School of Natural and Complementary Medicine defined a basic model of holism (see Figure 3.1). It was important in this defining process to acknowledge that this was only one way of perceiving the individual, hence the terminology a basic model. To remain semantically neutral the model was called 'A Basic Model of (W)Holistic Medicine'.

The model outlines a multidimensional approach to the individual, perceiving the individual as having physical, mental and spiritual dimensions that are fundamentally interrelated and inseparable. Physical is defined as the realm of matter; mental as the realm of thoughts and emotions; and spiritual as that dimension of

Figure 3.1 **A Basic Model of (W)Holistic Medicine 1999, School of Natural and Complementary Medicine, Southern Cross University**

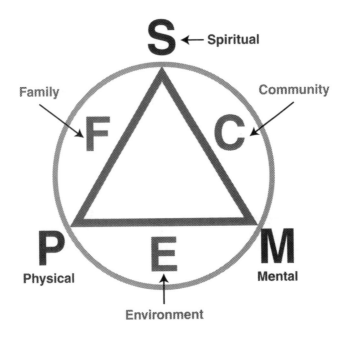

the individual that contains their core beliefs and values which gives rise to their 'life purpose', *joie de vivre* and 'will to live'. While the spiritual dimension of an individual may involve religion and religious beliefs, the concept is equally applicable to individuals who are agnostic or atheistic.

It is also important to recognise that the individual does not exist in isolation. In this model the individual is placed in a social and ecological continuum of family, community and environment. Here family is defined as all the important relationships in an individual's life; community as the broader social group or groups of which the individual is a part; and environment as the physical ecosystem in which the individual lives. In total six elements of whole-person care have been defined: (1) physical; (2) mental; (3) spiritual; (4) family; (5) community; and (6) environment.

The purpose of this model is to stimulate an understanding of the multidimensional nature of the individual and to describe a common language that can facilitate discussion and education. The educational goal of this model is to ensure that naturopathic students have a basic framework on which to base a whole-person practice, especially when making the difficult transition from being a student to a student clinician.

The therapeutic order

Clinical methods used by naturopathic physicians are applied in an ordered manner consistent with stimulating the healing power of nature, which directs maintenance of health and healing in the organism. The order of this application defines a hierarchy of healing, a therapeutic order. This order proceeds from least to most force, assumes an order of efficiency in integration of therapies and is determined by both the natural laws of healing and the patient's individual priorities and needs.

During the process of defining naturopathy in the United States many naturopathic physicians described the need to examine further the concepts of an innate order to the healing process. Today, this healing order has emerged from a deeper understanding of the core principle, the healing power of nature. This therapeutic order or hierarchy of healing is derived from concepts in Hippocrates's writings and those of medical scholars and nature doctors concerning the nature and laws of healing and provides a unifying theory of naturopathic medicine. Jared Zeff (1997) expressed these concepts as the 'Hierarchy of Therapeutics', which was modified by Snider and Zeff (Pizzorno & Snider 1999) into the Therapeutic Order. Faculties from North American naturopathic colleges contributed to this development (see below).

The Therapeutic Order
1. Re-establish the basis for health:
Remove obstacles to cure by addressing the determinants of health.

2. Stimulate the vis medicatrix naturae (healing power of nature):
Stimulate the inherent self-healing processes using techniques specific to individual modalities (including botanical, homœopathic, nutritional, hydrotherapy, psychological–spiritual medicine, Ayurvedic, Tibetan, Traditional Chinese Medicine, acupuncture).

3. Tonify weakened systems:
Use specific strategies from individual modalities (including botanical, homœopathic, nutritional, hydrotherapy, psychological–spiritual medicine, Ayurvedic, Tibetan, Traditional Chinese Medicine, acupuncture and others) to tonify weakened systems. Examples of tonification include: (i) strengthen the immune system; (ii) decrease toxicity; (iii) normalise inflammatory function; (iv) optimise metabolic function; (v) balance regulatory systems; (vi) enhance regeneration; and (vii) harmonise with the life force.

4. Correct structural integrity:
Use therapeutic exercise, manipulation, massage and other structural approaches to organise structure and promote healthy function.

5. Prescribe specific natural substances:
Use specific modalities or interventions for pathology, for example Tea Tree oil (*Melaleuca alternifolia*) for fungal infections and Saw Palmetto (*Serenoa repens*) for benign prostatic hyperplasia.

6. Prescribe specific pharmacological or synthetic substances:
Use modalities or interventions for pathology. Examples include antibiotics for infections and analgesics for pain.

7. Use higher-force interventions:
Use surgery, suppressive drugs, radiation, chemotherapy and other approaches.

The Patient
The actual Therapeutic Order may change,
depending on the individual patient's needs
for safe, effective care. The needs of the patient are
primary in determining the appropriate approach to therapy.

Source: Adapted from the original model developed by Zeff (1997) and modified by Pizzorno and Snider (1999).

Determinants of health

Naturopathic medicine is not primarily the diagnosis and treatment of disease with natural agents. It is a practice based upon the restoration of health. Although health is the natural state of being, it is affected by the interaction of the being with the environment, both internal and external. Health is a product of conditions which create health, and has specific determinants that can be studied and perceived in the patient. Naturopathic physicians address these important determinants as the first clinical step in the therapeutic or healing order (see Table 3.1).

Educational programs

Educational programs in Britain, the United States and Australia (see Table 3.2) reflect the differences between countries in the practice and regulation of naturopathy. In these countries, the last 10–15 years have seen naturopathic education move away from private college teaching and into private and government-subsidised universities. (Evans 2000).

Table 3.1   Determinants of health

Inborn
- Genetic makeup (genotype)
- Intra-uterine/congenital
- Maternal exposures
  —drugs
  —toxins
  —viruses
  —psycho-emotional
- Maternal nutrition
- Maternal lifestyle
- Constitution: determines susceptibility

Disturbances
- Illnesses: pathobiography
- Medical interventions (or lack of)
- Physical and emotional exposures, stresses and trauma
- Toxic and harmful substances

Hygienic factors/lifestyle factors: how we live
(Environment, lifestyle and psycho-emotional/spiritual health)
- Fresh air
- Exposure to nature
- Clean water
- Light
- Socioeconomic factors
- Culture
- Rest
- Exercise
- Nutrition
- Unadulterated food
- Loving and being loved
- Meaningful work
- Community
- Stress (physical, emotional)
- Trauma (physical, emotional)
- Medical interventions
- Spiritual, religious or inspirational life

Source: Developed by Zeff (1997) and modified by Pizzorno and Snider (1999).

Programs themselves reflect a change in the knowledge base of naturopathy. There is an increasing emphasis on scientific research as a tool for validating and exploring naturopathic practices. This has produced some controversy within the profession. Some argue that the movement away from the empiricism and traditional practices which have characterised naturopathy has resulted in the loss of a coherent philosophical perspective and the erosion of traditional naturopathic practice. Others make the argument that the use of scientific research to identify the safety and efficacy of traditional practices is what ensures the development of the profession as part of the current healthcare system worldwide (Hunter 2002).

Table 3.2   Major naturopathic training programs in Britain, North America and Australia in 2003

North America
Canadian College of Naturopathic Medicine (Toronto, Ontario)
Bastyr University (Washington)
National College of Naturopathic Medicine (Portland, Oregon)
South West College of Naturopathic Medicine and Health Science (Tempe, Arizona)
The University of Bridgeport College of Naturopathic Medicine (Bridgeport, Connecticut)

Britain
British College of Naturopathy and Osteopathy (London)

Australia
Australasian College of Natural Therapies (Sydney, New South Wales)
Australian College of Natural Medicine (Brisbane, Queensland)
Melbourne College of Natural Medicine (Melbourne, Victoria)
Nature Care College (Sydney, New South Wales)
Southern Cross University: School of Natural and Complementary Medicine (Lismore, New South Wales)
Southern School of Natural Therapies (Melbourne, Victoria)
University of Western Sydney (Sydney, New South Wales)

Upgrade qualifications
In addition to this a small number of universities (affiliated with private colleges) offer extension programs which enable practitioners with advanced diploma qualifications to earn bachelor degrees:

Charles Sturt University (Bachelor of Health Science—Complementary Medicine)
Southern Cross University (Bachelor of Natural Therapies)
University of New England (Bachelor of Health Science—conversion)
Victoria University (Bachelor of Health Science—Natural Medicine)

The most significant difference between courses offered in North America and those offered in Australia and Britain is that in North America naturopathic studies are post-graduate courses of four years' duration. Naturopathic medicine training in North America includes minor surgery and midwifery and graduates are able to prescribe orthodox pharmaceutical drugs. Their training includes herbal medicine, homœopathy, manipulative therapy, nutrition, hydropathy, lifestyle counselling, spirituality and health, natural hygiene and detoxification, physical medicine (including manipulation and electrotherapy) and exercise. On graduation practitioners are entitled to describe themselves as naturopathic doctors or naturopathic physicians. However, there are currently only thirteen states in America which permit the licensing of naturopathic practitioners. Licensing of naturopathic practitioners is a state matter and naturopathic practice falls under the definition of the practice of medicine, which is limited to medical practitioners.

In Australia and Britain naturopathic education is provided as an undergraduate degree or diploma. The programs in Australia include the study of nutrition, herbal medicine, tactile therapies and homœopathy. In Britain naturopathy is often taught without the inclusion of herbal medicine, nutritional supplements and homœopathy as therapies. Naturopathy may include hydropathy and osteopathy and is most likely to be based around dietary manipulation, fasting, remedial exercise and positive mental attitude. Natural medicine practitioners in both Britain and Australia are not trained to undertake surgery or to practise midwifery. Naturopaths in both Australia and Britain are self-regulated and although there are moves towards registration there are no minimum educational standards for practice in these countries.

Anecdotal comparisons of educational programs in these three countries seem to indicate that the United States maintains the strongest commitment to eclectic practice. This is combined with a training that emphasises a strong scientific base and the clinical skills to practise as a prime contact practitioner. In Britain naturopathic education is much closer to the traditional practice of naturopathy and in particular to the ideal of drugless medicine. In Australia a limited range of disciplines are taught within naturopathic programs and there is a strong emphasis on the importance of a scientific base but not at the expense of traditional naturopathic philosophy. In comparison with US programs Australian naturopathic education appears to have more depth in the modalities, while US programs have more depth in the biomedical sciences. This difference was marked in the 1980s; however, it had narrowed significantly by the turn of the millennium.

Models of naturopathic medicine

These different educational models give rise to different approaches to practising naturopathic medicine. North American naturopathic graduates are licensed to practise as primary care physicians and carry the sole responsibility for their patient's health. This responsibility includes making a western medical diagnosis as well as a naturopathic diagnosis, and undertaking the investigations that are required to confirm this diagnosis. In addition, naturopathic physicians can practise, in accordance with the laws in specific jurisdictions, minor surgery, assist in child delivery and prescribe certain plant-based pharmaceutical drugs (Smith & Logan 2002). Currently naturopaths are licensed in four Canadian provinces and twelve US states.

In Australia and Britain naturopaths practise under common law and currently no occupational regulation exists. In these countries naturopaths act as prime contact clinicians but not as primary care clinicians. Prime contact refers to the ability of a patient to present to a naturopath as their primary contact with the healthcare system. While not educated to be primary care practitioners, naturopaths need an appropriate level of education to be able to make critical clinical decisions about appropriate referral to other healthcare providers, most essentially orthodox medical doctors. In many instances patients are co-managed between a naturopath and general practitioner. However, one significant interprofessional challenge is that many patients do not tell their doctor that they are taking natural medicines due to concern about the orthodox medical practitioner's reaction. A survey by MacLennan *et al.* (2002) showed that 52.7 per cent of individuals who had used natural medicines in the previous year did so without their general practitioner's knowledge. This problem is not limited to Australia; in the United States 63 per cent of respondents ($n = 831$) who used orthodox and complementary medicine did not disclose at least one of their complementary therapies to their doctor (Eisenberg *et al.* 2001).

Another interprofessional challenge in Australia is the concerns that orthodox general practitioners have as registered clinicians in referring to unregistered health professionals. While cross-referral and interprofessional communication does take place, there is considerable work that needs to be undertaken to increase and strengthen the connection. In Australia, state health departments are looking at occupational regulation of naturopaths as part of a wider agenda of establishing standards within the field of complementary medicine. This will be a major step forward in the professionalisation of naturopathic clinicians.

The number of licensed naturopathic physicians is quite small in comparison to the North American population. There are approximately 3000 licensed naturopathic physicians in a population of 313 million (USA and Canada). This gives a practice to population ratio of 1 to 104 000 people. In contrast, in Australia approximately 3000 naturopaths are in practice in a population of 19.8 million, which gives a practice to population ratio of 1 to 6000, seventeen times the US figure. While these figures are approximations they reflect a real distinction between these two countries. In Australia the community exposure to naturopathy and the community under-standing of naturopathic practice is much greater, simply due to the number of naturopaths in the community. Six per cent ($n = 183$) of a randomly selected sample of the South Australian population ($n = 3027$) in 2000 had seen a naturopath in the previous year. This represented 3.3 per cent of males and 8.7 per cent of females interviewed (MacLennan *et al.* 2002).

Blending science and tradition

One of the critical arts of naturopathic medicine is blending science and traditional knowledge. Unlike other forms of traditional medicine, naturopathy includes biomedical science as part of its core belief structure. Physiology and biochemistry and an understanding of the physiological basis of health and disease are central to a discipline that has a focus on homœostasis and stimulation of the body's innate capacity to return to equilibrium. In addition to the inclusion of science, naturopathy has a long tradition and an evolved approach to practice that forms the basis of its philosophy and its clinical principles.

The modern naturopath walks a fine line between these two paradigms and works with both the scientific and the traditional knowledge. Ideally the naturopath needs to remain constantly vigilant and constructively critical, aware of the current science and its application to practice. At the same time, it is important to utilise and respect the traditional knowledge and remain mindful of the central tenets of naturopathic practice. While this might seem a difficult task to some outsiders, naturopathic graduates have generally become adept at successfully juggling these two paradigms after four years of intensive naturopathic education. Research in Canada on a sample of 41 students suggests that they enter naturopathic education with either the scientific or holistic world-view dominant and do not change this dominant world-view while studying naturopathy. However, what occurs is a new appreciation of the other world-view which Boon attributes to a socialisation effect (Boon 1998). In at least one educational institution this balancing of science and tradition is considered an essential graduate outcome and embedded into the educational curriculum.

Case studies in naturopathic treatment

The principles and practices of naturopathic medicine can best be summarised by examining the treatment approaches arising from two case studies.

Case 1

A 42-year-old man presents with upper abdominal pain and reflux. In addition he has mild hypertension (145/95) and mild hypercholesterolemia. At the time of his presentation his doctor is monitoring both with a view to medication if they are not reduced in the next two months. He has had a diagnosis of excessive stomach acid production and on gastroscopy there is some inflammation of the oesophagus. He is already taking an acid inhibitor but wants to know if there are other ways that his symptoms can be managed.

Further discussion reveals that the last year has been particularly stressful. He is a team manager in a large corporation and although he denies that his job is stressful there has been a recent restructuring which has required him to make redundant half of his staff. About nine months ago his grandmother, to whom he was particularly close, died. He and his wife have just had their first child who is currently twelve weeks old. In the course of the pregnancy foetal monitoring revealed the possibility of a genetic abnormality which required ongoing foetal testing throughout the pregnancy. Fortunately, the child was delivered normally and the predicted abnormality was not present.

The naturopathic consultation revolved around encouraging the patient (and his wife who was also present) to recognise the stresses that had been present in the last year. There was discussion of the nature of early parenting and its joys and difficulties and the patient was given a number of pieces of advice.

- **To exercise for 40 minutes to one hour three times a week.**
- **To eat slowly and when seated. He was also told to avoid coffee, alcohol, acidic foods (e.g. orange juice and tomatoes) and spices and to eat every three hours.**
- **His dietary advice emphasised a low-fat, low-salt diet and included deep-sea fish three times a week and other foods rich in essential fatty acids.**
- **His herbal medicines included *Matricaria chamomilla* (chamomile), *Viburnum opulus* (cramp bark), *Cynara scolymus* (globe artichoke), *Erythraea centaurium* (centaury) and *Glycyrrhiza glabra* (liquorice) (low dose).**

In two months his blood pressure was normal, his cholesterol was normal and his stomach symptoms were greatly reduced. Recognition of the underlying stresses in his life had given him a sense of control and by taking up exercise he had lost 5 kg and was significantly more relaxed.

Case 2

A 49-year-old woman presents with significant mood fluctuations especially premenstrually, menstrual irregularity with some menorrhagia of three months' duration and non-specific stiffness in the mornings. On further questioning she has experienced some heat at night and occasional hot flushes during the day, and her pre-menstrual symptoms include headaches, nausea and constipation in the week prior to her period. Recent hormonal tests reveal her FSH is not yet at post-menopausal levels. Her diet is based around meat as the major source of protein, and she eats few grains, little fruit and relies on chocolate for her mid-afternoon energy boost. She works for a large legal firm and has considerable responsibility and frequent deadlines. She is married and has three teenage children and a husband who is employed as a high school teacher.

The naturopathic consultation revolved around a discussion of menopause and the peri-menopausal hormonal changes and the symptoms that could be related to hormonal change. Many of her symptoms related to changing hormonal levels and the patient was reassured to recognise that although her hormone tests did not indicate menopausal status yet her clinical presentation was indicative of peri-menopausal changes. The patient was encouraged to discuss what she knew and didn't know about menopause. She welcomed some suggestions for reading about the menopausal process and what treatment options were available. A number of preventive health screens were discussed including cholesterol tests, mammograms, pap smear and bone density tests. The possibility of calcium supplementation depending on the outcome of bone density testing was considered.

Dietary recommendations included:

- **increased deep-sea fish intake (including tinned bony fish such as salmon and sardines) while reducing her red meat intake;**
- **a review of her calcium intake;**
- **inclusion of linseed, sunflower seeds and almonds as part of her daily breakfast;**
- **increased intake of phytoestrogen-rich foods including soy foods, grains and legumes.**

Her herbal prescription included ***Angelica chinensis* (dong quai)**, ***Cimicifuga racemosa* (black cohosh)**, ***Verbena officinalis* (vervain)**, ***Taraxacum vulgaris* (dandelion)** and ***Hypericum perforatum* (St John's wort)**. Other recommendations included a regular program of exercise based around weight-bearing activities such as walking, gym work and tennis. This patient was managed for the next three years during which time she moved through menopause. She was happy to use herbal and nutritional supplements to manage all her menopausal symptoms.

Future development

The marked increase in community utilisation of complementary medicine over the past three decades has led to a resurgence in the role of naturopathic medicine. In Australia educational programs have entered the university sector while in the United States one naturopathic college has made the transition to a federally recognised university. Smith and Logan (2002) consider that there appears to be a rapid professional evolution within naturopathic medicine. This is a view shared by those who have seen the changes taking place over the past decade. It is likely that naturopathic medicine, like other complementary medicine practices, is heading toward the mainstream. How this new integrated medicine will look is uncertain; however, it is fairly certain that there will be increased links between naturopathic and orthodox health professionals and their institutions and policy makers. Many challenges will need to be met by the profession. How naturopathic medicine rises to the challenges of this new integrated healthcare will shape its future. Those within the profession generally see the future as positive and the potential of their medicine and profession as immense. Long-time naturopathic physician and educational pioneer, Dr Bill Mitchel, summed up this potential poetically to a group of naturopathic educators at the annual meeting of the AANP in Salt Lake City in 2002 when he said, 'naturopathic medicine is a flower that is yet to bloom'.

Recommended reading

Pizzorno, J. and Murray, M. (eds) 1999, *Textbook of Natural Medicine*, 2nd edn, Churchill Livingstone, New York.

Newman Turner, R. 1984, *Naturopathic Medicine. Treating the Whole Person*, Thorsons Publishers, Wellingborough.

Jonas, W.B. and Levin, J.S. (eds) 1999, *Essentials of Complementary and Alternative Medicine*, Lippincott, Williams & Wilkins, Philadelphia.

4

Traditional Chinese Medicine
Corinne G. Patching van der Sluijs, Alan Bensoussan

Traditional Chinese Medicine (TCM) is a comprehensive, holistic oriental healing art that includes acupuncture, herbal medicine, massage, diet and exercise therapy. In the West, acupuncture and herbal medicine are the most commonly used TCM modalities. Acupuncture involves the insertion of fine metallic needles at defined locations. Herbal treatment constitutes injesting an empirically determined herbal formula often consisting of roots, berries, leaves or twigs. Even though this ancient medical system has developed in China over some 3000 years, TCM is enjoying a renaissance in occidental countries such as England (Chan & Lee 2002), the United States (Hui *et al.* 2002) and Australia (MacLennan *et al.* 2002).

One plausible explanation for this trend may be that TCM provides a viable treatment option for a variety of ailments. Well-designed clinical trials have demonstrated the effectiveness of TCM for a range of medical conditions, including acupuncture in alleviating primary dysmenorrhea (Helms 1987) and migraine headaches (Loh *et al.* 1984) and herbal medicine in reducing the signs and symptoms of Irritable Bowel Syndrome (Bensoussan *et al.* 1998) and atopic eczema (Sheehan & Atherton 1992).

After outlining the historical development of TCM, this chapter explores the basic theories of health and disease according to this medical practice. The case histories of two fictional patients, Mary and June, will be used as examples to explain TCM philosophy, pathology, diagnosis and treatment principles.

A brief history of TCM

The history of Chinese medicine extends back to before 2100 BCE when three legendary emperor-gods, Fu Xi, Shen Nong and Huang Di, were said to have lived. Fu Xi was credited with designing nine types of acupuncture needles at a time when acupuncture and moxibustion were first invented to relieve minor complaints. Shen Nong was the founder and instigator of agriculture, and was also reputed to have determined the functions and classification of hundreds of medicinal plants by tasting them. During this process he was said to have been poisoned daily (Zhang &

Rose 1999; Liu 1995). Finally, the first emperor Huang Di, along with his cabinet, developed medical techniques for the diagnosis and treatment of disease (Chan 2002).

The oldest extant literary classic which first conceptualised Chinese medicine was attributed to Huang Di. The *Huang Di Nei Jing* (*The Yellow Emperor's Classic of Internal Medicine*) was compiled by several authors during the Warring States period (475–221 BCE) as a series of questions asked by Huang Di of his Chief Physician, Qi Bo. The book is an early blueprint of Chinese medicine as it descibes definitions of health, the attainment of longevity and medical theories and practice (Zhang & Rose 1999). The book consists of two volumes, the *Su Wen* (*Simple Questions*), which discusses medical theory including terminology, physiology, pathology and philosophy, and the second volume, the *Ling Shu* (*Spiritual Axis*), which mainly focuses on the practice of acupuncture and moxibustion.

Herbal medicine thrived during the Han Dynasty (202 BCE to 220 CE). During this time many herbs from India and the Middle East were imported into China via the Silk Road along with an understanding of their actions and use. The culmination of this growth in knowledge resulted in the compilation of the first herbal text entitled the *Shen Nong Ben Cao Jing* (Zhang & Rose 1999).

Other classic texts written during this period include the *Mai Jing* (*The Classic of the Pulse*) by Wang Shu He and the *Shang Han Lun* (*On Cold Damage*) by Zhang Zhong Jing. The *Shang Han Lun* discusses the aetiology and treatment of febrile diseases and presents numerous herbal prescriptions that are still used today. In total, some 6000 medical texts detailing the theories and clinical experiences of medical doctors during the ages are still in existance today (Liu 1995).

TCM continued to flourish until the end of the nineteeth century when western medical ideas were introduced into China by Jesuit missionaries. This new medical system was favoured by the Nationalist Government and by '1929 the National Committee of Public Health had adopted a resolution to abolish TCM' (Zhang & Rose 1999: 167). However, since the founding of the People's Republic of China, the communists revitalised, modernised and encouraged the use of TCM. They understood that TCM offered low-cost basic healthcare that could cater for large numbers of people.

The formal integration of TCM with modern medicine began in the 1950s. Today, China, South Korea and Vietnam are some of the few countries in the world where traditional and western medicine are integrated and practised at every level of the healthcare system for the treatment of both acute and chronic conditions. Every major city in China has a hospital of TCM and most hospitals practising western medicine have a department of TCM. Approximately 40 per cent of China's healthcare constitutes traditional medical care (Hesketh & Zhu 1997). However, this figure climbs to a staggering 80 per cent if individuals who consume herbal preparations for both the treatment and prevention of disease are considered (Bensoussan & Myers 1996).

Introducing Mary and June

Mary is a 40-year-old career executive who directs several large client portfolios for a major international investment bank. Her job entails the management of significant sums of international money, which means frequent overseas travel liasing with clients. Even though Mary spends a lot of time away from her family she enjoys the challenges of her profession. Unfortunately, the stress of her work is taking a toll on her body.

Mary is a thin woman who is constantly on the move. She often feels tired, irritable and short tempered. Mary has trouble sleeping, but when she does sleep she has vivid dreams. Her eyes are often sore, and within her field of vision she has noticed black floating specks. Each month she experiences severe dysmenorrhea which leaves her exhausted and depressed. The dysmenorrhea is worsened with stress and she occasionally needs to take time off work. During times of stress Mary also suffers from alternating constipation and diarrhoea with cramping pains in the lower abdomen. Mary, however, is reluctant to see a doctor and be given medication.

During lunch one day her friend June suggested that Mary see a Chinese medical practitioner. June had experienced much relief from period pain after a course of treatments. Mary had never considered Chinese medicine but was willing to try as she knew her ill health was affecting her life. She made an appointment for the next week.

The basic theories of TCM

By observing and studying their environment, the ancient Chinese philosophers developed theories to help explain the nature and behaviour of phenomena within the universe. These theories expounded the principles of motion and change, concepts that were applied to the ancient sciences including medicine, agriculture, geography and astronomy (Liu 1995; Wiseman & Ellis 1996). The main theoretical tools applicable to Chinese medicine are the theories of Yin and Yang, the Five Phases, the Channels and progression of disease according to the Six Divisions (of the body). These theories help to explain health and disease within the human body. Importantly, like other scientific theories that have stood the test of time, these theories are based largely on observation and claim some predictive ability.

The theories of Chinese medicine not only describe medical ideas that are paramount to the philosophy of TCM but also those that can be applied to specific clinical contexts. This is not unusual in the history of science. For example, light may be described as electromagnetic radiation (of different wavelengths) in order to facilitate an understanding of diffraction, refraction and appearance of the colours of the rainbow. In different circumstances light may also be described as particles (quanta) capable of colliding with other particles and exhibiting momentum. Each theory more readily lends itself to an application in a specific context. The theoretical premises described in this chapter, therefore, might be best treated as tools used by TCM practitioners to help explain the relationship between symptoms and signs, and the progression or resolution of disease. They are arguably reliable tools in that they offer guidance toward designing intervention and have some capacity to predict clinical outcome.

Yin and Yang

It was observed by the ancient Chinese philosophers that all phenomena in the universe can be grouped into pairs of opposites or mutual complements, called Yin and Yang. The first reference to this theory was made in the *Book of Changes* written in 700 BCE (Maciocia 1995). These pairs describe how characteristics function in relation to each other, and explain the process of change (Freeman & Lawlis 2001).

The *Nei Jing* (Veith 1972) defines these opposite but complementary pairs in terms of fire and water. Phenomena which are Yang in nature exhibit the characteristics of fire, such as lightness, brightness, heating and activity, and have a tendency to move outwards and upwards. Yin phenomena exemplify water by being heavy, dark, cold and quiet. Their movement tends to be down and inwards. Fire is essential in sparking and maintaining physiological processes, whereas water is nourishing, moistening and cooling. For health to be maintained, a balance is needed between water and fire, that is, between Yin and Yang.

Each Yin and Yang component of a complementary pair is defined in relation to the other. For example, day is determined in relation to night and tallness defines shortness. Likewise, the anatomy of the body can be described in terms of Yin and Yang. The back is Yang in relation to the front, which is Yin; the chest is Yang when compared to the abdomen (Ni 1995).

Another premise of the theory of Yin and Yang is that no one phenomenon is absolutely Yin or Yang in nature. Within Yin or Yang there is a grain of its complementary opposite, allowing for the potential to change. This can be seen diurnally, whereby within the Yin of night lies the seed of Yang, allowing for the possibility of another day. Likewise the seasons: within the equinox of summer lies the potential for the solstice of winter. For all cycles of change there must be a dynamic balance to ensure a harmonious transition. Therefore, the theory of Yin and Yang can be applied to explain the dynamic relationships between phenomena during the processes of change.

From Mary's brief case history, a TCM practitioner would be able to determine her overall nature as being either one of Yin or Yang. Mary's condition exhibits more Yang-like qualities such as insomnia, a thin body type, always on the go and restlessness. A Yin-type person would tend to be cold, pale, move slowly and possibly be overweight. These are very broad categories and on their own are not enough for an adequate diagnosis.

The Five Phases or Elements

The Five Phases or Elements are represented by Wood, Fire, Earth, Metal and Water. The phases depict cyclical change associated with the seasons, growth and physical development. Categories of related functions, qualities and structures pertinent to Chinese medicine are also represented by each of the phases. Therefore, associated with each phase is a season, climate, Organ, body tissue, emotion, colour, smell and taste. These are called 'correspondences'. (The word 'Organ' refers to the TCM concept of 'organ' and is written with a capital 'O' to differentiate it from English and/or conventional medical meanings. This also applies to other TCM concepts such as Blood, Qi, Essence and Spirit.) The main correspondences are listed in Table 4.1, and they serve as useful tools for diagnosis.

Table 4.1   The main correspondences of the Five Phases

	Wood	Fire	Earth	Metal	Water
Season	Spring	Summer	Late Summer	Autumn	Winter
Climate	Wind	Heat	Dampness	Dryness	Cold
Developmental stage	Birth	Growth	Transformation	Harvest	Storage
Colour	Green	Red	Yellow	White	Black
Organ	Liver and gall bladder	Heart and small intestine	Spleen and stomach	Lungs and large intestine	Kidneys and bladder
Sense organ	Eyes	Tongue	Mouth	Nose	Ears
Tissue	Sinews	Blood vessels	Muscles	Skin	Bones
Emotion	Anger	Joy	Worry	Sadness	Fear
Taste	Sour	Bitter	Sweet	Pungent	Salty
Smell	Rancid	Scorched	Fragrant	Rotten	Putrid
Sound	Shouting	Laughing	Singing	Crying	Groaning

Two main dynamic relationships exist between the phases and these are used as models to explain harmony and disharmony within the body (refer to Figure 4.1). The first, the Generating Cycle, flows in a clockwise fashion. The preceding element, termed the 'mother', generates and promotes the ensuing or 'child' element. Therefore, pathology within an Organ may occur if a deficient child element demands nourishment from the mother, or if the mother element fails to nourish the

Figure 4.1   Dynamic relationships of the Five Phases

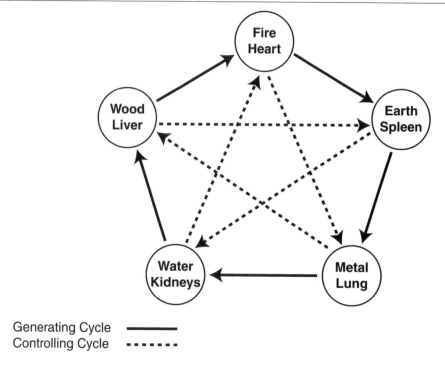

Generating Cycle ——————
Controlling Cycle ▪ ▪ ▪ ▪ ▪ ▪

child adequately. Treatment may entail tonifying the mother organ if the child is deficient (Liu 1995).

The Controlling or Restraining Cycle ensures that each phase controls and is controlled by another phase of the cycle. This cycle maintains balance within the body by preventing excessive energy build-up in any one Organ (Liu 1995).

The Generating and the Controlling Cycles are inseparable relationships that mutually support and restrain the system, ensuring stability and balance within the body. Due to all phases being interrelated, a pathological change within one Organ will impact on the whole system (Liu 1995). This will be explained further in relation to Mary's case history later.

Within a healthy organism, these dynamic but controlled relationships ensure a state of balance and harmony. The metabolic processes of homœostasis, which involve internal feedback mechanisms to ensure a state of equilibrium within the body, can therefore be represented by the relationships depicted by the Five Phases.

The Five Phases and homœostasis

Homœostatic processes ensure the internal environment within the body is kept relatively constant within narrow limits of physiological variation. Processes under homœostatic control include blood pressure, body temperature and blood glucose. The regulation of signals that maintain homœostatic balance are complex and may include positive, negative and mixed feedback control mechanisms (Bellavite *et al.* 1998).

The Five Phase model describes a homœostatic system with inbuilt regulatory controls. The promoting action of the Generating Cycle combined with the regulatory inhibition of the Controlling Cycle demonstrates the workings of a balanced system. The interrelated nature of each phase depicts a complex organism made up of a network of structures that depend directly or indirectly on the state and changes of the other components or phases (Bellavite *et al.* 1998).

All living organisms are able to self-organise, internally regulate and adapt to the external environment. In order to respond and adapt to external stimuli, the organism must function as an open system so that stimuli can be registered, internalised and then responded to appropriately. An open system also allows for healing to take place, as the organism is able to internalise an external stimulus, such as the manipulation of an acupuncture needle at an acupoint, to bring about balance via the relationships according to the Five Phases (Bellavite *et al.* 1998). Therefore, external environmental stimuli can affect the functioning and ultimately the health of an organism. This inseparability of the universe from the body is one of the basic philosophies of TCM.

The basic philosophies of TCM

The development of a science such as medicine depends on the pervasive philosophy of the culture of a society (Liu 2002). In this respect, the theories of TCM are rooted in ancient Taoist and Confucian thought. However, Chinese medicine as practised today has also culminated from the analysis, synthesis and integration of medical philosophical ideas and clinical observations generated over the past three millennia. This has resulted in a unique theoretical framework that describes the physiology of the body, the aetiology of disease and the diagnosis and treatment of the patient.

This section discusses the main philosophies of TCM. These include the holistic nature of the body, the unity of man and the universe, the uniqueness of the individual, the nature of disease and the concept of Qi.

The concept of holism

The concept of holism is fundamental to TCM diagnosis and treatment. Holism implies the complete integration of all functioning systems within the body creating unity. This is achieved by a network of energy pathways or meridians that connect all Organ systems, allowing for integration through communication and homœostatic regulation. Due to this network, a disorder in one component of the system can influence the functioning of the whole organism.

The dichotomy of body and mind does not exist in holism. The emotions have a bearing on the body in both health and disease. Excessive emotions or emotions not appropriately expressed can cause disharmony in the associated Organ. Likewise, disharmony within an Organ can cause emotional distress.

As holism implies that all components of an organism interrelate, the condition of the whole organism will be reflected in each part of the system. This is an important principle for diagnosis, as the condition of the skin, tongue or pulse reflect pathological changes that occur within the body (Maciocia 1995).

Holism also refers to the unity and integrity of the body with the universe. The body obtains its needs directly from the environment in the form of air, water, food, light and touch. In this way, the universe has a direct effect on the health and wellbeing of the individual. Other important environmental influences to consider when making a diagnosis are the impact of the seasons, climate, geography, social interactions, living conditions and workplace conditions (Liu 2002).

The close relationship of the body with the universe means that any seasonal or diurnal variations in energy will affect the circulation of Qi (vital life energy) and Blood within the organism. These subtle energetic changes can be felt in the pulse. During the most Yang season of summer, Qi and Blood flow toward the body's surface and this is reflected in a full and superficial Yang pulse. In winter, Qi and Blood flow inwards reflecting the Yin nature of the season. The pulse will be felt close to the bone (Ni 1995). During the day, Yang Qi circulates towards the exterior of the body, whereas at night Yang energy flows towards the interior.

Other external universal factors that impact on an individual include the social environment and economic influences. The social environment involves social interactions with friends, relations, neighbours and work colleagues. Uplifting and edifying relationships will strengthen an individual, whereas stressful relationships will impact negatively. Economic influences, such as job loss, war or depression, impact on living standards. These stresses can give rise to pathology or influence existing disease processes (Liu 2002).

Therefore, when treating a patient the TCM practitioner will consider the whole person and their universe. Mary, on visiting a TCM practitioner, will be asked about her relationships at work and home, her lifestyle habits and her emotional constitution. TCM philosophy sees the individual as a microcosm reflecting the workings of the external macrocosm: the body is a part of, and cannot be disassociated from, the universe.

Each person is unique

Each person is unique. This uniqueness reflects individual environmental influences and individual metabolic requirements. Therefore, even though two people present with the same condition, their diagnoses may be different.

Mary and her friend both suffer from dysmenorrhea. On detailed assessment their whole-person profiles paint two very different types of ailments.

About a week before her period is due, Mary feels irritable and tense and her breasts begin to feel distended and painful. The menstrual pain begins a day before her menses and is relieved several days later. She feels a cramping, heavy, dull-like pain in her abdomen. Her menses is generally regular with dark blood and very few clots. Mary has noticed that her period pain is worse after a particularly stressful time.

June presented with a different set of symptoms. She felt an intense cramping in the lower abdomen that occurred during the time of menstruation. Her menstrual flow was bright red with small dark clots. Each month her lower back ached and she felt cold and miserable. She found that the application of heat relieved her abdominal pain and backache to some degree.

As can be seen, these case histories demonstrate two different scenarios for dys-menorrhea. Mary's condition is exacerbated by stress and is typified by a feeling of stagnation as noted by her swollen breasts and cramping before menses. June, however, did not display signs of stagnation, and stress did not influence her condition. She felt cold during her period and her pain was relieved by warmth. These different case histories mean that the diagnoses and treatment approaches for these two women will not be the same. Acupuncture points and herbs that promote the movement of Qi to disperse stagnation will be given to Mary, whereas June will be prescribed warming herbs or moxibustion.

Disease is disharmony within the body

Western medicine has been argued to have a predominantly reductionist approach to health and disease, attempting to search for the cause of a symptom and the eradication of the causative agent (Weatherall 1997; Kaptchuk 1993). In contrast, the practice of TCM searches for relationships between the body, the presenting signs and symptoms and the environment.

During the diagnostic process, all signs, symptoms and relevant information is considered, analysed and meshed to determine the syndrome complex or 'pattern of disharmony'. Liu (2002: 39) describes a pattern of disharmony as a 'pathological generalisation of a group of closely related symptoms at a given stage during the course of the disease development'. The practitioner obtains the case history from the patient by asking, looking, listening, taking the pulse and reading the tongue. Therefore, the diagnosis is an explanation of the internal disharmony and guides the practitioner in their choice of treatment (Kaptchuk 1993).

Qi and the Vital Substances

Qi is the fundamental substance that makes up the universe (Liu 2002). In its most dense form Qi constitutes matter and in its most rarified form Qi becomes energy. Therefore, the condensation of Qi can be envisaged as being on a continuum with matter at one extreme and energy at the other. Furthermore, the energetic nature of Qi causes movement and change both within the universe and the human body. Therefore, Qi not only constitutes the physical manifestation of the body but also the vital energy or life force that flows thoughout the organism (Maciocia 1995).

Within the body Qi can be defined by its function. These actions include movement, warmth, protection from pathogenic invasion and the transportation and transformation of metabolic substances. Normal or undifferentiated Qi flowing throughout the body is derived from ingested food and drink, inhaled air and from Qi contributed by one's parents at conception. Normal Qi transforms into other bodily forms of Qi, such as Organ, Channel, Nutritive or Protective Qi (Maciocia 1995; Wiseman & Ellis 1996).

The Vital Substances are the basic materials of life. These not only include Qi, but also Blood, Essence, the Spirit and Body Fluids. These materials are different manifestations of Qi, with Essence and Spirit being rarefied and Blood being a dense form.

Essence

Jing, or Essence, is the 'seed' or basis of life. A new life is formed when the reproductive Essence contained within the ovum and sperm unite. This Essence constitutes the underlying material for the new organism and will be the source of change throughout life as evident by growth and reproduction (Wiseman & Ellis 1996).

The Essence received from one's parents at conception is termed Prenatal Essence and is stored in the Kidneys. Prenatal Essence determines the constitution of the individual, and regulates growth, development, reproduction and ageing throughout the lifespan. With ageing, Prenatal Essence is gradually depleted and this decline cannot be fully restored. Postnatal Essence is extracted from ingested food, drink and air, and supplements the Prenatal Essence. Moderate living with the intake of good quality food and drink over a lifetime ensures a slower depletion of Essence and the possibility of a longer life (Maciocia 1995).

Spirit

Within the Heart resides the Spirit, or *Shen*. The Spirit is responsible for human consciousness, a trait unique to human life. Therefore, the Spirit gives an individual an awareness and a personality, enabling the ability to think, reason and make decisions. *Shen* is also the vital force behind Qi and Essence (Kaptchuk 1993).

Blood

Blood is a dense form of Qi which nourishes and moistens the body. Blood is formed when Qi that is refined from food and drink by the Spleen combines with air Qi extracted by the lungs. The Heart pumps Blood around the body via the blood vessels in conjunction with chest Qi (Maciocia 1995). The amount of Blood flowing within the vessels is regulated by the Liver. During times of activity Blood flows freely in the vessels; with inactivity the Blood is stored in the Liver (Ni 1995).

Body Fluids

The Body Fluids include all fluids, other than Blood, that are produced and secreted by the body. These include saliva, urine, tears, gastric juices, sweat and mucus. Fluids moisten the skin, muscles and organs, lubricate the joints and nourish the brain, marrow and bones. Fluids are extracted from ingested food and drink and their metabolism involves many Organs. The transport and discharge of Fluids is mainly under control of the Kidneys (Maciocia 1995).

The Organ Systems and the influence of pathology

The Organ Systems make up the framework of the body. The TCM concept of the Organs differs from that of western medicine. Western medicine defines the function of an organ by its anatomical and physiological structure, whereas Chinese medicine is concerned with the functional activity of an Organ (Kaptchuk 1993). Each Organ is regarded as a system made up of an integrated functional network that includes the Organ's corresponding tissue, sense organ, emotion, mental activity, bodily function, meridian and environmental influence (refer to Table 4.1). In Chinese medicine these Organ Systems are known as the *Zang Fu*. The main functions of the internal Organs are to produce, replenish, transform and move the Vital Substances (Maciocia 1995).

The body consists of eleven Organs. The five Yin Organs are the Liver, Heart, Spleen, Lungs and Kidneys. These are considered to be solid, inferring that their main functions are to produce, transform, store and regulate the Vital Substances. The hollow Yang Organs are the Gall Bladder, Triple Burner, Small Intestine, Stomach, Large Intestine and Bladder. The Yang Organs transport and digest the remaining portions of food and fluids that are not transformed into Vital Substances. The impure by-products are excreted via these Organs (Ni 1995).

Several Yin Organs are involved in the pathology of Mary's case history, as outlined in Figure 4.2. The Liver ensures the free flow of Qi, Blood and emotions within the body, so that all physiological processes are smoothly regulated. Mary's symptoms strongly suggest a disharmony within the Liver. The long-term stress at work has resulted in the stagnation of Liver Qi. The monthly pre-menstrual tension with swollen painful breasts and cramping are signs that the Liver can no longer regulate the smooth flow of Qi before and at the time of menstruation. Stagnation of Qi within the Liver has also affected Mary's emotional state. The anger and depression that Mary expresses are emotions often connected to the Liver.

The eyes are the sense organ related to the Liver. Mary's vision is interrupted by black floaters and her eyes are often sore. These are additional signs that the Liver is involved in the pathology of Mary's condition. The disharmony within Mary's Liver has failed to nourish the Heart adequately via the Generating Cycle. Besides pumping the Blood throughout the blood vessels, the Heart also houses the Spirit, or *Shen*. However, because the Heart lacks adequate nourishment the *Shen* is not rooted or grounded within the Heart, leading to insomnia and vivid dreams.

The process of digestion is predominately carried out by the Spleen, Stomach and Intestines. The Stomach initiates digestion, while the Spleen extracts the pure nutritive substances from ingested food and fluids and transports these to the appropriate Organs for transformation into the Vital Substances.

For digestion to proceed smoothly balance must be maintained between the Wood and Earth elements. The Liver controls the activities of the Spleen and Stomach via the Controlling Cycle, and also ensures the smooth flow of Qi during the digestive process. However, the continued stress within Mary's life has caused excessive energy build-up (stagnation) within the Liver and a corresponding deficiency of energy within the Stomach and Spleen. During times of acute stress, this stagnation is exacerbated and rises to such a level that it spills over onto the weakened Earth element (Spleen and Stomach), causing over-restraint and disruption to the digestive process, as evident by constipation and cramping in the lower abdomen. When the stress subsides the over-control by the Liver slackens resulting in the descent of Qi, as manifested by diarrhoea. In addition, the inadequate nourishment of the Heart by the Liver means that the Heart cannot nourish its child, the Spleen, causing further disruption to the activities of the Spleen and Stomach. This complex interrelationship has been simplified in Figure 4.2 to show how the Five Phase theory can be used as a model to explain the pathology of Mary's condition.

The origins of disease

The six excessive climatic influences

The six external climatic influences that may invade the body to cause disharmony are: Wind, Cold, Summer Heat, Fire, Damp and Dryness. Even though the climatic factors are linked to a season they can occur any time during the year. These pathogenic influences only invade the body and bring about disharmony if the climatic influence is unusually excessive, abruptly changes into another or the body's resistance is too weak to accommodate these changes (Maciocia 1995).

Figure 4.2   The pathology of Mary's condition as explained by the Five Phase model

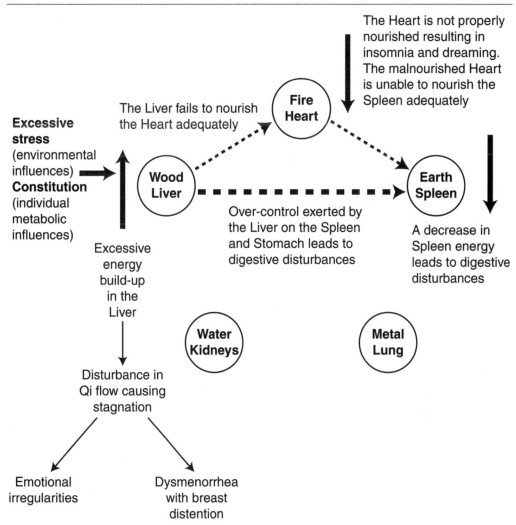

The climatic factors invade the body via the skin, mouth or nose. Symptoms typically arise suddenly and include aversion to the influence, fever, chills, body aches and tiredness. If the Protective Qi is strong the pathogen will be expelled and the patient will recover. However, if the Protective Qi is unable to ward off the influence the disease may go deeper into the body and affect the internal organs (Kaptchuk 1993).

June has just returned home from a barbeque at Mary's house. Even though it is summer the day and afternoon were unusually cool and breezy. The cool wind blew against the back of June's neck throughout the entire time. Right now, she does not feel well. She has chills and a slight fever, body aches, a slight headache, her face is pale and she feels cold. She blows clear, fluid-like mucus from her nose. She goes to the bathroom, fills up a waterbottle with warm water and snuggles up in bed under her blanket.

Even though Cold is attributable to winter an external attack can occur in any season, such as in the case of June during summer. June is susceptible to Cold because of a pre-existing internal condition towards Yang deficiency, as evident by feeling cold and pain being relieved by warmth. The signs and symptoms June is displaying are typical of an external pathogenic attack of Cold: sudden onset, feeling cold, chills, mild fever, headache, body aches and clear watery or white secretions. This pattern is similar to the initial onset of a cold or influenza. June would be prescribed a warming formula containing herbs such as cinnamon bark or ginger to expel the Cold.

The emotions

The emotions are an important internal cause of disharmony only if they are expressed excessively, restrained over a long period of time or arise suddenly with force. An internal disharmony within an Organ can also cause emotional imbalance (Kaptchuk 1993; Maciocia 1995).

The *Nei Jing* lists seven emotions that affect the body, and each one corresponds to one of the five Yin Organs. Joy is associated with the Heart, anger with the Liver, sadness and grief with the Lung, pensiveness with the Spleen and fright with the Kidney. An emotional disturbance disturbs the flow of Qi in a particular way, resulting in disharmony in the associated Organ as outlined in Table 4.2.

Table 4.2   The emotions and their corresponding Organs

Organ affected by emotion	Emotion	Effect of emotion on Organ
Liver	Anger	Anger makes Qi rise
Heart	Joy	Joy retards Qi movement
Spleen	Pensiveness, worry	Pensiveness and worry stagnate Qi
Lung	Grief, sadness	Grief disintegrates Qi
Kidney	Fright	Fright scatters Qi

The Heart and Liver are particularly vulnerable to emotional disturbances. Because the Heart houses the *Shen*, it is easily affected by emotional disharmony resulting in insomnia and disordered thinking. The Liver ensures the smooth expression of emotions. If Liver Qi becomes stagnated the emotions may become frustrated or the individual may express inappropriate and extreme mood swings, such as anger (Kaptchuk 1993).

Further factors that can precipitate illness

Other factors that precipitate ill health include diet, trauma, sexual activity and physical activity. Poor diet or irregularity in quantity of food can weaken the digestive processes of the Spleen and Stomach. Too much raw and cold food can cause internal Cold and Dampness resulting in diarrhoea, tiredness and abdominal pain. The intake of excessive amounts of fatty food can cause internal Heat and Dampness. Excess sexual activity weakens the Kidney while too much physical work can damage the Spleen, leading to Qi and Blood deficiency (Kaptchuk 1993).

Treating Mary and June

The treatments of Mary and June will aim to balance Yin and Yang and harmonise the activities of the Organ Systems, as outlined by the Five Phases.

Mary's consultation

Mary's condition is greatly influenced by stress. Mary is a company executive working under the pressure of time constraints and deadlines. Long working hours means little time with her family or for herself. This state of stress leads to muscle tightness and tension, causing the stagnation of Qi within the body and the Liver. Stagnation of Liver Qi causes the disruption of menstruation, digestion and emotional expression. In addition, deficiency within the digestive organs further impacts on her condition. In terms of Yin and Yang, Mary has a Yang-like constitution and pathology.

The practitioner examining Mary's pulse found it to be wiry and thin, reflecting a state of stress and anxiety. Her tongue was red along the sides, an area that corresponds to the Liver. These examinations confirmed that the primary aim of treatment should be to target the Liver, by calming the Organ and moving stagnated Qi. A secondary aim should be to strengthen the Spleen and Stomach.

Owing to the Five Phase interrelationship, treatment aimed at calming and balancing the Liver restores harmony within the Spleen and Heart. The Spleen ensures digestion proceeds smoothly, under the homœostatic control of the Liver. Sleep improves because the Heart receives nourishment from the Liver. The Spirit is housed. Further strengthening of the Spleen and Stomach produces adequate Qi and Blood for healing to take place.

During Mary's consultation, lifestyle issues were discussed and ways of reducing stress and finding balance in her life were explored. Reducing smoking and the consumption of alcohol and heating condiments such as chilli and garlic were advised to reduce internal agitation, heat and stagnation.

A basic herbal formula such as Chai Hu Shu Gan Wan, 'Bupleurum Pacifying the Liver Decoction', would be prescribed to Mary. The basic formula is made up of the following herbs:

- **Chai hu *(Radix Bupleuri)*; Zhi ke *(Fructus Citri aurantii)*; Xiang fu *(Rhizoma Cyperi rotundi)*: these herbs move Liver Qi stagnation and harmonise the Liver. Chai hu is an analgesic and sedative and Xiang fu inhibits uterine contractions and relieves spasm.**
- **Bai shao *(Radix Paeoniae lactiflorae)*: balances and pacifies the Liver. Bai shao acts as an antispasmodic to relieve pain.**
- **Chen pi *(Pericarpium Citri reticulatae)*: moves Qi and tonifies the Spleen. Chen pi acts as a stomachic by improving digestion through the increased secretion of gastic juices.**
- **Chuan xiong *(Radix Ligustici Chuanxiong)*: moves Blood and Qi. Chuan xiong inhibits uterine contractions and has a sedative and tranquillising effect.**
- **Gan cao *(Radix Glycyrrhizae uralensis)*: balances the formula and makes it more palatable.**

Additional herbs that may be added include:

- **Bai zhu and Shan yao to strengthen the Spleen and stop diarrhoea;**
- **Suan zao ren and Yuan zhi, sedating and hypnotic herbs that nourish the heart and improve sleep.**

Therefore, the basic formula would be modified to suit Mary's presenting signs and symptoms. The herbs may be given as raw herbs that are boiled as a decoction or as spray-dried concentrated granules which are dissolved in warm water.

The following acupuncture points may also be administered:

- **Liver 3 is calming and moves the Liver Qi.**
- **Pericardium 6 relieves stagnation of Liver Qi, regulates menstruation, calms the stomach and relaxes the mind.**
- **Liver 14 pacifies the Liver, harmonises Liver and Stomach.**
- **Spleen 6 invigorates the Blood, regulates menstruation and relieves menstrual pain.**

June's consultation

June's pattern of disharmony was due to internal Cold, or a deficiency of Yang. Signs of Yang deficiency, or a lack of physiological fire, are tiredness, feeling cold and a pale face. During her menses June felt especially cold and her body felt drained of energy. On inspection, her tongue was pale with a bluish tinge, indicating Cold. Her pulse was deep and slow, signifying an internal Cold condition. Her menstrual and back pain were not affected by stress.

June's was a long-term condition precipitated by exposure to Cold during puberty, as she had been an avid swimmer during her school days. As the body is growing and developing rapidly during puberty, it is vulnerable to the effect of pathogenic factors such as Cold (Maciocia 1998).

June's herbal prescription included herbs that warm the Uterus, expel internal Cold and move Blood. Cold causes stagnation, therefore Blood must be moved to prevent stasis. This ensures that the circulation of fresh Blood into the Uterus is maintained so that the Organ is nourished (Maciocia 1998). June was prescribed Wen Jing Tang, 'Warming the Menses Decoction', which included the following herbs:

- **Wu zhu yu *(Fructus Evodiae rutaecarpae)*; Gui zhi *(Ramulus Cinnamomi cassiae)*; Sheng jiang *(Rhizoma Zingiberis officinalis recens)*: these herbs expel Cold and warm the Uterus. They have a direct effect on the digestive process by increasing peristalsis and the secretion of digestive juices. Wu zhu yu can increase the body temperature.**
- **Dang gui *(Radix Angelicae sinensis)*; Chuan xiong *(Radix Ligustici Chuanxiong)*; Bai shao *(Radix Paeoniae lactiflorae)*: tonify and move the Blood. These herbs also decrease pain by relieving spasms and inhibiting contractions.**
- **Dang shen *(Radix Codonopsis pilosulae)*: tonifies Qi.**
- **Mai men dong *(Tuber Ophiopogonis japonici)*; E jiao *(Gelatinum Corii Asini)*: nourish Yin and the Blood.**
- **Mu dan pi *(Cortex Moutan radicis)*: moves Blood. Mu dan pi has a sedative and analgesic action.**
- **Ban xia *(Phizoma Pinelliae ternatae)*: balances the Uterus.**
- **Gan cao *(Radix Glycyrrhizae uralensis)*: balances the formula and makes it more palatable.**

The following acupuncture points may also be administered:

- **Stomach 36 tonifies Qi and scatters Cold.**
- **Conception Vessel 4 and Stomach 28 with moxa both warm the Uterus.**
- **Conception Vessel 6 with moxa moves Qi and expels Cold from lower abdomen.**
- **Spleen 6 invigorates the Blood, regulates menstruation and relieves menstrual pain.**

As can be seen from the case histories of Mary and June, dysmenorrhea can manifest as different syndromes when assessed by TCM diagnostic principles. The influence of the environment on individual metabolic requirements creates an internal condition unique to that individual. Herbal formulae and acupuncture treatments are consequently tailored to meet these requirements.

The future of TCM

Over the past two decades research on medicine has focused on the efficacy of a therapy and its application to clinical practice. This movement, termed evidence-based medicine (EBM), attempts to link clinical research with clinical practice. It is envisaged that proven therapies will be incorporated into medical care while ineffective therapies are discarded. The rules of EBM privilege certain kinds of evidence as having more weight in making decisions about the most suitable treatment.

The double-blind randomised controlled trial (RCT) was devised for testing the efficacy of drugs. This design attempts to reduce bias that could occur due to differences in experience not attributable to the medicine being tested. Inclusion and exclusion criteria, randomisation and the uniform treatment of subjects attempt to create similarity between treatment groups so that any measurable differences between the treatment and placebo group is attributable to the effects of the drug.

However, an attractive feature of TCM for consumers is that it offers an individualistic approach to patients. That is, patients with the same medical diagnosis may each receive very different herbal treatments depending on individual clinical manifestations. Tailored TCM diagnoses and treatments (although all patients have the same medical diagnosis) may be in conflict with the principles embodied in the concept of managed care. Practice guidelines and managed care implore the use of the 'best evidenced' treatment. If a new drug proves to be uniformly more effective than its predecessor, under the managed care system medical practitioners may be obliged to use the new drug. In contrast, the TCM argument is that each individual has their own 'best evidenced' treatment (although this still needs proving). The TCM argument continues that if individual diagnoses and treatments are of value to consumers, then is standardising care the best way to improve clinical outcome? In this sense there is concern that RCTs provide and encourage a group answer, that is, the standardised patient, and this may be in conflict with TCM practice.

Hence, as part of the future validation of TCM the claim that individualisation of treatment is important must be tested. EBM research needs to be applied intelligently to accommodate and test the nature of TCM practice. In this sense, an important aspect of validating TCM practice is to test not only the medicines themselves but also the theoretical tools used by practitioners. Therefore, researchers testing the efficacy of a TCM therapy need to design trials that are sympathetic to the practice demands of both western and eastern medicine.

Conclusion

This introduction to the practice of TCM provides brief insight into the experience, culture and philosophy of this longstanding medical practice. The basic theories of Yin and Yang and the Five Phases serve as models to guide the practitioner in understanding harmonious and pathological interrelationships between the Organ Systems. For a complete diagnosis the state of the Vital Substances, the functioning of the Organs and the impact of the environment on the constitutional makeup of the patient must be considered. Once obtained, this information is meshed and moulded to determine the 'pattern of disharmony', which also serves to guide the practitioner in the choice of treatment.

TCM is enjoying a surge in popularity of use around the world. This trend by consumers has led to an increased interest from health professionals for research into the safety and effectiveness of TCM as a viable therapeutic option for a range of conditions. However, research into the clinical effectiveness of TCM needs to incorporate the philosophies and principles of this form of medicine in order to truly elicit its full medicinal merit.

Recommended reading

Beinfield, H. and Korngold, E. 1991, *Between Heaven and Earth: A Guide to Chinese Medicine*, Ballantine Books, New York.

Bensky, D. and Gamble, A. 1993, *Chinese Herbal Medicine Materia Medica*, Eastland Press, Seattle.

Deng, T. 1999, *Practical Diagnosis in Traditional Chinese Medicine*, Churchill Livingstone, Edinburgh.

Maciocia, G. 1994, *The Practice of Chinese Medicine: The Treatment of Diseases with Acupuncture and Chinese Herbs*, Churchill Livingstone, Edinburgh.

Milburn, M.P. 2001, *The Future of Healing: Exploring the Parallels of Eastern and Western Medicine*, The Crossing Press, Freedom.

Ross, J. 1995, *Zang Fu: The Organ Systems of Traditional Chinese Medicine*, Churchill Livingstone, Edinburgh.

PART 2
Healing modalities

5

Acupuncture
Kylie A. O'Brien, Charlie Changli Xue

Acupuncture is a therapeutic approach that typically uses fine needles to stimulate specific locations on the body's surface. Acupuncture is one of the main treatment modalities of Chinese medicine and is practised widely in China, predominantly in hospital settings. In contrast, in western countries it is mainly practised in private practice by Chinese medicine practitioners and increasingly by other health professionals including western medical practitioners.

Acupuncture is the most recognised and practised traditional medicine technique in the western world (Eisenberg *et al.* 1998), dating back over 4000 years (Cheng 1987). The growing popularity of acupuncture globally is evidenced by increasing public demand, development of university-degree-level training, and by growing interest among orthodox medical practitioners. For example, an estimated 15 per cent of Australian general practitioners practise acupuncture (Easthope *et al.* 1998).

What is acupuncture?

Acupuncture is the practice of preventing ill health and treating illness by inserting very fine needles into the body surface at specific sites called acupoints that are chosen according to Chinese medicine theory, in order to elicit a therapeutic effect. Acupuncture is used in the treatment of a variety of clinical diseases and disorders and is also used in pain management.

An in-depth understanding of the Chinese medicine paradigm, philosophies and theories that guide Chinese medicine is essential in order for the practice of acupuncture to be mastered and the efficacy of acupuncture to be fully realised. A detailed examination of Traditional Chinese Medicine can be found in Chapter 4.

The practice of acupuncture encompasses a number of techniques that have in common the stimulation of acupoints on the body surface. Typically, fine needles are inserted into these acupoints and manipulated using a variety of techniques that have different therapeutic effects. Other types of acupuncture practices include ear acupuncture and scalp acupuncture. The use of electro-acupuncture, laser and magnets to stimulate acupoints are more modern applications.

The Chinese term for acupuncture, *zhen jiu*, actually means needling and moxibustion. Moxibustion is a technique used to treat and prevent diseases through the application of heat, in the form of a smouldering herb, to acupoints and other local points on the body (Cheng 1987). Each acupoint is associated with specific therapeutic properties. Acupoints are found along specific pathways called meridians and collaterals, or *jingluo*. Meridians and their branches, collaterals, may be thought of as the system of channels of the body in which Qi, commonly described in western literature as the vital energy of the human body, and Blood (another type of vital substance) circulate within the body (Cheng 1987; Kaptchuk 1983). Meridians, however, do not simply equate with nerves and blood vessels.

Meridians have both an external route along the body surface and an internal route within the body, connecting the organs in the interior of the body, known in Chinese medicine as 'zang-fu organs', with the external surface. This connection forms the basis of the traditional understanding of acupuncture: that stimulation of acupoints on the body surface affects the internal organ systems via the activity of Qi and Blood travelling through the meridians (Kaptchuk 1983).

Acupuncture treats a diversity of diseases using a variety of techniques. However, regardless of what technique is used in the treatment procedure, acupuncture is guided by the theoretical framework of Chinese medicine developed over many centuries.

History of acupuncture

The practice of acupuncture evolved in ancient China somewhere between 10 000 and 4000 years ago (Cheng 1987). The ancient precursor of the acupuncture needle was the 'bian stone', believed to be the earliest known medical instrument. It was oval-shaped or flat at one end with a semicircular edge for lancing lesions, with the opposite end being pyramid or awl-shaped for use as an acupuncture instrument and for bloodletting (Cheng 1987; Cai *et al.* 1995). Similar instruments of bone have also been unearthed.

Early evidence of the use of acupuncture and moxibustion has been found in the form of hieroglyphs inscribed on bones and tortoise shells from the Shang Dynasty (1600–1100 BCE). During this period, as more sophisticated materials developed, bronze needles began to appear. Then in the Warring States period, a time of much internal fighting (475–221 BCE), organised writings on acupuncture and moxibustion appeared including recordings of the earliest understanding of the theory of meridians and collaterals on silk scrolls (third century BCE) (Cheng 1987). *The Yellow Emperor's Classic of Internal Medicine* (*Huangdi Nei Jing*), thought to have been written between 770 and 221 BCE, described in detail the fundamental theories that continue to guide Chinese medicine and acupuncture, including Yin–Yang Theory and the Theory of Meridians and Collaterals (Yan 1984).

Over time bian stones began to be replaced by metal needles including those made from iron, silver and gold. Between 256 and 260 CE, the renowned Huangfu Mi compiled the *Systematic Classic of Acupuncture and Moxibustion* (*Zhen Jiu Jia Yi Jing*). This book was the earliest systematised book exclusively limited to acupuncture and moxibustion and historically one of the most influential acupuncture texts (Cheng 1987).

China became prosperous as a feudal society during the Sui (581–618 CE) and Tang (618–907 CE) Dynasties and acupuncture also flourished, being designated as one of five departments of the Internal Medical Bureau. At this time acupuncture knowledge began to cross cultural boundaries and was introduced to Korea, Japan and India in the sixth century CE (Cheng 1987). Medical exchanges also began to occur between China and other Southeast Asian countries such as Malaysia, Burma, Indonesia and Cambodia sometime after the fifth century CE (Cai *et al.* 1995). The refining of printing techniques during the period extending from the Five Dynasties (907–960 CE) to the Yuan Dynasty (1271–1368 CE) expedited the dissemination of Chinese medicine material still further (Cheng 1987).

During the Song Dynasty (960–1279 CE) a renowned acupuncturist, Wang Weiyi, revised the locations of the acupoints and their meridians (Cheng 1987). Wang Zhizhong, another well known scholar, devised the method and unit of measurement, the 'cun', used for measuring and locating acupoints (Cai *et al.* 1995). The Ming Dynasty (1368–1644 CE) saw the development of more than twenty combined techniques of manipulation and the idea of using a moxa stick in moxibustion, as distinct from using a moxa cone, was introduced. Existing works relating to acupoints away from the regular meridians were re-examined and a new category of 'Extra points' was formed (Cheng 1987).

It was not until the sixteenth century CE that acupuncture and moxibustion were introduced to Europe. Then in China itself, from the beginning of the Qing Dynasty (1644–1911 CE) including the Opium War period (1840 CE), Chinese herbal medicine became regarded by doctors as superior and acupuncture waned (Cheng 1987). In 1822 officials of the Qing Government abolished the Acupuncture—Moxibustion Department of the Imperial Medical College, declaring that 'acupuncture and moxibustion are not suitable to be applied to the Emperor' (Cheng 1987: 7). However, acupuncture still continued to develop. Liu Zhongheng wrote the *Illustration of the Bronze Figure with Chinese and Western Medicine* in 1899, in which he advocated the study of acupuncture through a combination of western and Chinese medicine (Cheng 1987).

With the introduction of western medicine into China, traditional Chinese medicine was eventually denounced, with acupuncture being defamed as 'medical torture' and the acupuncture needle named a 'deadly needle' (Cheng 1987: 7).

From 1914 the Chinese Government attempted to restrict the development and practice of Chinese medicine including acupuncture, and the practice subsequently began to decline. However, Chinese medicine and acupuncture continued as a folk medicine and many continued to protect and develop acupuncture and moxibustion, with electro-acupuncture being introduced in the 1930s (Cheng 1987; Cai et al. 1995).

The fate of acupuncture turned again in 1944 when the Communist leader Mao Zedong made a speech at a meeting of cultural and educational workers that inspired western medical practitioners to study and research acupuncture and moxibustion. In 1950, Mao recommended a policy to unite doctors of western and Chinese medicine (Cheng 1987). Chinese medicine and acupuncture regained popularity and status and continues to develop in the areas of research, practice and policy today.

Theoretical framework

The theoretical framework of acupuncture includes the following components:

1. **Philosophical basis, including:**
   Yin–Yang Theory
   Five Phase Theory
2. **Description of human physiology, including:**
   Zang-Fu Organ Theory
   Theory of Qi, Blood, Body Fluids
   Meridian Theory
3. **Understanding of aetiology and pathogenesis**
4. **Differentiation of syndromes**

This section will focus on describing Meridian Theory, which is particularly important in acupuncture. Meridian Theory, however, cannot be understood in isolation from the above theories and concepts. The Yin–Yang Theory, Five Phase Theory and Zang-Fu Theory and the concepts of Qi, Blood and Body Fluids have been described in Chapter 4, 'Traditional Chinese Medicine'. All are fundamental theories that guide the practice of Chinese medicine including acupuncture.

The understanding of aetiology and pathogenesis of disease in Chinese medicine is vastly different from that of western medicine, and the subcategorisation of a disease into pattern complexes or syndromes is a distinguishing feature of Chinese medicine that sets it apart from western medicine. These are described in detail in Chapter 4.

The term 'zang-fu organ' that will be used throughout this chapter describes the internal organ systems as understood in Chinese medicine. The function of zang-fu organs is conceptually different and broader than the western medical understanding, although there are similarities. Zang-fu organs are best thought of as functional systems understood according to Zang-Fu Theory.

Finally, Chinese medicine holds that there are four interdependent substances within the body that are fundamental to life: Essence (Jing), Qi, Blood and Body Fluids (Cai *et al.* 1995). These substances provide the material and functional basis of the human body. Dysfunction and/or inadequacy in one or more of these substances will result in dysfunction of various organs or systems in the body (see Chapter 4 for more details).

Meridian Theory

Meridian Theory studies the course and distribution, physiological functions and pathological processes of the meridian system and its interrelationship with the zang-fu organs (Qiu *et al.* 1993). It provides the basis for the understanding of physiology and pathology in the human body, and underpins the practice of acupuncture. It also underpins and guides the clinical practice of other modalities of Chinese medicine including herbal medicine, massage and qi gong (Cai *et al.* 1995).

Meridian system

The meridian system (*jing luo xi tong*) describes the communicating system of pathways in which Qi and Blood circulate within the body (Cheng 1987; Kaptchuk 1983; Xue & Yang 1990). It provides the basis for interconnection of the body's organs and tissues, the upper and lower portions of the body and the body's interior and exterior and thereby the basis for the physiological functioning of the body as an integrated whole (Deadman *et al.* 1998; Cai *et al.* 1995; Cheng 1987).

The meridian system is composed of meridians (*jing*) and collaterals (*luo*), collectively known as *jingluo*. *Jing* means 'pathway' or 'longitude' and *luo* means 'to attach'. Using the analogy of a tree, the meridians are likened to the trunk and main branches, running interiorly and longitudinally within the body and connecting to the zang-fu organs. The collaterals are likened to the fine branches of the tree. They are more superficial and run transversely from the meridians, connecting the meridians with the connective tissue and cutaneous regions (the leaves) (see Deadman *et al.* 1998; Qiu *et al.* 1993).

There are twelve main meridians, duplicated on the opposite side of the body, traversing the trunk, upper and lower limbs and head, called 'regular meridians'. There are also several other categories of meridians. In addition to the meridians, there are twelve muscle regions and more superficially distributed cutaneous regions where the Qi and Blood circulating in the meridians and collaterals nourish the muscles, tendons and skin (Cheng 1987). The existence of cutaneous regions overlying and connected to the superficial channels (collaterals) also provides the theoretical basis for explaining how exogenous pathogenic factors may invade the meridian system through the surface of the body (Deadman *et al.* 1998).

The meridian system also functions as a defence system against pathogenic invasion, in particular the Bladder meridian that courses over a large area of the body. Conversely meridians may serve as a route of transmission of pathogens when the body's Zheng Qi (antipathogenic Qi) is insufficient (Cheng 1987).

Twelve regular meridians

The twelve regular meridians are divided into six Yin and six Yang meridians. There are three Yin meridians of the hand and foot respectively, traversing mainly the medial aspect of the upper and lower limbs. There are also three Yang meridians of the hand and foot respectively, traversing mainly the lateral aspect of the upper and lower limbs (Cheng 1987). Several of the Yin meridians also course over the front of the body (abdomen and chest) while the Yang meridians course over the head and back (with the exception of the Stomach meridian which courses over the chest and abdomen) (Deadman *et al.* 1998). Each meridian is duplicated on the opposite side of the body.

There are 361 acupoints on the twelve regular meridians and the Du (Governing) and Ren (Conception) meridians on the body midline. Each meridian varies in the number of acupoints it contains, from nine acupoints on the Pericardium and Heart meridians to 67 acupoints on the Bladder meridian. Figure 5.1 shows the course of the meridians on the upper body.

Association of meridians with specific organs and sense organs

Each regular meridian is associated with a specific zang-fu organ and the name of the meridian is derived from the organ, the limb over which it travels and its Yin or Yang classification (see Table 5.1) (Deadman *et al.* 1998). According to theory, each zang organ, considered solid and more internal, is associated with a paired hollow fu organ, considered more external. It is the meridian system that provides the connection between these paired organs. This pairing of zang-fu organs and their meridians is described as an interior–exterior relationship. For example, the Lung (zang organ) is paired with the Large Intestine (fu organ). The paired organs and meridians are set out in Table 5.1. Clinically this pairing is the reason why points on one meridian may be used to treat disorders relating to its paired meridian's organ. The connection between meridians also allows zang and fu organs to affect each other pathologically in disease. (See Cai *et al.* 1995.)

The meridians connect each zang organ with a particular sense organ. For example, the Liver meridian links to the eyes. Eye diseases may result from pathology of the Liver system; in such cases, acupoints on the Liver meridian may be used in treatment of eye conditions. The other correspondences between zang organs and sense organs are: Kidney—ears, Heart—tongue, Lung—nose, Spleen—mouth and lips.

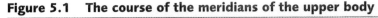

Figure 5.1   The course of the meridians of the upper body

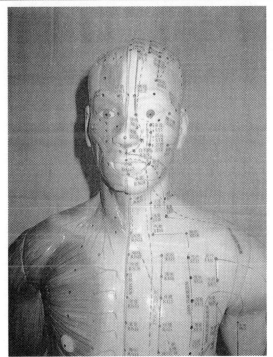

(Photo: Charlie Xue)

Cyclical sequence of Qi

The twelve regular meridians form a cyclical sequence beginning with the Lung meridian and ending with the Liver meridian (Cheng 1987) (see Figure 5.2). Each meridian is associated with a specific two-hour time period of the day in which the Qi is particularly active (see Table 5.1). This time period can be taken advantage of in the diagnosis and treatment of diseases associated with specific organs.

Clinical significance of Meridian Theory

Meridian Theory is clinically significant in three ways:

1. **explaining aetiology and pathogenesis of disease;**
2. **guiding diagnosis;**
3. **guiding treatment.**

Since the meridian system provides the connection between the zang-fu organs, the same system can allow these organs to affect each other pathologically in disease and can be the route of transmission of pathogenic factors in the body (Cai *et al.* 1995).

Figure 5.2   Meridian cyclical flow of Qi

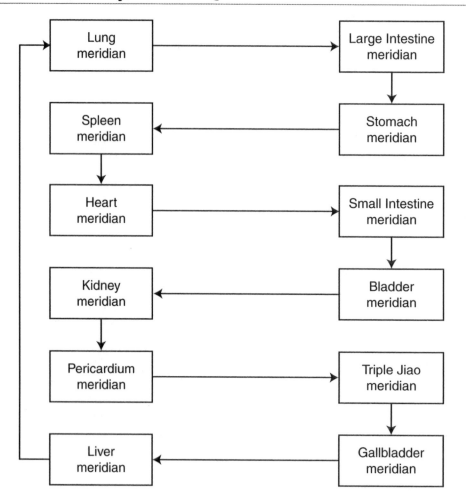

Diseases associated with different meridians and/or associated organs can manifest characteristic signs and symptoms or sign/symptom complexes. Therefore, by understanding the links between meridians and their organs and the characteristic signs and symptoms associated with disorders of the meridians and/or organs, one can locate the disease and understand the aetiology and pathogenesis.

In addition to the aforementioned, knowing the route of a meridian can aid in the diagnosis of disorders. For example, headaches at the vertex (of the head), where one of the internal branches of the Liver meridian traverses, are typically related to the Liver organ system. Certain acupoints on a meridian may be tender when there is a disorder of the associated zang-fu organ. In addition, there are extra points not

Table 5.1 Name, course, correspondence and time of peak Qi activity of the twelve regular meridians

	Course	Yin meridian (time of peak Qi flow/activity)	Pairing[a]	Corresponding Yang meridian (time of peak Qi flow/activity)
Hand meridians	Upper ←→ limbs[b]	Lung meridian of Hand Taiyin (3 a.m.–5 a.m.)		Large Intestine meridian of Hand Yangming (5 a.m.–7 a.m.)
	←→	Pericardium meridian of Hand Jueyin (7 a.m.–9 a.m.)		Triple Jiao meridian of Hand Shaoyang (9 a.m.–11 a.m.)
	←→	Heart meridian of Hand Shaoyin (11 a.m.–1 p.m.)		Small Intestine meridian of Hand Taiyang (1 p.m.–3 p.m.)
Foot meridians	Lower ←→ limbs[b]	Spleen meridian of Foot Taiyin (3 p.m.–5 p.m.)		Stomach meridian of Foot Yangming (5 p.m.–7 p.m.)
	←→	Liver meridian of Foot Jueyin (7 p.m.–9 p.m.)		Gallbladder meridian of Foot Shaoyang (9 p.m.–11 p.m.)
	←→	Kidney meridian of Foot Shaoyin (11 p.m.–1 a.m.)		Bladder meridian of Foot Taiyang (1 a.m.–3 a.m.)

Notes: [a] Paired zang and fu organs are found adjacent to each other in each row of the table above.

[b] The course of the meridians may extend onto the face and trunk of the body also.

associated with meridians that may show tenderness with certain internal organ diseases. For example, there is a point on the lateral lower leg that is often tender when there is appendicitis. In some cases, there may be changes in the skin overlying a meridian (Cai *et al.* 1995).

Acupuncture may be used when there is imbalance in the body to regulate the function of the meridians and the Qi and Blood and restore the balance of Yin and Yang (Cai *et al.* 1995; Qiu *et al.* 1993). Knowledge of Meridian Theory guides not only the selection of acupoints in acupuncture practice and massage therapy, but also guides Chinese herbal medicine treatment (Cai *et al.* 1995). Each herb has an affinity for particular zang-fu organs and reaches them via the meridian system (Bensky & Gamble 1993; Cai *et al.* 1995). Thus, each herb is said to 'enter' one or more meridians.

Acupoints

Acupoints (*shu-xue*) are specific points where the Qi of the zang-fu organs and meridians is transported to the external surface of the body (Cai *et al.* 1997; Li *et al.* 2000). The Chinese characters for acupoint translate to 'transportation' and 'hole' (Qiu *et al.* 1993). Each acupoint is associated with specific therapeutic properties and also shares general properties with other acupoints on the same meridian.

Fundamentally, the choice of acupoints is based on identification of the disease syndrome (sign/symptom pattern complex). In general, when a zang-fu organ or a meridian is diseased, points are chosen from the associated meridians to correct the imbalance. Each acupoint has specific functions as well as a general influence on a disorder of a meridian and/or its associated zang-fu organ. For example, the point Neiguan (Pericardium 6) on the inside of the wrist has a general effect on the Pericardium meridian but is specifically used to treat nausea and vomiting (Cheng 1987). Choice of acupoints will be discussed in more detail later.

Acupoints are generally divided into three main groups (Cai *et al.* 1997; Li *et al.* 2000):

- **Regular points: acupoints of the twelve regular meridians and the Ren and Du meridians (midline of body, front and back). There are a total of 361 regular acupoints.**
- **Extra (extraordinary) points: acupoints with specific names, locations and functions that do not lie on the regular meridians.**
- **Ashi points ('tender points'): points of local tenderness found on palpation that do not have specific locations and may or may not correspond with regular acupoints.**

Acupoints are often named by analogy to features of nature including water, mountains, animals and plants, or to architectural structures or household utensils (Cheng 1987). To facilitate learning by western students, the acupoints are labelled and numbered according to the meridian they belong to. For example, Yu Ji (which means 'fish border') is Lung 10, the tenth point on the Lung meridian.

The regular meridians have specific points that are common in terms of function. For example, each of the regular meridians has a 'Xi Cleft point' that is usually used to treat acute types of disorders. Each meridian also has a 'Yuan' or 'Primary point' that is often used to treat deficiency-type disorders associated with that meridian or its related organ (Li *et al.* 2000).

Empirical points are those with a historically established effect or indication. The function of such a point may not necessarily bear any obvious relationship with the meridian of which it is a part. For example, Tiaokou (Stomach 38) on the lateral lower leg is an important point for treatment of shoulder problems, but the Stomach meridian does not actually pass through the shoulder (Deadman *et al.* 1998).

Clinical practice: applications of acupuncture

Acupuncture is indicated for a wide range of clinical disorders including gynaecological disorders, musculoskeletal pain, ophthalmological disease, stroke, Bell's palsy, arthritis, asthma, common cold, urinary tract disorders and insomnia, to name a few.

Each acupoint has specific indications. For example, the indications of Neiguan (Pericardium 6) on the inside wrist include cardiac or chest pain, stomach pain, vomiting, nausea, palpitations, pain in the elbow and arm, motor impairment of the upper limb, unilateral migraine and insomnia (Qiu *et al.* 1993; Li *et al.* 2000; Cai *et al.* 1997).

Certain acupoints are contraindicated under certain conditions. Many acupoints are contraindicated in pregnant women for instance, including those that stimulate blood circulation and those on the abdominal and lumbosacral areas. In general, acupuncture is contraindicated in areas where there is infection, ulcers, tumours or scars and in patients who are prone to continuous bleeding after injury or spontaneous bleeding. Acupuncture should also be avoided on patients who are over-hungry, over-tired or very nervous. In the case of weak patients, acupuncture should be performed using gentle technique with the patient in a supine or prone position rather than sitting up. Care must be taken in needling of points overlying important viscera (see Qiu *et al.* 1993).

Steps in an acupuncture treatment

There are four main steps in an acupuncture treatment:

1. **diagnosis of disease and differentiation of syndrome;**
2. **formulation of treatment principle;**
3. **selection of acupoints;**
4. **needling.**

Diagnosis of disease and differentiation of syndrome

During a Chinese medicine consultation, a case history is taken and the patient's tongue appearance and pulse are recorded. A physical examination may also be part of the consultation. The signs and symptoms are then analysed according to complex Chinese medicine theory and the disease/disorder and syndrome identified. Acupoints may be used in diagnosis. For example, tenderness of specific acupoints may be associated with disorders of the related zang-fu organ or with areas of musculoskeletal tension. Tenderness of Extra points, those not located on meridians but having specific locations, may be pathognomonic of certain diseases. Based on the theory that the organs and parts of the body are mapped out on the surface of the ear, the ear may be inspected for changes in skin colouring, localised morphological changes (e.g. nodules and papules), flexibility and tenderness of acupoints as an aid to diagnosis (Qiu *et al.* 1993).

Treatment principles

An acupuncture prescription is individually formulated for the patient, based on the treatment principle that follows disease diagnosis and syndrome differentiation. For example, if a disease is due to Kidney Qi deficiency, the treatment principle will be to strengthen or tonify Kidney Qi. The acupuncture prescription is guided by Chinese medicine theory, the patient's age, constitution, gender, the season of presentation and strength of Zheng Qi.

An understanding of disease aetiology and pathogenesis is essential. Signs and symptoms may be reflective of secondary manifestations (termed *biao*) or the root cause (*ben*). Depending on the relative strength of the patient's Zheng Qi (antipathogenic Qi) and the pathogenic factor, the treatment principle may focus on treating the ben or biao or both.

Choosing the right point

Points are chosen according to Meridian Theory as well as other guiding theories of Chinese medicine including Zang-Fu Theory, Yin–Yang Theory and Five Phase Theory. Acupoints are also chosen according to their individual functions. Each acupoint has an effect on the meridian that it belongs to as well as one or more specific functions.

Points may be chosen according to their location. Local points are those overlying or very close to the diseased region while adjacent points are those located nearby. Distal points are located on the limbs, usually below the knees and elbows. Distal points are commonly chosen from an involved meridian to treat diseases of the head, chest, abdomen and back. Local, adjacent and distal points are commonly combined to treat pain, disorders of the zang-fu organs and meridian disorders (see Deadman *et al.* 1998).

There are many principles by which to select acupoints. For example, acupoints may be selected from:

- **the lower body to treat diseases of the upper body and vice versa;**
- **the back to treat the front of the body and vice versa;**
- **one meridian to treat its interiorly–exteriorly related meridian (Deadman *et al.* 1998).**

While points on the same side as the disease are commonly used, points on the opposite side of the body to the disease may also be chosen—this is called cross-needling (Deadman *et al.* 1998).

Empirical points may be selected for certain indications. In addition, empirical combinations of points have historically been found to be extremely effective. Combinations of acupoints may be selected, for example:

- **to treat the root cause of disease (ben) and its manifestations (biao);**
- **from the upper and lower body;**
- **from one meridian and its interiorly–exteriorly related meridian (Deadman *et al.* 1998).**

Needling techniques

Acupuncture needle insertion and manipulation techniques are many, each with its own therapeutic effect. Speed of needle manipulation, time of retention and method of withdrawal all have therapeutic significance. Angle and depth of needle insertion and needle choice varies for each acupoint and depends on location and other factors including musculature of the patient.

When the needle is inserted, the patient often feels a sensation termed 'De Qi' or 'arrival of Qi'. It may be a sensation of distension or numbness or heaviness around the point or a sensation travelling along the course of the meridian. The practitioner often feels a sinking or tight sensation under the needle tip. The thera-peutic effect of acupuncture is closely related to the achievement of the 'arrival of Qi' (Li *et al.* 2000).

Filiform acupuncture needles vary in length and thickness. Most are made from stainless steel and are single-use, disposable needles. In addition, there are other types of needles including the 'dermal hammer', a hammer-like instrument, the head of which contains many short, fine needles, tapped against the skin to cause a localised area of redness and bleeding and relieve stagnation of blood. It is typically used in the treatment of musculoskeletal disorders.

Cupping

Cupping is a technique in which a glass (or sometimes bamboo or pottery) cup is placed on the skin after a negative pressure is created within the cup by use of a flame. The cup is applied on an area of abundant muscle and left on the body for a specific time depending on the condition. Cupping may be used alone, precede, follow or be used in conjunction with acupuncture, where the cup is placed over an inserted needle. In 'mobile cupping', the skin is lubricated with massage oil first, then the cup applied and moved or pushed over the surface of the body. It is usually used on large muscle areas found in the back, buttocks and thighs (Qiu *et al.* 1993). Indications for cupping include musculoskeletal problems, arthralgia, common cold, abdominal pain and diarrhoea (Cai *et al.* 1997; Qiu *et al.* 1993).

Moxibustion

Moxibustion is a technique that uses the application of heat in the form of a smouldering herb to areas of the body. The material used is 'moxa-wool' which is typically made up of the Chinese herb 'Ai ye' (*Artemisia vulgaris*), in the form of a cone or stick. Moxa has a warming function that encourages the flow of Qi in the meridians and Blood in the vessels and helps expel cold (cold in the body is thought to impede the smooth flow of Qi and Blood in the body). An ignited stick of moxa may be held near the acupoint or local area, or a piece of moxa is attached to the handle of the acupuncture needle. Alternatively, a moxa cone may be placed either directly on the skin and ignited (direct moxibustion) or indirectly on the skin resting on top of an insulating material such as a slice of ginger (see Cheng 1987).

Specific types of acupuncture

Ear acupuncture

According to ear acupuncture theory the body parts and organs are mapped onto the surface of the ear in the pattern of an inverted foetus (Qiu *et al.* 1993). The regular meridians connect (directly or indirectly) with the ear, linking the zang-fu organs with the ear. When there is disease in the body, it may be reflected in the corresponding areas on the ear. Therefore, examination of the surface of the ear and reactiveness to stimulation may be used as a diagnostic tool. Needles may be used to puncture specific acupoints. Alternatively, small seeds may be taped to ear points with sticky plaster (this is called ear taping). These are stimulated by manually pressing a few times per day. Ear acupuncture may be used in both the prevention and treatment of disease (Qiu *et al.* 1993).

Scalp acupuncture

According to scalp acupuncture theory various areas on the scalp (as opposed to specific points) relate to different areas of the brain. These areas are more specifically lines of approximately 2–4 cm in length that generally relate anatomically to the region of brain they represent. Areas include a motor area, a sensory area and a speech area. These areas are strongly stimulated by rotating the needle rapidly at a frequency of approximately 200 times per minute. Alternatively, electro-acupuncture may be used (Cai *et al.* 1997; Qiu *et al.* 1993). Clinically they are often used in the treatment of disorders of cerebral origin, for example in the treatment of post-stroke sequelae, paralysis, numbness and chorea (Cai *et al.* 1997; Qiu *et al.* 1993).

Laser acupuncture

Laser acupuncture is a modern adaptation of acupuncture that uses a laser instead of a needle to stimulate an acupoint. It has advantages in the treatment of patients averse to needles, including children, and is easily portable for off-site visits. The efficacy of laser acupuncture in comparison to traditional acupuncture has not been fully investigated.

Electro-acupuncture

In electro-acupuncture tiny electrodes are attached to the handles of the acupuncture needles inserted in the skin and a current applied. Electro-acupuncture is used to stimulate nerves and muscles, alleviate muscular spasm and promote circulation of blood and relieve pain. Different waveforms are used to treat different conditions (Cai *et al.* 1997). Clinical applications include treatment of arthritis, pain, neuritis, post-stroke sequelae and Bell's palsy and it is often used in scalp acupuncture.

Acupoint magnetic therapy

In this form of therapy a magnetic field acts on meridians and acupoints. Magnets, available in varying strengths of magnetic field intensity, may be used in the form of a magnetic sheet or bead that is applied directly or indirectly to an acupoint or area of pain. Two magnetic sheets may also be placed so that opposite or similar poles face each other (e.g. one on either side of the limb) in order to drive the magnetic force deeper into the tissues. There are also electric magneto-therapy devices that allow an electric current to pass through an electromagnetic coil or electromagnet to produce a constant or alternating magnetic field. Magnetic therapy is indicated for diverse conditions including arthralgia, swelling and pain due to trauma or sprains, hypertension, coronary heart disease, sciatica, asthma, gastrointestinal dysfunction and headache (Cai *et al.* 1997).

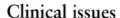

Clinical issues

Infection control

Adherence to infection control guidelines including the use of aseptic technique is of vital importance in the practice of acupuncture in order to protect the patient and practitioner. Blood-borne diseases including hepatitis B and C and HIV/AIDs may be spread via contaminated needles. Practitioners should adhere to national and state health regulations and infection control guidelines.

Choice of instruments

The use of single-use disposable acupuncture needles and sharps is recommended to decrease the risk of occupational exposure for the practitioner. Acupuncture needles and other instruments used in an acupuncture practice should comply with the requirements of the relevant regulatory authorities. In Australia this body is the Therapeutic Goods Administration (TGA) and TGA approval will be indicated on packaging.

Prevention and management of acupuncture accidents

Occasional problems such as a stuck needle or bent needle may arise if the patient moves or is nervous or there is an incorrect needling technique (Qiu *et al.* 1993). Broken needles can occur but are uncommon. Training in the correct needling technique including management of such problems is important. Needle inspection prior to insertion, care during manipulation and insertion and ensuring that the patient remains still during treatment will help prevent such problems (Qiu *et al.* 1993). Fainting can also occur and care should be taken with first-time patients, particularly those who are very nervous. Haematoma, swelling around the acupuncture site due to subcutaneous bleeding, and bleeding at the acupuncture site can occur and is usually avoided by pressing the acupoint with a sterile cotton swab or ball following removal of the needle (Qiu *et al.* 1993).

Acupuncture research

Chinese medicine and acupuncture has developed for hundreds of years on the basis of experiential evidence. The value of such empirical evidence to guide practice should not be underestimated. In more recent times there has been a move towards evidence-based medicine demanding that effectiveness of a medicine or therapy be adequately demonstrated using appropriate research methodology. This has seen an increase in research into acupuncture.

In the past, much acupuncture research has suffered from poor methodological design and inadequate sample size (Vincent & Furnham 1997; Filshie & White 1998; Linde *et al.* 2001). Acupuncture has posed some particular problems in research design including the identification of an adequate placebo. Sham acupoints, acupoints at non-classical sites, have been shown to be an unsuitable control for a number of reasons including the fact that analgesia can occur at these sham sites (Vincent & Furnham 1997). Research that uses sham acupoints as the control will only produce information about the relative effectiveness of particular sites of needle insertion but 'not about the specific effects of acupuncture' (Vincent & Furnham 1997: 182) including the efficacy of the acupoint or combination of acupoints tested in treating disease. However, research designs with more appropriate placebos have now been developed and there are increasing examples of good studies (Vincent & Furnham 1997).

Acupuncture research has been aimed at what effects it has, how it works and whether it is efficacious in the clinical treatment of specific disease.

Research into the effects and mechanism of acupuncture

Three main areas of research into the effects of acupuncture are the:

- **analgesic effect;**
- **regulatory effect; and**
- **immunological effect.**

Analgesic effect of acupuncture

Acupuncture analgesia is a complex process involving complicated neural pathways, neurochemical transmitters and pain mediators. Various attempts have been made to explain the mechanism of acupuncture anaesthesia, the most well-known theory being the 'Gate Theory'.

Research has shown that during analgesia, mediation occurs at different levels of the central and peripheral nervous systems, including the brainstem and thalamus and the posterior horns of the spinal cord grey matter, with the peripheral nerves being the afferent nerves involved in transmission of the acupuncture signal (Qiu *et al.* 1993). Central neurotransmitters including 5HT, catecholamine (CA) and acetylcholine (ACh) and morphine-like substances are thought to play an important role (Qiu *et al.* 1993). Acupuncture has also been found to decrease the concentration of pain-inducing mediators such as histamine and bradykinin in the peripheral blood system (Qiu *et al.* 1993).

The effect of needling on the peripheral nervous system has been examined. One model proposes that the reason acupuncture is able to help many conditions including chronic pain is that for many conditions the common underlying problem is radiculopathy and that acupuncture helps by restoring the normal function of the peripheral nervous system (Gunn 1998).

The Australian National Health and Medical Research Council (NHMRC) Working Party report on acupuncture concluded that pain relief using acupuncture was valid and explainable in neurophysiological terms (NHMRC 1989). It is worth noting, however, that in Chinese medicine the way in which acupuncture is perceived to work is couched in Chinese medicine theory: by treating the underlying disorder and factors that have caused the pain including Qi and Blood stagnation (Cheng 1987).

The regulatory effect of acupuncture

In Chinese medicine, acupuncture is used in order to restore the balance of Yin and Yang in the body. The concept of balance of Yin and Yang is akin to that of homœostasis. Acupuncture has a regulatory effect on organs and tissues of the body including the heart, respiratory system, gastrointestinal system, gallbladder, biliary tract, liver, kidney and bladder. For example, acupuncture research in patients with cardiac arrhythmias and premature heartbeats has shown a positive regulatory effect (Qiu *et al.* 1993). Research into the use of acupuncture in treatment of bronchial asthma has shown positive results and is postulated to work by down-regulating (or decreasing) the tone of the vagus nerve and up-regulating (or increasing) sympathetic excitation. This leads to a relaxation of the smooth muscle and relief of bronchial spasm, and an increase in blood vessel constriction in the bronchial mucous membranes and reduction of oedema (Qiu *et al.* 1993).

A number of reports in the literature lend support to the notion that acupuncture has a regulatory effect on gastrointestinal function, including motility, secretion and electrical activity (Qiu *et al.* 1993). Interestingly, the effect of acupuncture and moxibustion has shown a 'biphasic' regulatory effect for certain conditions or functions. For example, acupuncture has been shown to lower blood pressure in hypertensives and raise it in hypotensives. Acupuncture has also been shown to have a biphasic regulatory effect on the secretion of gastric acid and on gastric peristalsis (Qiu *et al.* 1993).

Immunological effect of acupuncture

Acupuncture and moxibustion can increase the body's resistance and prevent illness. They can be used to treat viral diseases including the common cold, mumps and hepatitis, bacterial diseases including dysentery, and acute and chronic inflammatory diseases including gastritis, chronic pharyngitis and mastitis (Qiu *et al.* 1993).

How acupuncture and moxibustion regulate immune function has been the subject of much research, particularly in small animals. For example, animal research has also shown that (Qiu *et al.* 1993):

- **moxibustion can promote the function of the humoral immune system;**
- **acupuncture has a significant anti-inflammatory effect;**
- **acupuncture can activate the phagocytic function of the hepatic reticulo-endothelial system.**

Research in humans has also shown that acupuncture can increase the phagocytic function of leucocytes in patients infected with *Staphylococcus aureus* (Qiu *et al.* 1993).

Evidence of clinical efficacy

Studies have shown that acupuncture is effective in treatment of problems as diverse as nocturia in elderly patients (Ellis *et al.* 1990; Ellis 1993), gastrointestinal dysfunctions (Ghaly *et al.* 1987; Qiu *et al.* 1993; Filshie & White 1998), seasonal allergic rhinitis (Xue *et al.* 2002), dysmenorrhea (Helms 1987) and back pain (Strauss & Xue 2001). Several studies on acupressure, pressing of acupoints either digitally or using pressure studs (applied, for example, with a wrist band), have reported positive results in the treatment of conditions such as morning sickness and vomiting during pregnancy (Filshie & White 1998). The treatment combination of acupuncture and Chinese herbal medicine has also been shown to be effective in, for example, hemiplegia (Xue 1993, 1998). Moxibustion of the acupoint Zhiyin (Bladder 67, posterior to the nail of the fifth toe) in pregnant women with foetuses in breech presentation has been shown to increase foetal activity during the treatment period and increase the number of cephalic presentations (i.e. head first) compared with the control group (Cardini & Huang 1998). The evidence for efficacy of acupuncture in management of chronic pain is somewhat equivocal (Lewith & Vincent 1998). Similarly, controlled clinical trials of acupuncture treatment of headache have been inconclusive (Hester 1998).

A systematic review of acupuncture studies in 2001 found convincing evidence for the use of acupuncture to treat post-operative nausea and that the limited evidence available suggests that acupuncture may have positive effects in treatment of fibromyalgia, temporomandibular joint dysfunction, stroke rehabilitation and chemotherapy-induced nausea (though results were equivocal for morning sickness). Acupuncture trials for treatment of tinnitus and weight loss, however, did not show important effects (Linde *et al.* 2001).

Future research directions

More research is needed to assess the efficacy of acupuncture in the treatment of many diseases or disorders, either as a mode of primary treatment or in conjunction with western medical treatment.

In establishing the efficacy of acupuncture, the differences in 'medical acupuncture' or 'western' acupuncture compared to traditional acupuncture should be kept in mind. The relative efficacy of traditional acupuncture and 'medical acupuncture' has not been established. Traditional acupuncturists carry out diagnosis and treatment according to Chinese medicine theory whereas western acupuncturists do not necessarily do so. Practitioners of western acupuncture often use manual stimulation with or without needle retention or periosteal acupuncture where the needle tip very briefly touches the periosteum (Hester 1998). They also tend to use more trigger points (very tender points in a muscle) (Hester 1998).

Clinical studies that incorporate the theories upon which acupuncture is based are necessary so that research can guide clinical practice and importantly help build the bridge of knowledge between Chinese and western medical cultures. Future research needs to include economic analyses of acupuncture (e.g. cost–benefit or cost effectiveness) to ascertain the potential of acupuncture to save governments and insurance companies money.

Attempts to explain how acupuncture works are dependent upon the paradigm under which it is analysed. Most attempts, particularly those in relation to the action of acupuncture in pain reduction, have used a mechanistic approach favoured by modern science and knowledge of neurochemical pathways and mediators. However, there are emerging paradigms based on quantum mechanics and holographic principles that describe phenomena in terms of energy fields or energetic systems that have been applied to how acupuncture works and merit further exploration (see Gerber 1988).

The World Health Organization (WHO) defines health as not merely the absence of disease but a positive state of mental, physical and social wellbeing (WHO 1986). The potential of acupuncture to prevent ill health and promote better than average health in the sense of the WHO definition deserves further exploration. Chinese medicine and acupuncture have the potential to bring new approaches to prevention and treatment of illness to western medical culture. The future challenge in development of medicine and Chinese medicine research will be to accept change and make the shift in thinking that is required.

Recommended reading

Cai, G., Chao, G., Chen, D. *et al.* (eds) 1995, *State Administration of Traditional Chinese Medicine, Advanced Textbook on Traditional Chinese Medicine and Pharmacology*, Vol. I, New World Press, Beijing.

Cai, J. *et al.* 1997, *State Administration of Traditional Chinese Medicine, Advanced Textbook on Traditional Chinese Medicine and Pharmacology*, Vol. IV, New World Press, Beijing.

Cheng, X. (chief ed.) 1987, *Chinese Acupuncture and Moxibustion*, Foreign Languages

Press, Beijing.

Deadman, P., Al-Khafaji, M. and Baker, K. 1998, *A Manual of Acupuncture*, Journal of Chinese Medicine Publications, East Sussex, England.

Kaptchuk, T. 1983, *Chinese Medicine: The Web That Has No Weaver*, Rider, London.

Qiu, M.L., Zang, S.C., Yu, Z.Q. *et al.* 1993, *Chinese Acupuncture and Moxibustion*, Churchill Livingstone, Edinburgh.

6

Aromatherapy
Mark A. Webb

Many textbooks on aromatherapy state that as a healing modality it is many hundreds, if not thousands, of years old, dating back to the times of the ancient Egyptians, Mesopotamia and ancient China. Certainly, the reverence and use of aromatic substances such as unguents, incenses, spices, herbs and macerated oils have been well documented and were prevalent in these cultures. Yet while the distillation of plant essences has its birth in Islamic alchemy, aromatherapy as practised today has a much more recent history. Renée Gatefosse, a French perfumery chemist, coined the term *aromathérapie* in 1937 to describe the use of volatile oils to effect a therapeutic response to various conditions and diseases experienced by humans.

The essence of aromatherapy

Without the advent of steam distillation there would be no aromatherapy today. Steam distillation uses water in its vapour form, steam, to vaporise the volatile aromatic compounds found in various parts of aromatic plants. Once vaporised the steam and volatile aromatic oil vapours are channelled into a condenser (heat exchanger), where cold water flows around the hot vapour-filled pipes. This quick cooling of the vapour returns both the steam and volatile oil back to liquids. Volatile oil is predominantly composed of hydrocarbons and oxygenated hydrocarbons; these very non-polar components and the polar water do not mix. By placing both within a separator the two are easily separated, usually with the volatile oil floating on top of the water (due to lower specific gravity) where it can be easily drawn off. This simple form of extraction allowed human beings to produce highly concentrated aromatic substances from plants. These volatile aromatic substances are called 'essential oils'. Essential oils have many advantages over their parent plant material, in that being highly concentrated they can be more easily transported, stored and used in a wide variety of ways, from culinary to medicinal. Essential oils are derived from the fragrant components of aromatic flowers, grasses and trees. They are also referred to as volatile oils because if left in the open air they will quickly evaporate. Essential oils are stored by the plant within small oil glands or sacs that occur in different parts of the plant depending on the plant family involved. Plant families rich in essential oils include the Lamiaceae (mint), Apiaceae (carrot and parsley), Asteraceae (daisy), Myrtaceae (eucalyptus and tea tree) and Rutaceae (citrus fruits).

It is important to note that essential oils are not the only components of modern aromatherapy practice. Other aromatic substances commonly used within aromatherapy include:

- **Expressed oils—These are citrus oils that are produced by maceration of the fruit, which ruptures the cells containing oil. These cells are called flavedo and are found within the outer layers of the rind.**
- **Absolutes—These are aromatic substances usually extracted from flowers such as jasmine, rose, neroli, mimosa and boronia for the fragrance and perfumery industry, using petrochemical solvents which do not damage the heat-sensitive aromatics.**
- **Carbon dioxide extracts—Some aromatics are extracted from dried plant material using hypercritical carbon dioxide at great pressure (20 atmospheres) and low temperature. This is a form of 'solvent' extraction that requires expensive technology to produce very pure and highly concentrated extracts.**

Today, within complementary therapies, aromatherapy has a broad base. Unfortunately the term 'aromatherapy' has also been subverted by the corporate world to market products with often less than natural origins. This subversion has been one of the major reasons why the orthodox medical community and the general public alike do not take aromatherapy seriously. Such a view is unfortunate, as modern aromatherapy is in fact a rigorous medical modality.

Much has been discovered since Gattefosse's time and there is now a greater understanding of the chemical structures and the therapeutic properties of the constituents of essential oils. This understanding has emerged from the empirical use of the oils by practitioners to treat a wide variety of conditions and diseases, combined with knowledge gained from analysis of the oils by chemists. Arising from this understanding are several distinct modern approaches to aromatherapy.

Contemporary aromatherapy

The first of these approaches came from the work of a French doctor, Jean Valnet, who used essential oils during the Crimean War to treat the wounded, when medical supplies were exhausted. His work built upon the discoveries of Gatefosse and showed the effective antimicrobial and wound-healing properties of essential oils. The tradition of using essential oils in this very medical sense continues in France to this day. The French doctor Daniel Pénoël has done much to popularise the French method of aromatherapy in the English-speaking world and is thought of as the father of the worldwide 'Aromatic Medicine' movement.

Across the channel in England, however, a different approach to aromatherapy exists. The predominant paradigm of aromatherapy in England began when the work of Valnet inspired Marguerite Maury, a French cosmetologist, to pursue the uses of essential oils in beauty therapy. It was this work that set the stage for using low concentrations of essential oils in vegetable oils as carriers to nurture the skin. Later in 1959 at a beauty therapist conference Maury met Micheline Arcier, who went on to develop the popular massage technique used by aromatherapists. The 'Micheline Arcier technique' (MR), as it is known, combines the modalities of Swedish massage, lymphatic drainage, polarity therapy and acupressure with aromatic oils. When performed correctly, the MR massage technique is gentle yet has profound effects in lowering client stress levels. MR massage is the cornerstone of English aromatherapy but the final part of the English puzzle came when Robert Tisserand published his fundamental text *The Art of Aromatherapy* in 1977. This work not only popularised aromatherapy with the general public, but also catalysed the formation of the English aromatherapy industry as a whole. The English 'popular aromatherapy' model quickly spread to America and Australia where it was initially taken up by beauty therapists as a method for introducing a pleasant smelling relaxation massage to their clients. Later various schools and colleges started to teach certificate and diploma courses in aromatherapy, predominantly following the English model.

The third style of aromatic use comes from Germany and involves the inhalation of aromatics to treat psychological and emotional disorders and diseases. 'Aromachology', as it has become known, has shed light upon the powerful effects aromatics have upon the unmediated pathway that olfaction has to the human brain.

With the turn of the twenty-first century there has been much progress around the world in the reintegration of all forms of aromatherapy. Today in countries like Australia, England, New Zealand and the USA popular aromatherapy is being practised alongside clinical aromatherapy. As acceptance by orthodox practitioners and regulatory authorities grows and industry experience and the practitioner knowledge base expands, there will be the advent of 'aromatic medicine' in these countries. Many aromatherapy practitioners are already upgrading their skills and knowledge in the areas of anatomy and physiology, chemistry, pharmacology, toxicology and the uses of new essential oils. Networking with other complementary therapists, such as remedial massage therapists, reflexologists, Bowen Technique therapists, naturopaths, herbalists and flower essence practitioners to name a few, is also becoming more commonplace as practitioners realise the benefits of these strategic alliances. Orthodox medicine is also beginning to use the knowledge and skills of aromatherapists in areas such as childbirth, palliative care and aged care. Integration of aromatherapy with other medical practice has seen improvement in patient outcomes by relieving physiological and psychological stresses as well as improving quality of life.

The science of aromatherapy

The explanatory theories of how and why aromatics work on human physiology and psychology closely parallel the development of orthodox medical rationales and discoveries. The evolution of this understanding began with the earliest studies of gross anatomy in the Renaissance by Leonardo da Vinci and has continued through to the current advances in cellular research. Scientific techniques and methods of analysis have provided many useful tools in discovering the complex chemical interactions between human physiological systems and essential oils. Organic chemistry, for example, has provided essential oil researchers with a chemical roadmap to understanding the chemical constituents of essential oils: 'A more detailed understanding of the actual chemical components of essential oils began with the work of chemist Otto Wallach between the years 1880 and 1914. Wallach was an assistant to the eminent F.A. Kekule, the first to accurately describe the chemical structure of the benzene molecule' (Schnaubelt 1999: 88). Benzene is the basic structure of many cyclic aromatic compounds within aromatic chemistry such as phenols and ethers (see Figure 6.1).

Figure 6.1 Benzene, thymol and anethole molecules

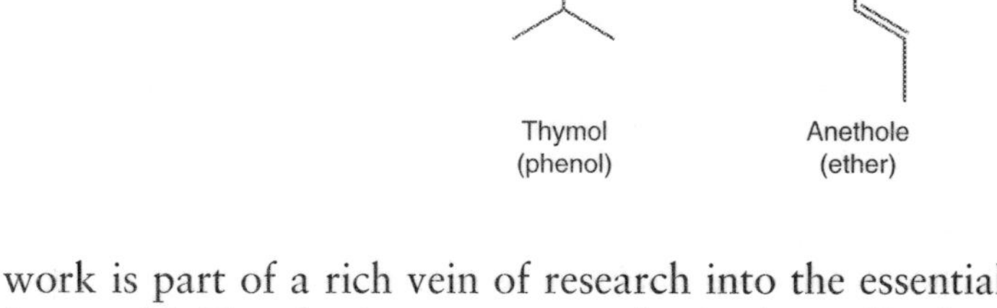

C_6H_6 Benzene · OR · Thymol (phenol) · Anethole (ether)

Wallach's work is part of a rich vein of research into the essential oils of plants throughout the world. To take just one example, in Australia there has been an exponential growth in the cataloguing and analysis of native Australian plants and their constituents, including essential oils, over the past century by many scientists including:

- **Richard T. Baker and Henry G. Smith in the early 1900s to 1920s: these plant chemists used empirical analytical techniques to determine the constituent makeup of many _Callitris_ and _Eucalyptus_ species before the advent of gas chromatography and mass spectrometry.**
- **A.R. Penfold in the 1940s to 1950s: a major researcher in essential oils at the then Museum of Technology, Sydney, Penfold and his colleagues were responsible for discovering and analysing many new Australian aromatic species.**
- **D.J. Boland, J.J. Brophy, E. Lassak and I.A. Southwell have been a few of today's productive researchers who have since the late 1970s been rechecking much of the original research conducted by previous scientists. They have also contributed research on many new species in the Myrtaceae family and other Australian genera.**

Other scientific and historical antecedents have also provided foundational and empirical knowledge to the field of aromatherapy. These contributions come from activities ranging from indigenous use of plant materials to herbalism. Activity in these fields, in combination with the ability to analyse chemically the constituents found within aromatic substances, has advanced theories of aromatherapy exponentially. Two important examples of the use of modern scientific method being applied to aromatherapy oils are gas chromatography (GC) and mass spectrometry (MS). GC separates the essential oil into individual chemical constituents and MS identifies those constituents by their molecular structure. 'In combination gas chromatography and mass spectrometry is a very powerful, complex and expensive tool for essential oil research' (Schnaubelt 1999: 151). Increasingly, however, GC–MS analysis is not overly expensive as there are many private and government laboratories which will conduct analysis under contract for a modest fee, thus allowing growers of aromatic plants to benefit from this modern analytical technique.

These methods of investigation have led to greater understanding of the constituents found within aromatic compounds and how those constituents may affect human physiology. Current knowledge of human anatomy and physiology allied with the chemical constituents of essential oils make it possible to postulate and attempt to prove clinically the efficacy of aromatherapy as a healing tool.

Aromatic chemistry

Aromatic chemistry is concerned with explaining the actions of functional groups and their interaction with human physiology. Functional groups are small parts of aromatic molecules which give that molecule its effect. Take for instance the –OH (hydroxyl) group of alcohols and phenols which is anti-bacterial. Aromatic constituents are categorised by the number of carbon atoms in the molecule and by their functional groups. Strictly speaking monoterpenes (C_{10}) and sesquiterpenes (C_{15}) are not functional groups but the hydrocarbon chains to which functional groups are attached. They do, however, have therapeutic actions and are included in discussions on this subject.

Most aromatic constituents found within essential oils can be placed within one of the following groups:

- **Monoterpenes**
- **Sesquiterpenes**
- **Monoterpenols**
- **Sesquiterpenols**
- **Phenols**
- **Aldehydes**

- **Ketones**
- **Esters**
- **Ethers**
- **Oxides**
- **Lactones**
- **Coumarins**

By using the example of lavender it is possible to illustrate functional groups and the biological impact of aromatic chemistry. From this analysis it will be evident that understanding essential oils from this perspective allows practitioners to choose an oil based on its physiological and/or psychological effects on the body.

Case study—lavender

To appreciate the overall effects and the actions of the components of essential oils, it is helpful to look at one plant as a case study. In this instance, lavender is a wise choice as it is a herb and a fragrance that has never gone out of fashion and has enjoyed widespread use from historical times to the present day (Johnson 2003). There are many species of lavender grown worldwide, each with unique properties, but there are some broad conclusions that can be drawn. Tables 6.1 and 6.2 give the chemical constituents and major functional groups of lavender respectively.

The research supporting the physiological effects of essential oils and their constituents is extensive. For lavender it is appropriate to begin with a now famous piece of research from the University of Vienna wherein mice were exposed to Lavender essential oil and two of its main constituents, linalool and linalyl acetate, to ascertain their sedative effects (Buchbauer *et al.* 1991). The researchers found that mice that were exposed to and inhaled lavender and its constituents showed a significant decrease in activity, and this decrease was closely related to exposure time to the oils.

The sesquiterpenes of lavender, with several double bonds, are reputed to have anti-inflammatory actions that are effective in reducing inflammation caused by stings and bites (Bowles 2000). Monoterpenols have been shown to have strong anti-bacterial and antifungal properties. Carson and Riley (1995) found that terpinen-4-ol, linalool and alpha terpineol are active against *Escherichia coli, Staphylococcus aureus* and *Candida albicans*. Terpinen-4-ol was the only constituent tested which was active against *Pseudomonas aeruginosa* (Bowles 2000). Bowles also reports studies that show linalool from Lavender oil has a spasmolytic effect on smooth muscle (Lis-Balchin & Hart 1999) while lavender ketones can kill papilloma and the herpes virus (Pénoël & Franchomme 1990). Research by Ulmer & Schott (1991) at the Ruhr-University Bochum, Germany, supports the understanding that oxides have expectorant properties and Jurgen *et al.* (1998) suggest that 1,8 cineole exhibits anti-inflammatory effects in bronchial asthma by inhibiting inflammatory leukotrienes and prostaglandins.

Tisserand (1997) states that lavender inhibits mycobacterium *Tuberculosis, Staphylococcus, Gonococcus*, Eberth's *Bacillus* (typhoid) and Loeffler's *Bacillus* (diphtheria) and when vaporised is effective against *Pneumococcus* and haemolytic *Streptococcus*.

Physiological principles

In discussing human physiology and aromatherapy the primary concern is with the pharmacokinetics of essential oils. This is the study of the absorption, distribution, metabolism and excretion of essential oils in the body. It can incorporate issues such as the physiological and physiochemical factors which influence the rate of absorption, distribution, metabolism and excretion. Take, for example, Thyme and Thuja essential oils (Thuja being a highly toxic oil). Oral ingestion of large amounts of Thyme or smaller amounts of Thuja oil instantly places a huge burden on the liver, due to their hepatotoxic constituents. However, dermal absorption of a similar dose may cause little concern and olfactory application will have no toxic effects whatsoever.

Olfaction theory

The most obvious piece of human anatomy connected with aromatherapy is the nose. The sense of smell and the process of olfaction is one of the most interesting aspects in the use of aromatics therapeutically. Olfaction has been described thus:

> The sense of smell is a primal sense for most humans as well as animals. From an evolutionary standpoint it is one of the most ancient senses. Olfaction allows for vertebrates . . . to identify food, mates, predators and provides both sensual pleasures as well as warning of dangers. For both humans and animals it is one of the important means by which our environment communicates to us (Leffingwell 1999).

Table 6.1 Chemical constituents of lavender (botanical name *Lavandula angustifolia*; family Lamiaceae/Labiatae)

Constituent	Percentage (%) present in essential oil	Group
linalyl acetate	40	ester
linalool	31.5	monoterpenol
(Z)-beta-ocimene	6.7	sesquiterpene
beta-caryophyllene	5.16	sesquiterpene
lavandulyl acetate	4.2	ester
terpinen-4-ol	4	monoterpenol
3-octanone	1.5	ketone
lavandulol	0.7	monoterpenol
1,8 cineole	0.69	oxide
camphor	0.3	ketone

Table 6.2 Lavender's major functional groups

Functional group	Therapeutic properties
Ester: number of carbon atoms 10 + acid	Antispasmodic Sedative Possible immuno-modulator
Sesquiterpene: number of carbon atoms 15	Anti-inflammatory Possible hormonal effects
Monoterpenol: number of carbon atoms 10	Anti-infectious Vasoconstrictor Tonic and general stimulants Sedative
Ketone: number of carbon atoms 10 (mono) 15 (sesqui)	Mucolytic properties Wound healing Anti-haematomal properties Anti-viral
Oxide: number of carbon atoms 10 (mono) 15 (sesqui)	Exocrine gland stimulant Expectorant

Bowles describes the process of olfaction as being when

> odorous substances are breathed in through the nose, dissolve in the olfactory
> mucosa and may stimulate the olfactory nerves which have fine hair-like endings
> called cilia embedded in the mucus. They may stimulate the trigeminal nerve,
> which is a branched nerve responsible for detecting pain, touch, temperature in
> many parts of the face and head, including the nasal epithelium (Bowles 2000:
> 95–6).

The olfactory system is classified as a chemoreceptor because it responds to
chemicals in solution. This is similar to the sense of taste and in fact contributes
greatly to that sense. When a person has a head cold for instance, their sense of
taste diminishes owing to the corresponding reduction in the sense of smell. To
understand this complex process it is best to examine what happens physiologically
when an odour is perceived.

The receptors for olfaction are found in the nasal epithelium (*Regio olfactoria*) of
the superior and medial nasal conchae. The olfactory receptor cells are modified
neurons with fine hair-like extensions called cilia. The human olfactory system
contains approximately 100 million of these specialised cells. The cilia, which cover
the conchae, are themselves continuously covered in a layer of mucus which is
exuded from the anterior glands. In order for an odour/aroma to be detected it must
be dissolved in this watery mucus and this is why the sense of smell is recognised as
chemoreception. The cilia detect these dissolved chemicals and initiate nerve signals.
The olfactory nerve (first cranial nerve) transmits this signal up through the cribiform
plate, which has approximately twenty holes (foramina) to facilitate this passage. The
cribiform plate forms part of the ethmoid bone of the cranium. (See Figure 6.2.)

The structure of these olfactory nerves is similar to the general anatomy of nerve
structures. They possess dendrites and cell bodies but differentiate and terminate
in the highly specialised olfactory vesicle. Each odour/aroma or sensation of
odour/aroma is then transmitted by an unmyelinated nerve fibre (axon) which
connects with other receptor cells. These nerves then synapse with nerves within
the olfactory bulbs.

The olfactory bulbs are ovoid in shape and are extensions of the brain that are
positioned superior to the nasal cavity. This connection to the brain is known as
the olfactory tract. Each set of olfactory nerves connects to specialised cells in the
olfactory bulb called mitral cells. One hundred axons from the olfactory nerve
contact with each mitral cell in groupings known as glomeruli (Etherington *et al.*
2000). There is a complex interplay within the olfactory bulbs because interneurons
link the glomeruli with each other and they also connect the two olfactory bulbs with
each other. These form two areas of the brain called the medial and lateral olfactory
areas. These areas are connected to the limbic system in the brain.

Figure 6.2 The anatomy of olfaction

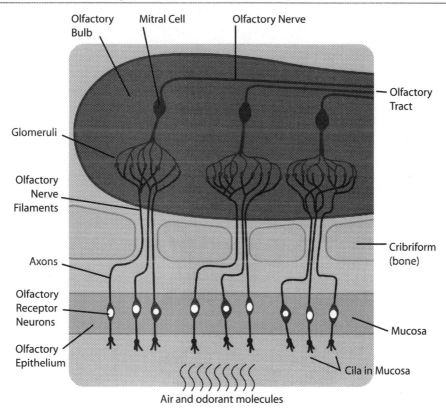

Air and odorant molecules

Olfaction and the limbic system

Anatomically, the human sense of smell is strongly linked to the generation of emotion.

> The olfactory bulbs are directly connected to the hippocampus and the amygdala in the limbic system, which is important for memory and emotion. This is why smells are evocative of past places and feelings. Some smells stimulate the limbic system to activate the hypothalamus and pituitary gland, which triggers the release of hormones associated with appetite and emotional responses including pleasure, fear and sexual drive (Etherington *et al.* 2000: 655).

> The human response to aromas is associated with olfaction naturally. The neurons in the olfactory system, which are the chemical sense of the body, rest in the section of the midbrain known as the limbic system. The structures of the limbic system extend from the midbrain through the hypothalamus into the basal forebrain, which is not only concerned with visceral functions but

also with emotional expression. The cortical and medial nuclei of the amygdala, a body situated within this system, receives information from the olfactory system. The basolateral nuclei are involved with the expression of emotion (Shepherd 1983: 8).

The limbic system is a collection of nuclei and tracts in the brain that are involved in the creation of emotions, sexual behaviours, fear and rage, motivation and processing of memory. These components of the limbic system are primarily located as a border point where the cerebrum is connected to the midbrain. This includes the rim of gyri around the corpus callosum. Also forming part of the limbic system are the mamillary bodies, which are reflex centres for olfaction and protrude from the base of the hypothalamus posterior to the pituitary gland. The hypothalamus, which is found at the base of the diencephalon, is responsible for visceral regulations such as body temperature and homœostasis. The hypothalamus is also the part of the limbic system that regulates many motivations, drives and emotions.

The amygdala is another vital part of the limbic system and is located in the temporal lobe just anterior to the hippocampus. The amygdala is connected to the ability to process chemical signals from the olfactory system, hippocampus, cerebral cortex and hypothalamus in the expression of emotions. In turn, the hippocampus is found deeply interior in the temporal lobe and is connected to the cortex on the interior base of the cerebral cortex. The hippocampus's function is the formation of new memories. Damage to this region of the brain renders people unable to form new memories but old memories remain undamaged.

Lastly, the septal area of the limbic system is believed to be responsible for the recognition of pleasure and reward. It is located beneath the anterior of the corpus callosum and is connected to the hypothalamus, hippocampus and amygdala (Etherington *et al.* 2000; Marieb 2000).

These components comprise the limbic system (see Figure 6.3), which is thought to be a primitive area of the brain because it is responsible for many autonomic visceral functions. However, the interconnectedness of this system and its role in mood, behaviour, emotions, motivations, sexual drive and memory make the limbic system an integral aspect of human physiology and psychology. That this brain system is linked to the olfactory system in many ways makes the use of essential oils via olfaction a fascinating area of research. The mapping of the neural pathways from olfaction throughout the limbic system is just beginning.

Implications of olfaction for aromatherapy

Unlike other human senses smell has no gatekeepers and in effect has an unmediated impact on the brain. As the olfactory system is linked physiologically with the limbic system, the lexicon of aromas collected over a lifetime can have a profound effect. For example, the smell of freshly baked bread may cause the physiological

Figure 6.3 The limbic system

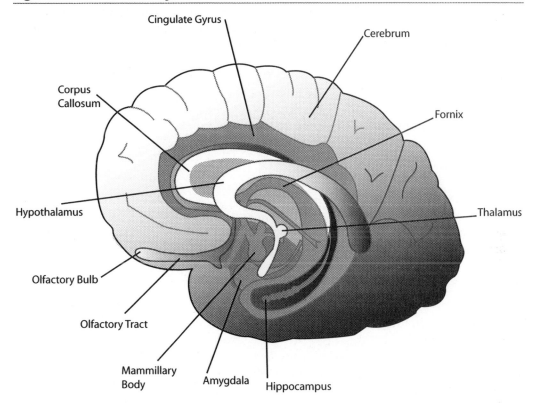

response of an increase in saliva production. This response to aroma is unmitigated by the higher functions of the brain. So it can be concluded that essential oils, being highly aromatic substances, will have an effect on the human physiology. This may be for two reasons. First, that the person smelling an essential oil has that aroma already in their memory via the limbic system and has associated it with a pleasurable experience. Therefore it is an act of recollection activating long-term memory and exciting neural pathways in the limbic system, specifically the septal region. Second, the aromatic molecules having passed through the million cilia in the nasal passage, through the cribiform plate and epithelium, have chemically interacted with the nerves, synapses and neurotransmitters and entered the limbic system. Thereby the oils have caused an alteration of brain chemistry which elicits the brain's own neurotransmitters, producing sedating, arousing, pleasurable or excitatory responses.

Odour stimuli in the limbic system or olfactory brain release neurotransmitters among them encephalin, endorphins, serotonin and noradrenaline . . .

within the limbic system resides the regulatory mechanisms of our highly explosive inner life, the secret core of our being. Here is the seat of our sexuality, the impulse of attraction and aversion, our motivation and our moods, memory and creativity as well as our autonomic nervous system (Fischer-Rizzi 1990: 26–7).

The brain centre for smell is closely related and connected to the limbic system. This centre is in turn closely in communication with the hypothalamus which is of course a reflex point through the nerve pathways with the autonomic nervous system (ANS) and via chemical messengers with the pituitary gland and other glands in the body (Noonan 1997).

The interaction of the olfactory and limbic systems may go some way to explaining the powerful relationship between human physiology and essential oils. Much research is still needed to be done to ascertain, map and understand this complex aspect of human brain chemistry. It is known that the entire body is capable of receiving chemical information from essential oils but the olfactory system and limbic system are the only parts of the central nervous system that allow for direct contact with the external environment. Hence these systems are integral to individual personalities and that makes these systems extremely important in a therapeutic context.

As a therapist it is important to know and understand the complex structure and chemical communications that comprise olfaction. However, as with all aspects of human physiology there are variables that can impact on the sense of smell in a client presenting for aromatherapy treatment. Has the client had a stroke or other nervous system injury that may have damaged the region of the brain relating to smell? Does the client smoke cigarettes or use other medical or illegal inhalants which can also impair this brain region? If the client is female, she will have a heightened olfactory sense during ovulation. Additionally, not all aromas will evoke a positive response. The limbic system being associated with both olfaction and memory may, on some occasions, trigger a negative physiological/psychological response. As an example it is helpful to review the following case study.

Case study

Jane is a 45-year-old corporate executive who, due to her busy lifestyle and work schedule, is suffering from a stress-related skin disorder. An aromatherapist may decide to use Lavender essential oil (for its well-documented calming and sedative properties) in the treatment of this condition. Upon offering Jane a sample of Lavender essential oil to smell the therapist discovers that she cannot stand the smell, in fact it causes the opposite response expected. What is evidenced is an increase in Jane's heart rate and blood pressure. After calming down Jane reveals that as a small child she was often forced to stay with her grandmother, who mistreated her. The grandmother wore lavender and the aroma immediately transported her back to being that small, scared child.

The sense of smell is, as this example illustrates, a profound memory key that can strip away years of cognitive thought in an instant. Conversely, if Jane's grandmother had been a sweet, loving person Jane would probably have enjoyed the smell of lavender, as there would be many positive associations attached to this scent. This is just one of the many reasons why taking a thorough medical history from a client is very important. Aside from the various physical contraindications there may be psychological and/or emotional issues that aromatic stimuli may trigger when used within a treatment.

Dermal absorption theory

The olfactory route is not the only way in which essential oils can impact on human physiology. The integumentary system is a highly complex body system and it is one of the traditional methods of applying essential oils via massage. Skin protects the deeper tissue from either mechanical (bumps) or chemical (acids and bases) damage, bacterial damage, ultraviolet radiation, thermal damage and desiccation. Further, skin aids the body in heat loss and retention, excretion of urea and uric acid and synthesis of vitamin D. This multifunctional organ is composed of three layers: the epidermis, dermis and subcutaneous.

In an aromatherapy massage the application of essential oils in a base oil/cream can be used for a number of possible outcomes. The practitioner may be treating a disorder of the skin itself but more commonly it is used as a method for essential oil uptake into the bloodstream. Essential oil constituents can in turn circulate through the entire body exerting physiological effects before being excreted via urine, faeces, lungs, lymph or the integumentary system itself.

Aromatherapy research

Olfactory aromatherapy research

Research conducted at Columbia University, New York, by Zhang and Firestein (2002) has identified a surprisingly large family of genes in rats that appear to code for odour receptors. This gene family is one of the largest ever discovered, programming 500 to 1000 different types of receptors. Scientists think this large and diverse group of genes is what helps animals detect such a huge variety of odours.

In rats and mice the olfactory lining is divided into four zones, each containing neurons with different odour receptors. Neurons expressing the same receptor genes within each zone appear to be randomly arranged. In the olfactory bulb, however, fibres from neurons with the same gene receptor converge on just one or a few glomeruli, specialised structures in which olfactory neurons connect with other types of neurons (see above). Research suggests that an individual odour molecule stimulates several types of receptors, each of which responds to a part of the molecule's structure. Brain mapping techniques have shown that the pattern of glomeruli activated by each odour forms a map or code that the brain may recognise as a unique scent (Zhang & Firestein 2002).

By studying how olfactory neurons establish connections with other neurons in the adult brain, researchers hope to learn how nerve fibres connect in other brain regions. Unlike most neurons, olfactory neurons that die can be replaced by new neurons that serve the same function.

> Olfactory information travels not only to the limbic system . . . but also to the brain's cortex or outer layer where conscious thought occurs. In addition, it combines with taste information in the brain to create a sensation of flavour. Learning more about these links will help explain how odours affect our thoughts, emotions and behaviour (Leffingwell 1999).

There has been a recent increase in clinical studies into the effects of essential oils in this field. A placebo controlled study from the University of Southampton, England, exposed fifteen patients with severe dementia to diffused Lavender oil for ten repeat sessions (Holmes *et al.* 2002). The results showed a significant improvement in agitated behaviour when using diffused Lavender oil when compared to the placebo. Another randomised, controlled trial was conducted at the University of Miami upon 40 adults to test the effects of the inhalation of two well-known essential oils, Lavender and Rosemary (Diego *et al.* 1998). Subjects who inhaled Lavender essential oil showed increased beta power on EEG patterns, suggesting increased drowsiness; they reported feeling more relaxed with less depressed mood. Their maths computations were faster and more accurate upon testing after the inhalation. Subjects who were tested with Rosemary oil showed decreased alpha and beta power on EEG patterns, suggesting increased alertness. They also reported less anxiety, and felt more relaxed and alert. Their maths computations were faster but not more accurate following the inhalation.

Dermal aromatherapy research

There have been claims made by researchers investigating aromatherapy that dermal absorption does not occur and that the effects of essential oils are mainly due to olfactory effects or absorption into the bloodstream via the lungs. These theories have since been proven to be incorrect. Clinical studies on dermal application of essential oils are few but some evidence is emerging in support of dermal absorption as an effective approach to aromatherapeutic treatment.

In a trial conducted at the University of Bradford, England, Williams and Barry (1991) tested the theory that various terpene compounds would enhance the dermal penetration of a polar molecule 5-fluorouracil (5-FU). Their finding revealed that various essential oil constituents had differing effects upon the rate of absorption, with 1,8-cineole (oxide) increasing absorption by 95 times.

A later study from Bradford by Cornwell and Barry (1994) showed that sesquiterpenes also increased dermal absorption, with nerolidol (found in Nerolina oil) being the most effective with an increased absorption of twentyfold. The sesquiterpenes were also noted for being extremely difficult to remove from the skin once applied, which adds to their use as fixatives/base compounds within blends.

For stress-related hypertension, for instance, the therapist may use dermal application as part of a treatment regime. One study conducted in Vienna found that the topical application of Western Australian Sandalwood (*Santalum spicatum*) essential oil has been clinically proven to lower stress levels and systolic blood pressure (Hongratanaworakit *et al.* 2000). (Note: face masks were worn by the test subjects to prevent the olfactory pathway from influencing the results.)

A 1998 randomised, double-blind, controlled, seven-month trial (with follow-ups at three and seven months) was conducted in Scotland to investigate the effects of essential oils upon alopecia areata (hair loss) (Hay *et al.* 1998). The test group had essential oils of Thyme, Rosemary, Lavender and Cedarwood diluted in jojoba and grapeseed oils massaged into their scalp daily. The control group had just the carrier oils jojoba and grapeseed massaged into their scalp daily. The study showed an improvement of 44 per cent for the test group compared to 6 per cent for the control group. The authors concluded that the essential oils were a safe and effective treatment for hair loss.

Methods of application

There is a wide variety of application methods for the use of aromatics from personal perfumery to massage, aromatic bathing, inhalation or even in foods and beverages. Each of these is mentioned in some detail throughout this chapter. The different methods are diverse and within each of these are variations that depend largely upon the expertise of the practitioner and the desired outcome. For example, the method of aromatic bathing ranges from simple to advanced in its application. At the simple end of the scale is the 'English' low-dose method using a few drops of essential oils for a soothing, relaxation bath. Alternatively, higher doses (up to 50 drops, when properly emulsified in the water) are used.

Additionally, application procedures for essential oils are always evolving. Aromatic profusion is a relatively new technique drawn from the clinical and aromatic medicine area of aromatherapy, whereby the therapist applies a single, relatively large dose (10–15 mL) of a neat essential oil blend to the client's body in the treatment of acute viral or bacterial infections. This is far removed from the low-dose model found in popular aromatherapy and relies on considerably more skill in areas of aromatic chemistry, pharmacology and therapeutic blending.

Indications

As diverse as the methods of applying essential oils are, the conditions for which they are effective are even more so. Some of the main ailments that will benefit from aromatherapy treatment are listed below.

Wounds

As modern pharmaceutical medications become less effective against the various resistant strains of microbes, research into the traditional uses of essential oils is being put into practice in the area of wound care and management. In the area of aged care, many bedridden clients develop skin tears and bed or pressure sores from prolonged pressure against their unmoving, fragile skin. Many nurses around the world who are trained in aromatherapy have been using essential oils within this framework (with due client and medical consent) in instances where pharmaceutical medications have consistently failed to rectify the condition(s) for individual clients over time. More recent research into wound healing has been conducted, showing that significant improvements in wound healing are made possible by the use of essential oils and herbal extracts (Kerr 2002; Primmer 2002).

Skin conditions

Aromatherapy is useful for a variety of other skin conditions, including acne and minor infections. As an example, the use of the very toxic Thuja (*Thuja occidentalis*) essential oil in the topical treatment of warts has been recommended by a number of sources. The effectiveness of this treatment can be seen in the illustrative case of an eight year old with a plantar wart. Neat Thuja oil was applied in the dose of a single drop per day directly to the wart over a period of a week. The tissue surrounding the wart darkened slightly, the wart died and was shucked off after approximately three weeks with no damage to the surrounding tissues and no recurrence of the condition.

Inflammation

A number of essential oils containing significant amounts of sesquiterpenes and sesquiterpenols have been shown to act as inflammatory mediators. For an insect bite, for instance, the application of a drop or two of neat Tea Tree or Lavender essential oil is well known to prevent infection and reduce inflammation and the pain of the bite. Applying a high concentration oil (up to 100 per cent) over relatively small areas of the skin will generally give a localised response in the tissues covered. Essential oils that truly stand out in this area are German Chamomile (*Matricaria recutita*), Nerolina (*Melaleuca quinquinervia* CT nerolidol/linalool) and Western Australian Sandalwood (*Santalum spicatum*). Research into the biochemical pathways responsible has revealed that Western Australian Sandalwood oil appears to inhibit inflammatory response by blocking enzyme 12-lipoxygenase and both cycoloxygenases COX1 and COX2 (Gearon 2002).

Pain

Pain management has recently become a favoured topic among aromatherapists, as many are now working in areas other than relaxation massage and are finding that client health needs revolve around quality of life, which for some is based upon pain management. Aromatherapy massage is particularly suited to the treatment of pain due to its soothing and calming qualities. Massage and the application of oils via this method can be localised to concentrate on the area of pain or to achieve general relaxation. While traditionally oils such as Wintergreen, Rosemary and Lavender have been used to help mediate pain, there are also newly discovered and commercially released oils available. One example of these is the previously little known Australian Kunzea (*Kunzea ambigua*) essential oil. This oil is showing promising effects in relieving the pain of arthritis and muscular sprains and strains. Ongoing research into how this and other oils mediate pain is currently being conducted by the author.

Respiratory illness

Aromatherapy is particularly appropriate to ease the discomfort of respiratory illnesses. Colds, flu, sinus infections and bronchitis respond to the anti-inflammatory, decongestant and antimicrobial qualities of certain oils. The inhalation method and aromatic bathing methods are both suitable for the treatment of conditions of the respiratory tract. Thyme and Eucalyptus oils are often employed in treatment of respiratory illnesses but there is a wide range of essential oils that can be used and blended to alleviate symptoms in such conditions.

Rheumatic conditions

Aromatic bathing may be used to treat a variety of conditions such as rheumatic joint complaints and aching muscles. Many commercial bath products utilise the beneficial effects of essential oils in their formulations. Lavender and Wintergreen are known for the relief they can yield in arthritic states. Sports people will relate to the smells of certain essential oils like Peppermint, Wintergreen and Basil that can be used in ointments or oil blends for sore muscles.

Other conditions

Just a few further conditions that respond well to aromatherapy treatment include:

- **bruises**
- **colic**
- **cracked skin**
- **dandruff**
- **flatulence**
- **fluid retention**
- **foot odour**
- **genito-urinary infections (cystitis and vaginal thrush)**
- **headache**
- **insomnia**
- **ringworm**
- **stress and tension**
- **tinea**

Practice issues

When essential oils enter the human body they have varying effects, depending upon the pathway and dosage. Paracelsus, the father of toxicology, stated that 'The dose makes the poison . . .'. By this he meant that all substances are poisonous depending on the dosage given; for some the toxic amount is quite low and for others very high. Oral ingestion of essential oils such as Thuja or Thyme essential oils, for instance, places a huge burden upon the liver, due to their hepatotoxic constituents, while dermal application of a similar amount may cause no concern whatsoever. Understanding the key differences between dermal and oral toxicity and between the therapeutic dose and the toxic dose forms the necessary knowledge base in aromatic pharmacology. With this knowledge therapists can safely prescribe and use higher concentrations and doses of essential oils in treatments than are normally used in popular aromatherapy.

In aromatherapy today there are two levels of treatment dosage rates. Clinical aromatherapy uses high-concentration essential oils (up to 100 per cent) and doses measured in millilitres for the treatment of physical diseases and illnesses such as acute influenza. By contrast popular aromatherapy employs low-concentration oils (1–5 per cent) and doses measured in drops for the treatment of psychological/emotional conditions such as stress.

At high dosages essential oils act like any other drug, with all of the benefits and associated dangers. At lower dosages, however, essential oils appear to have neuro-transmitter and/or hormonal-like properties, for example the apparent phytoestrogen effects upon women of anethole-rich essential oils such as Sweet Fennel or Aniseed Myrtle. When these oils are applied topically to the lower abdomen and back in a relatively low dosage of 2–5 per cent they have been found to ease menstrual cramping. For older female clients the same dosage will, over a period of a few months, help to mediate peri-menopausal signs and symptoms.

In a clinical setting knowledge of olfaction, the limbic system and brain chemistry is a valuable asset for the therapist. This is especially true for acute conditions, which require immediate attention, such as the lowering of high blood pressure or the reduction of a bipolar/depressive or anxious psychological state. Bearing in mind that referral may be necessary in extreme cases, the inhalation of the appropriate essential oils which are known to have sedating or calming effects are particularly useful in these conditions. Again, a well-trained therapist who is knowledgeable about the chemical constituents of essential oils will be able to select those essential oils most suited to the outcome required.

In the case of a client suffering depression, for example, inhalation of essential oils to interact positively with the limbic system can form part of a treatment regime. An oil blend in this instance may include Bergamot, Spikenard, Lavender and Rose. In a sound aromatherapy practice, these oils will have been chosen with the chemistry and effect of each oil clearly understood by the therapist.

Contraindications

There have been many instances in far too many books on aromatherapy where contraindications have been listed for essential oils when none were warranted, based on the chemical constituents and toxicology of the oils involved. Many of these warnings were based upon the incorrect interpretation of herbal lore and lack of clear scientific data (Guba 2000).

Today there is a far better understanding of the issues surrounding aromatic toxicology thanks to the work of researchers such as Guba, Tisserand and Balacs. In their seminal work *Essential Oil Safety—A Guide for Health Care Professionals*, Tisserand and Balacs clearly discuss many relevant issues within this important area of aromatherapy. Ron Guba has also done much to refute and debunk unwarranted fear-based warnings and his article on toxicity myths is of equal importance.

Some important and basic examples of toxicity issues in aromatherapy are:

- *Anticoagulants* Using Wintergreen oil (98 per cent methyl salicylate) with clients taking anticoagulant medication, such as warfarin, has the ability to potentiate the anticoagulant effects, thus causing internal haemorrhaging.
- *Pregnancy* There has been much misinformation regarding the potential dangers to both mother and child during pregnancy. Much of this caution has been ethically based, but much is also not based upon science. Reviewing the toxicological data it appears that very few commonly used essential oils are dangerous at any stage of pregnancy. Nevertheless, oils with a toxicity rating of 2 (LD_{50} between 1 and 2 g/kg) should be avoided in the first trimester; this is dose dependent and oils such as Basil (rich in ethers) should be avoided, due to the detoxification load placed upon the liver by such oils. Having said this, certain oils are used with good effect to relieve pregnancy symptoms like fluid retention and nervous tension. The emphasis in pregnancy must therefore be that aromatherapy should always be administered either by, or in consultation with, a qualified practitioner.
- *Epilepsy* There are many listings for essential oils that may trigger an epileptic fit; when the data are reviewed there are no documented cases of essential oils causing an epileptic fit. Oils high in toxic ketones should be avoided, but commonly accused oils such as Rosemary appear to be safe at popular aromatherapy dosage rates.
- *Dermal irritation* Certain essential oil constituents are known to be irritant to dermal and mucous membrane tissues. Aldehydes such as cinnamon aldehyde have a reputation for being irritant in this manner. The effects of most essential oil constituents causing dermal irritation can be negated to a large degree by blending with other constituents known to 'quench' the irritancy effects.
- *Phototoxicity* Certain expressed citrus oils such as Bergamot, Bitter Orange, Lemon, Lime and Angelica contain a particular type of furocoumarin, bergaptene, which can cause serious phototoxic effects to skin when applied with subsequent exposure to sunlight or ultraviolet radiation.

Quality issues

The quality of the aromatics on offer within the essential oil, food and flavouring and aromatherapy industries varies greatly depending upon their end use. How does an aromatherapist choose their aromatics and determine whether an aromatic has been stretched, adulterated or reconstituted from synthetic constituents?

As part of their professional training aromatherapists should be exposed to many varying qualities of aromatics. They need to experience synthetic and isolated constituents to allow them to build an aromatic memory (in a similar way to wine appreciation) for what makes an outstanding, therapeutic-grade aromatic. Most aromatherapists rely upon trust, trust in their teachers, peers and specialist industry suppliers who themselves are often working aromatherapists, to keep them informed and supplied with quality aromatics. Reliable suppliers of aromatics to the aromatherapy industry will generally have years of experience, be informative and have quality assurance standards in place.

Items to look for on quality aromatic packaging and literature include:

- **common and botanical names;**
- **specific chemotype (CT) for some species such as thyme and rosemary;**
- **country of origin;**
- **part of plant used and extraction technique;**
- **batch coding and best before or use-by date; and**
- **dark glass bottle (for neat aromatics) with appropriate-sized flow-restriction dripper.**

Percentage constituent analysis charts (from GCMS) should also be available on request for the knowledgeable therapist to make their own assessment of the aromatic. A therapist's nose is, however, still the cheapest and most reliable tool for assessing quality as previously mentioned. A well-trained nose can detect the subtle differences between a quality aromatic and an average or below-average one. Along with the supplier's reputation, this is generally regarded as sufficient precaution in choosing aromatics.

Patient compliance

As with all forms of therapy, if the client is not compliant and leaves the aromatic blend in its bottle little benefit will be achieved from aromatherapy. Fortunately within aromatherapy there tends to be high levels of client compliance as the client is not ingesting medicines with a disagreeable taste, as is often the case in herbal medicine for instance. Rather, the client is asked to undertake the pleasant tasks of applying aromatic oils, lotions and creams to their bodies or taking aromatic baths. Through judicious combination of oils, the skilled aromatherapist can make even the most medicinal smelling component oils blend into a pleasant mix and thus reduce the likelihood of client resistance. Non-pharmacological issues such as diet, exercise and other lifestyle changes are often much harder to achieve, but are equally if not more important to the client's continued wellbeing.

Aromatherapy and the medical community

Aromatherapy is slowly making its way into mainstream medical establishments in areas where it is not regarded as a direct threat to pharmaceutical medicine. Unfortunately, many times the first step into complementary medicine is as a last resort, when orthodox medicine has all but given up on a positive outcome for a client. Some remarkable examples of wound management and ongoing care of the aged have already been illustrated in this chapter. Future areas of focus will be in the use of essential oils in the field of infectious control and even palliative care, when quality of life is one of the most important issues to be encountered. Worldwide it is nurses, in particular, who are championing the cause of aromatherapy as a complementary medicine. Nurses recognise the therapeutic and holistic issues surrounding quality of life. By using aromatherapy they can provide a level of personal care that is often missing in a clinical environment. As the broader knowledge and scientific understanding of essential oils increase, there is likely to be an increase worldwide in the use of essential oils in hospital settings to mediate pain, reduce stress, assist in wound-care management, pain management, reduce nausea and reduce rates of infections.

The 'English' or 'popular aromatherapy' is the most prevalent style of aromatherapy worldwide but aromatherapy practices do vary from country to country. This variation is in part due to the fact that the practice of aromatherapy is dependent on each country's legal and educational requirements for certification. It is in France, where it more closely follows the biomedical medical model in its administration (see above), that aromatherapy is best accepted by the orthodox medical community.

Limitations of treatment

Aromatherapy in all its forms has many uses and applications; it is not, however, the cure-all that it is sometimes purported to be. Popular aromatherapy can provide real benefits in many areas of stress management and in dealing with emotional issues. Clinical aromatherapy can be helpful in many areas including infectious disease control, chronic-condition care, pain management and wound care. Yet aromatherapy in all its forms should not be viewed as a substitute but as a complement to orthodox healthcare. A prime benefit of aromatherapy knowledge is that it can be shared with patients to enable patients themselves to obtain relief from symptoms of some minor conditions. As more practitioners in all forms of medicine gain greater understanding of what is available there will be closer cooperation and networking, which will only improve patient outcomes and quality of life.

Conclusion

Aromatherapy in a range of modes is widely used around the world. New plant species are being identified for use, research into traditional practices continues and methods of extraction and application are developing. The methods by which essential oils can be administered range from the low concentrations via massage typical of the English aromatherapy school, to the high concentrations taken internally of the French aromatherapy, to the inhalation method of German aromatherapy. In the modern usage, however, people tend to avail themselves of an eclectic combination of administration forms featuring massage and inhalation in particular.

At the centre of all aromatherapy, though, is the synergy that exists between human physiology and plant biology. However aromatherapy is practised, understanding the chemistry of aromatic molecules is vital to the correct usage of essential oils in clinical practice. This knowledge enables the aromatherapy practitioner to select, blend and administer essential oils in the most effective manner. Olfaction and the sense of smell are theoretically the most interesting avenues of administering essential oils as smell is a primal sense with no mitigating influences in the body. The interaction of the olfactory nerves with the limbic system of the brain, which is involved in the creation of emotions, is of vital importance to the practice of aromatherapy, but dermal absorption also offers exciting potential.

Human beings have long understood the benefits of plants as food and medicine and with today's scientific analysis these historical practices are being validated. Each country has its unique aromatherapy practices that have developed in line with the attributes of the plants and the people who cohabit with them. Humans, in this instance, are not removed from their environment but are tied by the practice of aromatherapy to the ecosystem in which they live. The increasing interest in aromatherapeutic plants has implications for the future of farming and crop development, environmental sustainability and cultivation of plant species. Modern aromatherapy faces challenges but the growing evidence of its gentle efficacy ensures that it will be a significant part of the healthcare systems of the future.

Recommended reading

Mojay, G. 2000, *Aromatherapy for Healing the Spirit*, Gaia Publications, London.

Pénoël, D. and Franchomme, R. 1998, *Natural Home Health Care Using Essential Oils*, Osmobiose, La Drome.

Tisserand, R. and Balacs, T. 1995, *Essential Oil Safety—A Guide for Health Care Professionals*, Churchill Livingstone, Edinburgh.

Valnet, J. 1985, *The Practice of Aromatherapy*, C.W. Daniel Co., Essex.

Webb, M. 2000, *Bush Sense—Australian Essential Oils and Aromatic Compounds*, B-in-Print, Sydney.

7

Chiropractic
Phillip S. Ebrall

Chiropractic is a healthcare profession concerned with the diagnosis, treatment and prevention of mechanical disorders of the musculoskeletal system and the effects of these disorders on the nervous system and general health. There is an emphasis on manual treatments, including spinal manipulation or adjustment (World Federation of Chiropractic 1999).

Chiropractors are comprehensively trained providers of primary healthcare based on the defining principle that pathomechanical change in a functional spinal unit may affect related neurologic function, which in turn may be restored by correction of that mechanical change (Ebrall 2001). Altered neural function equates to changes in the optimal expression of health and wellbeing for an individual and this is perceived and/or measured as a change in health status. Chiropractors refer to these changes in the spine as a subluxation, a small but detectable change in the anatomical and/or physiological function of a joint or joint complex within the spine.

One of the more recognised approaches used for the correction of a subluxation is the chiropractic adjustment. This is the controlled delivery of a high-velocity, low-amplitude (HVLA) manual or mechanically assisted force into the joints of the spine at the level of subluxation. Its purpose is to restore normal movement and thus normal neurological function. The patient typically perceives this as a 'cracking' of the spine, back or neck as the adjustment is usually accompanied by audible sounds of joint cavitation. In simple terms, chiropractors use a refined form of manipulation to normalise spinal structure and restore normal neurologic function for the purpose of restoring and maintaining health. There are many different types of adjustment and this reflects the diverse nature of the subluxation as it is found in different patient populations and demographics.

The concepts of 'subluxation complex' (SC) and the 'adjustment' are central to the profession of chiropractic and are enshrined in both the World Federation of Chiropractic's (WFC) definition of chiropractic and the Association of Chiropractic College's (1996) position paper on chiropractic. Chiropractors typically conduct a full health assessment of the patient and then direct their attention to identifying levels of subluxation in the spine and to selecting the most appropriate therapeutic intervention to correct them. Other spinal therapists speak of subluxation as being a functional spinal lesion, a somatic lesion or a spondylogenic reflex syndrome, among other terms (Rome 1996), and apply a variety of manual means other than the chiropractic adjustment as their treatment protocol.

There are various elements of the subluxation complex (see Figure 7.1). Chiropractors will look for kinematic (movement) change within a particular spinal motion unit (SMU). Evidence of changes to the neurologic dimensions of the particular spinal level, the musculature both intrinsic and extrinsic to that level and the connective tissue and vasculature associated with that spinal level will also be sought.

The history of chiropractic

The concept that changes in the function of the spine are associated with changes in health is as old as antiquity. Precise descriptions of the nature of this dysfunction and its clinical consequences began to appear in the medical literature in the early nineteenth century (Harrison 1820; Terrett 1987). Yet it was not until a rather remarkable Canadian magnetic healer, Daniel David Palmer, practising in Davenport, Iowa, in the late nineteenth century, integrated the neurological and medical concepts of his day that the formal discipline of chiropractic was born in 1895.

At the time of Palmer a mechanical view of the spine prevailed with controversial mechanical treatments being promoted for disorders such as scoliosis. During this period, science in medicine was recognised as important by some but abused widely by many and the medical literature of the day demonstrated multifarious concepts of health and disease. The mode of intervention advocated by Palmer was remarkable in that, first, it did no harm, unlike much other intervention of the day, and, second, it was based on principles which held currency within the mainstream of medical thought (Ebrall 1995a).

Palmer demonstrated extensive knowledge of neurology and his concepts were well within the mainstream of thought in 1895. There was abundant literature at the time describing clinical and pathological features of diseases of the spinal cord and the concepts of 'nerve energy' and 'tone' were promulgated along with theories of inhibitory mechanisms which controlled the 'nerve force'. Nerve compression was thought a valid precursor of neural inflammation, and visceral disease was identified as referring pain and tenderness. In this context, Palmer's precepts and approach were well founded and somewhat conservative (Ebrall 1995b).

Palmer was assertive of the concept of tone, so much so that the title page of his seminal collection of writings stated that chiropractic is 'Founded on Tone' (Palmer 1910). His writings emphasised the importance of appropriate tone for optimal human functioning, and the principle of *too much or too little tone* can be seen as the extension of the founding principle of chiropractic (Ebrall 2001). His notion of tone provided a hypothetical bridge between the theory of vitalism and the manifestation of subluxation. 'Tone' also encompassed the dual concepts of either an increase or a decrease in functional tension within the nerve (Keating 1992).

The first formal text of the new chiropractic profession, *Modernized Chiropractic*, described 'a subluxated vertebra' as differing 'from normal only in its field of motion', suggesting 'its various positions of rest are differently located than when it was a normal vertebra and its field of motion may be too great in some directions and too small in others' (Smith *et al.* 1906: 24–6). The essential concepts at this time included small changes in vertebral position, small changes in movement of a vertebra and an impact on the proper functioning of the nervous system.

The first edition of another early text, *Principles and Practice of Chiropractic*, was written by the Professor of Symptomatology and Diagnosis at the National School of Chiropractic and published in 1915 (Forster 1920). Forster specifically addressed the theoretical, anatomical and physiological basis of chiropractic (pp. 6–46) and wrote in detail on the physiology and functioning of the nervous system and the manners in which it may be compromised, resulting in various clinical presentations. He thus introduced the concept that subluxation had dimensions other than just altered movement causing nerve impingement.

In 1927 the Palmer School of Chiropractic published *The Chiropractic Textbook* with a second edition some twenty years later (Stephenson 1948). Stephenson defined subluxation as 'the condition of a vertebra that has lost its proper juxtaposition with the one above, or the one below, or both; to an extent less than a luxation; and which impinges nerves and interferes with the transmission of mental impulses' (p. 320). A causative role for ligaments and muscles was identified with the concept that an abnormal disc offered 'considerable resistance to adjustment' and tended to 'misplace the vertebra again'. Further, it was stated that abnormal ligaments about the SMU 'do not assist much in keeping the vertebrae in normal position, when they are adjusted, until enough time is allowed for them to regain their normal form and texture'; and that 'the muscles are the means of subluxations occurring' (Stephenson 1948: 314–15).

The prevailing concept at the midpoint of chiropractic's first 100 years was that vertebral subluxation was a disrelationship between two adjacent vertebrae; however, it was considered that the nature of the altered relationship ranged from 'minute' (Firth 1948) to 'extreme' (Janse 1948). The need for organised research into the putative clinical entity was clear. An agenda was set to improve knowledge of postural distortions; the degree of permanency of distortions seen on X-ray; the nature of any corrective effects produced by various adjustive procedures, using before and after radiographs; and the correlation of individual and multiple distortions with change in function.

These developments occurred in the times when D.D. Palmer's charismatic son, Bartlett Joshua ('BJ') Palmer, had established himself as the chiropractic profession's most vocal spokesperson in the 1920s and 1930s. While advancements were made in understanding and developing the original concepts of Palmer, Firth and others as the profession spread around the globe, 'BJ' remained insistent there was only one constant of chiropractic philosophy. In his final volume, *Our Masterpiece*, published after his death in 1961, he maintained that 'dis-ease is only two kinds', either a decrease in the quantity of nerve flow or the inability of the body to function adequately with a decreased flow (Palmer 1966: 29). He maintained that the constant of 'chiropractic philosophy principle' was that a vertebral subluxation occluded an opening.

We now know that the neurophysiological mechanisms associated with subluxation are infinitely more sophisticated than this simplistic 'bone on nerve' belief and chiropractic has advanced well beyond that monocausal concept. The contemporary model of the subluxation complex (see Figure 7.1) grew out of the productive European school of chiropractic science (Gillet 1972; Wardwell 1992) which had re-established contact with American chiropractors following World War II. The model incorporates their mechanical view with the neurophysiological understanding of Janse (1948) and Homewood (1981) to name but two.

In the 1990s Gatterman and other participants in the Consortium for Chiropractic Research drove a consensus process designed to attain an acceptable level of agreement on subluxation terminology and usage (Gatterman 1992, 1995a, b, c; Gatterman & Hansen 1994). The outcomes encapsulated Lantz's work with the construct of the vertebral subluxation complex (VSC) (Lantz 1989) and led to the publication in 1995 of what is now accepted as the most articulate understanding of the functional spinal lesion, the VSC (Lantz 1995b).

The model depicted in Figure 7.1 has its genesis in these historical models and integrates the contemporary appreciation of the impact of biopsychosocial factors (Waddell 1998). The VSC must be considered as now being a firmly established clinical model and while many have contributed over time to the contemporary version it will continue to evolve to reflect expanding knowledge and understanding. Equally important milestones in the educational and legislative dimensions of the profession ran parallel with these developments in the clinical science and art of chiropractic. They are summarised in Table 7.1 and have underpinned the growth of chiropractic to become the third largest primary healthcare profession in the western world after medicine and dentistry (Chapman-Smith 2001a). There are now some 70 000 practitioners in the USA, 6000 in Canada, 3000 in Australia, 1600 in Britain and 100–500 in each of Belgium, Denmark, France, Italy, Japan, Norway, South Korea, Sweden, Switzerland, New Zealand, South Africa and the Netherlands (Chapman-Smith 2001a).

Table 7.1   Milestones in the history of chiropractic

Year	Milestone
1897	The Palmer School of Chiropractic, the first chiropractic educational institution, opened.
1905	Barbara Brake becomes the first chiropractor to commence practice in Australia. She was trained at the Palmer School (Peters & Chance 1996).
1913	Kansas becomes the first jurisdiction to recognise and license the practice of chiropractic.
1916	The first US-trained chiropractor commenced practice in Japan.
1923	Alberta becomes the first Canadian province to license chiropractic.
1939	The Canton of Zurich, Switzerland, becomes the first jurisdiction outside North America to license the practice of chiropractic.
1944	The Foundation for Chiropractic Education and Research (FCER) is established and becomes the profession's foremost agency for funding postgraduate scholarship and research.
1964	Western Australia becomes the first Australian state to enact chiropractic legislation.
1969	The first post-war US-trained chiropractor commenced practice in Japan.
1974	The US Council on Chiropractic Education (CCE) is recognised by the federal US government as the accrediting agency for schools of chiropractic and this leads to the development of affiliated accrediting agencies in Australia/New Zealand, Canada and Europe.
1975	Formal chiropractic education commences in Victoria, Australia, as the International College of Chiropractic. This program becomes the world's first program to be included within the government-funded tertiary education system (1981/82).
1976	Formation of the Australian Spinal Research Foundation (ASRF), a significant funding agency for chiropractic research.
1987	Final judgment in the *Wilk v. American Medical Association* case is entered and the way is opened for closer cooperation between chiropractic and medical doctors in education, research and practice.
1988	The World Federation of Chiropractic (WFC) is formed and now represents professional chiropractic associations in over 70 countries.
1993	The 'Manga Report' is published in Canada as the first government-commissioned report by health economists looking at the cost-effectiveness of chiropractic. It recommends a primary role for chiropractors with back-pain patients on the grounds of safety, cost-effectiveness and patient preference.
1994	Government-sponsored expert panels develop guidelines for the management of patients with back pain in the United States (Agency for Health Care Policy and Research) and Britain (Clinical Standards Advisory Group).
1996	US Government commences official funding support for an ongoing agenda for chiropractic research.
1997	The WFC is admitted as a non-government organisation (NGO) to the World Health Organization (WHO).
1998	The second 'Manga Report' is published and quantifies the direct annual savings which would flow from doubling the proportion of Ontario public who visit chiropractors for musculoskeletal disorders.
1999	The European Parliament accepts the 'Lannoye Report' which recommends the coordination of laws across member countries for the recognition of chiropractic and other complementary healthcare disciplines.

The General Chiropractic Council (Britain) opens its register for formal licensure of chiropractic practice, five years after the passing of *The Chiropractor's Act.*

2000   The House of Lords Select Committee on Science and Technology Report on Complementary and Alternative Medicine accepts that chiropractic is a leading discipline complementary to medicine with an important role in the British healthcare system.

2001   The Canadian government funds the first permanent Chair of Chiropractic Research through the Canadian Institute for Health Research. The Chair is at the University of Calgary.

Adapted from Chapman-Smith, D. 1998, 'Chiropractic history: the evolution to acceptance', in *The Chiropractic Report*, Toronto, with permission.

Theories of chiropractic

Palmer's founding theory of chiropractic was that the subluxated vertebra caused nerve interference, which could be corrected by using the spinous process to restore normal vertebral position. As the profession developed during its first 50 years the theories underpinning chiropractic came to revolve around the 'the supremacy of the nervous system', the 'influence of subluxation', and the 'role of spinal adjustment to correct subluxation and restore health'. In essence, these notions are reflected in the one theory that pathomechanical change in an SMU may affect related neurologic function, which in turn may be restored by correction of that change.

The anatomical, physiological, physical, clinical and neurological theories of chiropractic further developed on this foundation theory by hypothesising that subluxation led to impingement of the structures (nerves, blood vessels and lymphatics) passing through the intervertebral foramen, and that, as a result, conduction of the nerve impulses was impaired. The theories culminate with the hypothesis that such impairment results in abnormally altered innervation to certain parts of the organism so that such parts become functionally or organically diseased or predisposed to disease. The corollary is the theory that adjustment of a subluxated vertebra removes the impingement and restores normal innervation to diseased parts, thus rehabilitating them both functionally and organically (Janse *et al.* 1947).

These theories establish the science of chiropractic as being concerned with the relationship between structure, primarily the spine, and function, primarily the nervous system of the human body, as that relationship may affect the restoration and preservation of health (Vear 1981). The theories of chiropractic all revolve around the prime concept of kinematic change in the spine, usually in the smallest functioning unit, the SMU, which typically consists of an intervertebral disc and two facet joints. The reason such change is considered important is found in the chiropractic paradigm of the supremacy of the nervous system. Chiropractors maintain that homœostasis of the body is dependent on the normal function of the

Figure 7.1   A contemporary model of the vertebral subluxation complex

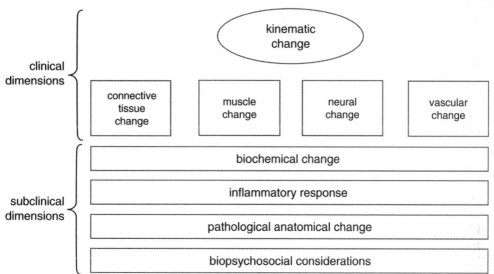

Source: Ebrall, P.S., *Assessment of the Spine* (in press).

nervous system, and herein lies the essential difference between chiropractic and other disciplines.

Orthodox western medicine attempts to replace homœostatic mechanisms through pharmacological intervention. From the eastern traditions acupuncture (see Chapter 5) restores balance between the Ying and the Yang by needling meridians and Traditional Chinese Medicine (see Chapter 4) restores balance by using herbal extracts as either pills or infusions. Among the component modalities of complementary medicine naturopaths use the least possible amount of natural intervention to have the most effect in restoring homœostasis (see Chapter 3) and homœopaths (see Chapter 11) use the law of similars to restore balance and health. Chiropractic is unique in its emphasis on the primacy of the nervous system to the homœostatic process.

Osteopathy is the closest discipline to chiropractic, being founded just a few years earlier in the same mid-western region of the USA. The British and Australian practice of osteopathy has parallels with chiropractic as it remains true to the role of manipulation in restoring and maintaining health; however, osteopathy as practised in the USA is essentially western medicine. Its practitioners are fully licensed for the use of drugs and surgery and this has significantly de-emphasised the value of manipulation (see Chapter 14 for more information on the practice of osteopathy).

The concept of kinematic change relates to the clinical fact that mechanical derangement in an SMU can generate pain. This principle is not disputed by any group of practitioners who work with the spine. Differences between groups, however, do arise when treatment for such frank pain is considered. Nerve root pain which may accompany disc protrusion is an obvious example. The surgeon may favour surgical removal of the fragments of the disc to remove the cause, while the chiropractor may favour conservative care to restore normal movement to the involved spinal level and facilitate natural healing of the disc, thus normalising the cause. There is, of course, a cross-over between the two extremes and there are times when surgery is the only option, but in the vast majority of patients with back pain, with or without disc involvement, the conservative approach is known to demonstrate excellent clinical and financial outcomes (Meade *et al.* 1990; Ebrall 1992a).

The validity of the theory of kinematic change or dyskinesia becomes increasingly important to the chiropractic paradigm as the size of the change diminishes. While the idea of early bone-setters and others was that of a 'bone out of place', the essential chiropractic paradigm arises from very small changes in functional positioning between vertebral segments. Research is now starting to show that these small changes do, in fact, cause significant and measurable outcomes (Adams & Hutton 1980; Briggs & Chandraraj 1996; Dolan & Adams 2001).

The generation of pain in cases of small kinematic change is multifactorial, ranging from irritation of tissues about the SMU by inflammatory metabolites to muscle hypertonicity arising in an attempt to guard or protect a malfunctioning SMU. While this theory has clinical plausibility and provides ample explanation for entities such as mechanical low back pain, it does not explain the myriad of clinical conditions which are empirically observed to respond to spinal adjustment. Several additional theories are useful in these cases, including dysautonomia, dysafferentation, dysponesis and diaschisis.

Dysautonomia relates to the concept that the autonomic nervous system may be affected by kinematic change in an SMU. The mechanisms postulated include bi-directional reflexes between somatic and visceral structures of the body. Ample evidence supports the theory that somatic stimulation has an identifiable and measurable effect on visceral function (Sato 1992; Budgell & Sato 1996; Budgell *et al.* 1997, 1998; Fujimoto *et al.* 1999; Budgell 2000; Budgell & Suzuki 2000; Budgell & Hirano 2001).

Dysafferentation refers to the principle that numerous centres in the brain rely on mechanoreceptive input in order to retain correct functioning (Seaman & Winterstein 1998). These centres respond to painful mechanical stimuli by varying the secretion of catecholamines and other substrates that affect cardiac output, blood pressure, insulin levels and other functions. It is theorised that mechanical changes at certain levels of the spine may have an effect on the function of specific organs through pathways mediated via the brain.

It is also possible that dysafferent input may affect the motor and pre-motor areas of the cortex, leading to a state of dysponesis manifested as inefficient movement patterns and behaviours. It is theorised that subluxation presents an imbalance of symmetry within the spine and this is reflected in mechanical changes in other parts of the body, such as altered posture (Smart & Smith 2001).

The theory of diaschisis refers to the loss of function and electrical activity caused by cerebral lesions in areas remote from the lesion but connected to it by the nervous system. This is the basis of the cerebral dysfunction theory (Terrett 1995) which relates symptoms such as visual disturbances and loss of concentration to a decrease in cerebral blood flow occurring secondary to cervical subluxation which causes vasoconstriction in the blood vessels supplying the brain (Budgell & Sato 1997).

While diaschisis helps to explain functional changes the question of pain referral from cervical structures to the head is explained by the mechanism of 'nociceptive convergence'. This mechanism leads to both a loss of somato-sensory spatial specificity (Piovesan *et al.* 2001) and the projection of pain to distant structures through second-order neurons. In the clinical situation it is appreciated that stimulation of a nerve arising from the upper segments of the spinal column (the greater occipital nerve) may induce increased excitability of the sensory nerves of the covering of the brain (Bartsch & Goadsby 2002). There seems to be a functional continuum between the nerve centres in the upper spinal cord and the nerves of the upper cervical segments which links to those nerves involved in cranial nociception. This would explain why subluxation within the cervical spine may generate pain perceived as headache by the patient. Conservative therapies such as manipulation are recommended as the treatment of choice for such headaches (Jull *et al.* 2002).

The evidence for chiropractic

During the twentieth century western medicine moved from the heroic to the informed. During the last decade of that century chiropractic started its significant shift from the believed to the known. Science has long been the driver for biomedicine; it has continually refined and developed diagnostic methods and therapeutic interventions and medicine has followed science into the new capacities created by these technologies.

On the other hand chiropractic practice has always been ahead of scientific justification and science can be considered as lagging behind the profession's theories and principles. Chiropractic has developed as an experiential profession driven by clinical results and patient satisfaction. From the time Palmer first codified his empirical experiences science has struggled to explain the clinical outcomes. This is not to say science has little to offer in explaining chiropractic. In fact more and more scientists from diverse fields are reporting findings which reflect the chiropractic paradigm.

In essence, the hypothesis that 'the structure of the spine governs the function of the body' is yet to be tested. However, the collective understanding of how the spine and its components integrate and function has accelerated over the past decade to the point where there are sufficient pieces of the puzzle to allow the development and testing of chiropractic-specific hypotheses.

Recent neurological evidence demonstrates that stimulation of nerves within the disc will elicit reactions in the multifidus and longissimus muscles (Indahl *et al*. 1997). Also, a direct relationship by autonomic nerves has been established between the receptors in ligaments about the SMU and the multifidus muscles (Solomonow *et al*. 1998). These muscles are important stabilisers of the spine and assist with position sense. The repositioning accuracy of human subjects assuming the sitting position is altered by applying vibration to the multifidus muscles to distort their proprioceptive sensors (Brumagne *et al*. 1999). Brumagne *et al*. (2000) also found this vibration induced a muscle-lengthening illusion that resulted in healthy subjects undershooting the target position.

These findings suggest an active role for paraspinal muscle spindle afferents in controlling spinal position and a sensitivity of the lumbar spine to changes in position. Further, spinal stability has been reported to decrease with fatigue (Taimela *et al*. 1999). Proprioception about the thoracolumbar spine is also altered in subjects with pain (Koumantakis *et al*. 2002). The size and direction of this repositioning error is variable and seems dependent on whether the spine is in flexion or extension (Newcomer *et al*. 2000).

Chiropractors have long argued that the correct functioning of the spine is crucial to the correct functioning of the body (health) and now there is evidence for a bi-directional flow of proprioceptive and other information among the elements of the spine including its supportive musculature. Nerves capable of monitoring proprioceptive and kinesthetic information are abundant in the disc, capsule and ligaments (Holm *et al*. 2002). The structures of the spine are well suited to monitor sensory information and control spinal muscles at each particular level. Holm *et al*. (2002) suggest they probably also provide kinesthetic perception to the sensory cortex.

Further, the spine sends information on movement and posture to the central nervous system (CNS) by taking neural signals from the ligaments of the spine into the spinal cord and on to ascending pathways and skeletomotoneurons (Sjolander *et al*. 2002). This allows continuous control of muscle activity through feed-forward, or preprogramming, mechanisms and supports the chiropractic argument that neurologic input from the spine is essential for normal health and wellbeing.

The above is just a sampling of the new information being generated by basic and clinical scientists and how this knowledge demonstrates there is substance in the theories of chiropractic. In addition, the question of chiropractic's value in health-care in terms of efficiency and cost-effectiveness has also been well demonstrated in the literature.

The cost of chiropractic management of low back pain in workers' compensation schemes is significantly less than medical management (Jarvis *et al.* 1991; Ebrall 1992a). Similar savings are evident with common musculoskeletal disorders in a general health insurance scheme (Stano 1993). It is known that chiropractic costs can be controlled (Jarvis *et al.* 1997) and its cost differential strengthened (Stano 1994). An independent Professor of Health Economics, Pran Manga, found compelling evidence that chiropractic management of patients with low back pain was significantly superior to conventional care in terms of effectiveness, safety, cost-effectiveness and patient satisfaction (Manga & Angus 1993). This came from a report that was commissioned by the Ontario Ministry of Health.

A second report by Manga (Manga & Angus 1998) argued that doubling the proportion of the Ontario public who visit chiropractors for musculoskeletal disorders from 10 per cent to 20 per cent would lead to direct annual savings of $348 million for the Ontario healthcare system, with indirect savings of some $1.85 billion per year (Chapman-Smith 1998). Other evidence-based arguments that chiropractic deserves serious considerations as a gatekeeper in public health exist in the literature (Stano & Smith 1996; Smith & Stano 1997).

Finally, the issue of the safety of the chiropractic adjustment, particularly in the cervical spine, is one which must be considered in terms of the risks and benefits to the patient. An authoritative review of the research evidence supporting behavioural and physical treatments for headache concludes 'manipulation is effective in patients with cervicogenic headache' (McCrory *et al.* 2001). A review of the literature estimates the risk to be between five and ten events per ten million manipulations (Hurwitz *et al.* 1996) and an authoritative assessment can be drawn from the records of the National Chiropractic Mutual Insurance Company, largest insurer of chiropractors in the USA. Their estimate of a serious complication such as a vertebrobasilar stroke causing permanent neurologic deficit following cervical manipulation is approximately one in two million procedures (Chapman-Smith 2001b). In medical terms this is extraordinarily low.

Cerebrovascular ischaemia following manipulation is unpredictable (Haldeman *et al.* 2002a) and random (Haldeman *et al.* 2002b) and the literature does not assist in identifying the patient at risk (Haldeman *et al.* 1999). A simple cause and effect relationship does not exist between neck manipulation and subsequent patient injury (Terrett 2002).

The internal forces sustained by the vertebral artery during skilled spinal manipulation are known to be almost an order of magnitude lower than the strains required to disrupt the artery mechanically (Symons *et al.* 2002). Chiropractors are highly skilled in the delivery of manipulation and there seems no question that the risk–benefit ratio of chiropractic spinal adjustment is acceptable (Haldeman *et al.* 2001). This is especially so in patients for whom the history and examination lead to a working diagnosis which includes cervical subluxation with or without headache.

The practice of chiropractic

Chiropractic care seeks to restore normal neurologic and physiologic function and thereby help to improve the health of the individual. The doctor of chiropractic is concerned about the 'whole person' and counsels patients in areas such as nutrition, proper exercise and diet, lifestyle changes and general health matters (Sportelli 2000). The initial consultation with a chiropractor includes an assessment of all body systems as well as the exploration of the presenting complaint. Chiropractors are trained in general diagnosis and the initial health examination may reveal underlying medical conditions such as hypertension, diabetes or unexplained weight loss which require referral to a medical practitioner for further investigation. Depending on the findings, the patient may be subsequently managed by a medical practitioner, co-managed by both the chiropractor and medical practitioner or retained for ongoing management by the chiropractor.

Studies of the chiropractic case-mix in Australia (Ebrall 1993), the USA (Hurwitz *et al.* 1998), and Europe (Hartvigsen *et al.* 2002) are remarkably similar. The findings show that the presenting complaint is back pain in about half of all new patient visits to chiropractors, with neck pain and/or headache accounting for most of the remainder. While it is apparent that the majority of patients attend with complaints of a musculoskeletal nature (Coulter *et al.* 2002), there is also a small representation of extremity pain and dysfunction and a very small percentage (less than 4 per cent) with complaints which may not be overtly musculoskeletal. The diagnostic questions therefore pursued by chiropractors are mostly those of a differential nature to ensure that the presenting complaint of the patient is indeed musculoskeletal in nature and is not an underlying problem more suited to medical or surgical intervention.

Chiropractic services are largely provided outside the state healthcare system although provisions may exist in different countries which allow patients to be funded by the state for care under various circumstances, such as for work-related injury, traffic accidents and services required by war veterans. In most countries where private health insurance schemes exist they typically include insurance tables which reimburse for chiropractic care. A number of clinics are evolving where a variety of healthcare providers join together with the chiropractor to offer a wider mix of services to the community and there are some instances of chiropractors being granted hospital privileges.

The overwhelming majority of chiropractors practice in a typical community setting, either as a sole practitioner or in association with one or more other chiropractors or related practitioners such as myotherapists. Chiropractors recognise the supportive value of specific exercises and the beneficial effects of other disciplines such as Pilates, Yoga, Alexander Technique and therapeutic massage. In the same manner in which medical practitioners may refer a patient for physiotherapy, a chiropractor may recommend the inclusion of the appropriate ancillary service in the overall management plan for an individual patient.

The chiropractic management plan takes into account the findings of the initial health examination and the specific spinal examination. The general findings provide a context for the specific spinal findings and may require changes to be made in the patient's lifestyle or work environment to maximise the benefits of the spinal treatment. During the spinal examination the chiropractor will use a variety of tests and procedures, including manual palpation, to determine the levels at which a sub-luxation complex may be suspected. In many cases the spine is X-rayed to identify the presence of any pathology or mechanical change which may preclude or modify manual intervention. The initial consultation includes a presentation of findings and a recommended management plan which typically sets out the projected frequency and duration of treatment with suggestions for supportive behaviour and therapies as needed.

The frequency and duration of care is dependent on a combination of the presenting signs and symptoms and the patient's desires and expectations. In broad terms, chiropractic management may be stratified as:

- **Type 1 care, where a precipitating or causative event can be identified, such as a fall or a lifting injury, and the presenting pain and dysfunction is associated with that event. This is an example of evidence-based care with quantifiable parameters.**
- **Type 2 care, where pain and dysfunction is present and, while no specific precipitating or causative event can be identified, the clinician is able to identify indicators for treatment. This is a transition model between evidence-based care and maintenance care.**
- **Type 3 care, where no specific precipitating or causative event can be iden-tified and the patient may not report pain or demonstrate dysfunction but the clinician is able to identify indicators for treatment. This is the essence of maintenance or supportive care and is validated when the patient returns to a state of pain and/or dysfunction in the absence of treatment.**
- **Type 4 care, where no specific precipitating or causative event can be identified and the patient does not report or demonstrate dysfunction but the clinician is able to perceive indicators for treatment. This is the essence of preventive or wellness care.**

The spine is generally very responsive to adjustment and manipulation and with Type 1 care frequently reaches an asymptomatic state after three to fifteen treatments over several weeks. After a period of Type 1 or 2 care the patient may consider Type 3 or maintenance care, which is typically ongoing over a longer period of time at an individual frequency which prevents relapse.

The most controversial aspect of chiropractic is the Type 4 or preventive care, provided in the belief it will maintain a certain level of wellness in the patient. While ample evidence exists which demonstrates the value of chiropractic in the first three types of care, the question of 'wellness', especially over a longer period of time, is much more difficult to study. In the absence of published evidence, practitioners tend to rely on marketing devices to create an awareness of this type of care and this in turn raises questions about the ethics of such practices. A governing principle of all complementary medicine particularly applies in this situation, namely that if the patient is informed and consenting and if the practitioner is licensed and competent, then the doctor–patient relationship should be a private and individual matter.

Chiropractic practitioners themselves are known to have a relatively high level of practice satisfaction (Coulter et al. 1996). Repeated surveys show that chiropractic patients also have a high level of satisfaction with the nature of the care they receive (Kassak & Sawyer 1993; Jamison 1996; Hayes & Gemmell 2001; Long & Hawk 2001; Coulter et al. 2002). This possibly reflects the humanistic and holistic attributes reported to be evident in the manner in which chiropractors interact with their patients (Gatterman 1995b, 1997).

Patient satisfaction seems to be further influenced by patients' characteristics, patients' previous experience with healthcare, patients' expectations (Sigrell 2002) and the communication of advice and information to the patient (Hertzman-Miller et al. 2002). A study of new patients with current low back pain of more than two weeks' duration found high agreement on the expectations that the chiropractor should find the problem and explain it to the patient. They also expected to be given advice about training and exercise. Most patients (80 per cent) either expected to be substantially better in one to two treatments or did not know how long it would take to get better. The majority (56 per cent) of chiropractors expected that it would take three to five chiropractic treatments before substantial improvement was felt (Sigrell 2002).

The profession of chiropractic

Chiropractic education in North America is largely delivered by private, non-profit-making institutions dependent on student tuition for funding (Coulter 1999). In contrast, the formal chiropractic programs in other countries (Australia, Brazil, Canada, Denmark, Japan, Mexico, South Africa, South Korea and Britain) are within the university system. Australia led the way when a chiropractic program established in Melbourne in 1975 became the world's first within the government-funded tertiary education sector in 1981–82 (see Table 7.1).

Common international standards of education have been achieved through a network of accrediting agencies that began with the Council on Chiropractic Education being recognised by the US Office of Education in 1974 (see Table 7.1)

(Chapman-Smith 2001a). Entrance requirements vary according to the country and it is not uncommon for commencing students to hold a previous university degree. In the USA a minimum of two years' university credits in qualifying courses is mandatory although a number of colleges require four years.

Typical chiropractic education programs range between four and five years of full-time academic study and either include extensive clinical training or are followed by postgraduate clinical placement and/or licensing exams. Government inquiries have affirmed that chiropractic undergraduate training is of equivalent standard to medical training in all pre-clinical subjects. In at least one program (University of Southern Denmark) chiropractic and medical students take the same basic science courses together for three years before entering separate streams for clinical training (Chapman-Smith 2001a).

The entry of graduates into professional practice and the related issue of licensing or registration is typically a state jurisdictional matter. Common licensing examinations are conducted in North America by the National Board of Chiropractic Examiners. In Europe the Board of Education conducts a structured twelve-month Graduate Education Program and a mandatory internship leading to assessment before registration. Licensing authorities exist in all countries where chiropractic is established and in those countries where chiropractic is developing the various professional associations are working towards this goal.

National associations of chiropractors from more than 70 countries form the voting membership of the WFC. The goals of the WFC include promoting uniform high standards of chiropractic education, research and practice; developing an informed public opinion among all peoples with respect to chiropractic; and acting with national and international organisations to provide information and other assistance in the fields of chiropractic and world health. The WFC was admitted by the World Health Organization (WHO) as a non-governmental organisation in 1997 and under this important relationship delegates have attended WHO annual meetings in Geneva and various regions of the world since 1989. Chiropractors within the WFC have met with WHO officials, national ministers of health and their senior staff members on many projects and issues of mutual interest.

The future of chiropractic

Almost every society in history has had some form of manual, spinal healthcare. Over the past century the world has seen one mode of this type of care formalised as chiropractic; however, despite its high level of public acceptance chiropractic is still limited in the proportion of the community to which it provides care. For chiropractic to expand its role as a high-touch, low-tech healthcare discipline in the western world it must seriously explore its place in the somewhat paradoxical environment of economic rationalism. On the other hand, chiropractic's low-tech approach is especially appropriate in less wealthy, developing countries.

A number of challenges lie ahead for the profession. While an expanded role for chiropractors as primary-care providers has been identified (Bowers & Mootz 1995; Hawk *et al.* 1996; Gaumer *et al.* 2001) there are barriers to achieving this. Not the least is the self-perception by a portion of the chiropractic profession that, as neuromusculoskeletal system specialists, they are either uninterested in or ill-prepared for providing primary care (Gaumer *et al.* 2002). Further, the role of a chiropractor as a health education resource for patients requires clarification and a degree of standardisation (Jamison 2002). It is known that the provision of written advice at the initial consultation to patients with back pain can be a contributory factor to better outcomes and potential health gain (Roberts *et al.* 2002).

A second challenge arises when the broad diversity in styles of chiropractic practice and utilisation (Ebrall 1992b) is taken to extremes by a small minority. Typically these practitioners claim they require a high frequency of visits over a long duration to achieve correction of an asymptomatic problem. They may or may not use a mantra of preventive chiropractic or increased chiropractic awareness and may or may not require the patient to pay a lump sum upfront for an extended period of care. This style of practice is aggressively assertive towards the patient and presumptuous that its frequent intervention will, on average, do more good than harm.

A third challenge lies in the science and politics of clinical guidelines and the need for chiropractic to be included as a stakeholder to ensure the validity of such documents. For example, a total of eleven sets of guidelines for the management of low back pain were published in North America, Europe and Australia between 1984 and 2000 (Koes *et al.* 2001). Those guidelines that were based on strong methodology and prepared by a multidisciplinary committee representing all major professional groups (including chiropractors) who treated patients with low back pain recommended skilled spinal manipulation as a modality. On the other hand, guidelines developed by committees in Australia, Germany, Israel and the Netherlands that lacked any chiropractic/osteopathic/physical therapy input did not recommend skilled spinal manipulation (Chapman-Smith 2002). In one case the national professional association itself withdrew guidelines (Lawrence 2002) it had developed through consensus methodology (Chance 1996; Ebrall 1996a, b, c). This is in stark contrast to the chiropractic profession in both the USA and Canada, which has produced clinical guidelines which are now accepted for the practice of chiropractic in those jurisdictions (Haldeman *et al.* 1992, Henderson *et al.* 1994).

Chiropractic continues to evolve as a well-accepted form of complementary medicine. Research from many disciplines is validating the theory and practice of chiropractic and is bringing spinal manipulation out of the investigative category to become one of the most studied forms of conservative treatment for spinal pain (Rosner 2002). A combination of this research and the paradigm shift in the thinking of today's healthcare consumers will continue to drive chiropractic towards fulfilment of its valuable and appropriate role in the healthcare systems of the world.

Further reading

Sportelli, L. 2000, *A Natural Method of Healthcare: An Introduction to Chiropractic*, 10th edn, Practice Makers, Palmerton PA.

Chapman-Smith, D. 2000, *The Chiropractic Profession*, NCMIC Group Inc., West Des Moines.

Coulter, I.D. 1999, *Chiropractic. A Philosophy for Alternative Health Care*, Butterworth Heinemann, Oxford.

Gatterman, M.I. (ed.) 1995, *Foundations of Chiropractic: Subluxation*, Mosby, St Louis.

Haldeman, S. (ed.) 1992, *Principles and Practice of Chiropractic*, 2nd edn, Appleton & Lange, Norwalk.

8

Counselling
Stephen Andrew

Life problems impact on all facets of an individual's 'being'. The pain of living can be felt in the body, the mind, the soul and the spirit. While counselling can assist those with pain in all four of these areas, the primary focus of counselling, or psychotherapy, is on the mind and the soul. This assistance may be offered as 'counselling' in a formal setting by a psychologist or counsellor, or less formally as 'health counselling' delivered as an adjunct or companion stream to another healing discipline. Inevitably, good health is a holistic entity and is not possible unless the 'invisibles' of existence, thoughts and feelings, are attended to. Similarly, formal counselling, without reference to the physical and the spiritual needs of the client, may be an exercise of diminished efficiency and efficacy. This chapter will consider the nature of counselling as a modality as well as its place in the broader medical community.

As with many of the other disciplines covered in this book, counselling has hosted an ongoing debate as to whether it is a science or an art. The field's founding father Sigmund Freud declared that the new discipline must embrace and adhere to the scientific paradigm (Freud 1937). The most influential post-Freudian, Carl Jung, also spoke of the scientific nature of psychological work (Jung 1966). Both men, however, worked in ways that were often outside the strictures of science. Over a century later the uncertainty continues. Present-day departments of counselling and psychology can be accommodated within schools of science or schools of humanities. Academics within these departments write papers that follow strict positivist scientific delineations but turn out graduates who routinely disavow the scientific ethic (Rowan 1992).

While the location of the field of counselling practice is uncertain, the discipline's label also lacks universal agreement. 'Counselling', 'therapy', 'psychotherapy', 'psychology', 'analysis' and (less charitably) 'head-shrinking' all vie for top definitional billing. (The words 'counselling' and 'psychotherapy' will be used interchangeably throughout this chapter.) Practitioners of counselling may be known as 'counsellors', 'therapists', 'psychotherapists', 'psychiatrists', 'advisers', 'psychologists' (of various persuasions), 'pastoral carers', 'social workers' and so on. Length and type of training for each of these disciplines vary enormously. Many health practitioners not formally trained in counselling use some of the skills and theories of psychotherapy in their work. This may be offered on a one-to-one basis between the practitioner and the client as 'health counselling', or via referral to a counsellor. Rather than looking for a static, definitional point, it is useful to view counselling as a vast, multidimensional metaphorical map. The topology includes areas both known and unexplored (but probably 'inhabited'). There is still a lot to learn about the land already charted, but perhaps infinitely more to understand in the undiscovered terrain. Some of this landscape can be seen, much of it is hidden and no vantage point reveals all there is to take in. Some observers even doubt the existence of the central feature of this map, the soul, or psyche, as there is no record of an empirical sighting. To complicate matters further, this map is 'alive', largely because it is generated by the cartographic duo of client and counsellor. In good counselling these protagonists jointly create a map of the unseen real. And while there are common, perhaps universal, features in all these maps, each is unique.

Counselling defined

Below is a compilation of possible definitions of counselling, drawn from different therapists and therapeutic orientations, across time. There is a logic and a beauty in this sometimes chaotic variety of approaches. Therapy is a creative endeavour, even at the definitional stage. The reader is invited to critically construct a personal definition.

The very act of defining psychotherapy has been judged as difficult (McLeod 1998), imprecise (Corsini 1989), disputatious (Kovel 1978) and 'misleading' (Szasz 1974: 11). Corsini asks 'What is psychotherapy?' before declaring 'Frankly, I don't know whether I can define the term' (1981: xi).

In practice, counselling takes the form of a 'deliberate . . . systematic' (Caplin 2001: 2) interaction between two or more people. It is an invention, an artificial and ritualised relationship complete with rules, expectations and ethical principles. Key components of the counselling relationship might include 'empirical investigation, reality testing and problem solving' (Beck & Weishaar 1989: 285), 'enthusiasm' (Jung 1960: 248), 'truth' (Feltham 1999: 3), 'awareness' (Latner 1976: 156), 'intimacy' (Akeret 1997: 17) and 'love' (Peck 1996: 186).

The process may aim primarily for 'change' (Geldard & Geldard 2001: 7), 'development' (Latner 1976: 154; Ivey 1988: 9), to 'manage . . . problems of living' (Egan 1998: 7), to offer 'an alternative life' (Akeret 1997: 15) or to 'realize, to understand, to see with greater clarity, deeper meaning and insight, to bring the pieces together into a comprehensible whole' (Moustakis 1967: 14). Counselling may seek to foster in the client qualities of 'eccentricity' (Hillman 1992b: 35) or 'spontaneity, release, naturalness, self-awareness, impulse awareness, gratification [and] self-choice'

(Maslow 1987: 61). It may attempt to 'activate the unconscious' (Grof 1988: 116), to make this unconscious material conscious (Freud 1926) and 'assist the counselee to find his[/her] true self, and to help him or her to have courage to be this self' (May 1989: 28).

Grof has described the vast range of psychotherapeutic ideas as a 'hopeless labyrinth of conflicting and competing systems' (1985: 138). However, it is possible to take a more positive view of this diversity. The abundance of definition reflects the richness of the field. The field, in turn, mimics the multitudinous complexity of the human beings it seeks to interact with and assist.

The act of counselling is, at bottom, a synthesis of some fundamental human activities: listening, talking and 'being there' for and with the 'other'. These activities are ageless, essential and utterly human. They coalesce and manifest as something between a dialogue and a monologue. The traditional slurry of a counselling session (problems, concerns, troubles, issues, sadness, disorientation, anxiety, confusion, grief, fear, loneliness, hate) can also carry the sought-after treasures of peace, relief, contentment, hope, joy, revelation, centredness, groundedness, inspiration, eudemonia, balance, fortitude and love. The fundamentals at work here are deeply mysterious and instinctively familiar.

Health counselling

The discipline of counselling can take on many forms. Health counselling is a subdiscipline of formal counselling. In colloquial terms it is counselling for non-counsellors: allied health professionals, teachers, social workers and clergy without formal training in psychotherapy but who are assisting people with psychological issues. Like all counselling, health counselling can be practised in increments. One may employ a technique from a particular counselling school, or embody an attitude of listening or asking questions in a way that echoes mainstream counselling practice.

In theory 'all counseling is health counseling' (Litwack *et al.* 1980: 19). In practice it differs from formal counselling in that it operates with an eye for other modalities of healing, seeks to broaden formal counselling's focus on the individual and embraces a holistic attitude that seeks to address 'emotional, intellectual, physical, social, and spiritual health' (Litwack *et al.* 1980: 19). The differences in emphasis between these two ways of working are small when compared to their similarities. Given the broad commonality between counselling and health counselling, formal counselling skills and theories can be easily incorporated into health counselling practice. The humanistic ideas of Carl Rogers (discussed in detail later in this chapter) move particularly gracefully between these two ways of counselling, partly because Rogers saw no correlation between the level of psychological training and psychotherapeutic effectiveness (Rogers 1973).

History of counselling

A brief look at the history of counselling provides more definitional clues. It is reasonable to assume that the antecedents of counselling emerged during human pre-history, alongside the rise and recognition of consciousness and the formulation of language. 'Human consciousness created objective existence and meaning' claimed Jung (1983: 285). With this separation from the subjective whole, some form of existential anxiety undoubtedly arose, which can be invoked today when one revisits the earliest myths and legends. These stories were created to reflect life's experiences and mysteries and were conveyed via spoken word. Themes and elements of uncertainty, anxiety, pain, triumph, exploration, explanation and experience inherent in these stories suggest little difference between tales told in human pre-history and those conveyed in a counsellor's consulting room. Thomas Moore declared: 'For me therapy is a deeply engaging pursuit of mystical knowledge. It requires . . . a willingness to enter into eternal mysteries described in the great myths and religious stories' (Moore 2002: 160).

In the fifth century BCE, the rise of Greek philosophy heralded a new type of human thought that questioned, conceptualised and offered answers in ways previously unknown. The nature of the universe, the world, life, death and all the perennial themes of western philosophical thought were discussed and debated. The idea of the soul, or psyche (the etymological basis of 'psychotherapy'), emerged as an entity separate from the body. A psychology, embryonic but recognisable as such today, was being outlined and contoured. 'Psychology, without the name, had become the focal point of philosophic thought' (Hearnshaw 1989: 18). The histories of psychology and philosophy continued to mirror each other until the mid-nineteenth century when psychological methodology attempted to become more scientific (Heil 1995).

Counselling in theory

There is no 'theory' of counselling, instead literally hundreds of 'theories'. These theories reside in a multitude of schools or orientations, are informed by various philosophies and ideologies, encapsulate differing skills and techniques and are promulgated by languages that sometimes approximate regional dialects. The adherents of each school passionately declare their theory's superiority over rival schools. While no theory works for all clients and all situations, most have something profound to say about the human condition. Against this background one can appreciate the comparisons made between psychotherapy and religion (Ouspensky 1978; West 2000).

No one is sure exactly how many psychotherapeutic approaches exist. Snyder *et al.* (2000) believe that there are more than 500 differing approaches. Spinelli

(1999) suggests over 400 varieties while Feltham (1999) offers up a similar number. Corsini (1981) lists over 240 different types of counselling, thirteen of which are considered major (Corsini & Wedding 1989). What these figures hide is the further diversity existing in practice as few practitioners could be classed as theoretical 'purists'. In addition, the personalities of clients and their presenting issues mirror the range inherent in humanity. Good counsellors respond to these differences and alter their practice accordingly. Many counsellors label themselves as eclectic therapists, constructing individual theoretical systems out of pieces of different theories (Norcross 1986).

If one were to view the range of diverse orientations from an elevated position, the differences in detail would appear to coalesce into three major schools of thought: the psychoanalytic/psychodynamic, cognitive-behavioural and humanistic approaches. Known respectively as the first, second and third forces in psychotherapy, these three genres cover much of the counselling landscape, incorporating many of the approaches alluded to above. Each of these main theories will be addressed in turn.

Psychoanalytic/psychodynamic therapy

Sigmund Freud, founder of the psychodynamic orientation and inventor of psychoanalysis, is the father (and father figure) of modern counselling. Freud was a pioneer without peer. He is one of a small number of psychotherapists whose reach extends into the general community. He saw his own impact on society on a par with that of Copernicus and Darwin (Freud 1916–17). He introduced into everyday parlance concepts like ego, id and super-ego, childhood psycho-sexual stages, dream analysis, Freudian slip, introspection, the pleasure principle, the death instinct, penis envy, Oedipus complex, projection, repression and sublimation. His belief that personalities and behaviours are largely driven by unconscious energies continues to shock and outrage the general populous. He remains a controversial, unnerving and much talked about figure. 'It is a shattering experience for anyone seriously committed to the Western traditions of morality and rationality to take a steadfast, unflinching look at what Freud has to say' (Brown 1970: 11).

While his general historical impact is huge, Freud's imprint on psychological thought and practice is also enormous. There resides in most counselling his idea that unseen or unconscious forces affect our happiness and wellbeing. That these forces have their roots in our childhood is another idea received from Freud. The name of his invention, 'psychoanalysis', reflects the need to look closely at the invisible forces of the psyche if we are to live well. Freud saw the mind as a battleground where the primitive, animalistic urges of the id are pitched against the moralistic and punitive power of the super-ego, with the ego desperately mediating between these two forces and the demands of the outside world. This quarrelsome *ménage à trois* resides within the self and causes its greatest problems when interacting with other humans also carrying similar psychical structures. All this is made even more tumultuous by the unknown or unconscious nature of this turmoil. Psychoanalytic counselling attempts to reduce the effects of this battle by bringing this unconscious material into awareness (Freud 1926).

According to psychoanalytic theory, intrapsychic conflicts are fuelled by childhood events. These early experiences are often linked to infantile sexual desires. Freud caused public and professional outrage with his observations that 'sexuality' encompassed experiences beyond that of genital pleasure to include bodily sensations in general and the emotions of love (Freud 1986). Criticism escalated to almost hysterical dimensions when Freud posited that these libidinal energies were present in children (Gay 1998). The instinctual desire to express these energies (focused sequentially around the oral, anal and phallic areas) and the corresponding oppositional demands (both internal and external) lead to these feelings being repressed. These unconscious 'id energies' would later reassert themselves over the ego in a variety of painful, maladaptive ways.

'It is easy now to describe our therapeutic aim,' said Freud. 'We try to restore the ego, to free it from its restrictions, and give it back the command over the id which it has lost owing to its early repressions' (Freud 1926: 205). Psychoanalytic therapy increases both the awareness of one's inner emotional turmoil and the ability to work with this conflict in a rational manner. The process is often long, requiring catharsis, a form of highly charged emotional release. Psychoanalysis employs various techniques to aid in the healing process such as introspection, free association (saying whatever comes into your mind), dream and fantasy analysis and interpretation. During therapy the counsellor also watches the relationship closely looking for resistance to the process and interpersonal dynamics between the therapist and client (transference), believing that occurrences in the therapeutic hour mimic the client's interactions with the world.

Freud's charismatic brilliance drew many great minds toward him. Carl Jung was the most prominent of the theorists to be invested into and then later exiled from Freud's inner circle. Jung expanded Freud's levels of consciousness to include a social or collective unconscious and introduced the idea of archetypal forces operating within the psyche (Jung 1934/1954). His influence in the practice of counselling today can be seen in the return to favour of spirituality in counselling (ridiculed and banished by Freud) and the use of notions of typological biases (introvert/ extrovert/feeling/sensing) (Jung 1921). Jung was probably the first western psychotherapist to recognise the richness that eastern philosophy could bring to counselling (Jung 1949). Other important analytic or 'post-Freudian' figures include Alfred Adler, Karen Horney, Anna Freud, Melanie Klein, Otto Rank, Sandor Ferenczi and Wilhelm Reich (Brown 1979). Present-day practitioners continue to reinterpret and modify the writings and practices of Freud and his followers.

Much of the controversy that surrounded Freud continues today, more than 60 years after his death. He attracts believers and defilers of equal passion and conviction. Prominent critics such as Masson (1988) and Szasz (1977), both originally trained in psychoanalysis, demonstrate a curious modern-day repetition of earlier post-Freudian dissent. Feminists (Maguire 1995; Worell & Remer 2003) have been critical of Freud's view of women ('a dark continent', Freud 1926: 212), while others have been offended by his pessimism. Statements like '[t]he aim of all life is death' (Freud 1920: 246) and '[a]ccording to Freud, the history of man is the history of his repression' (Marcuse 1974: 11) are examples of this attitude.

Cognitive-behavioural therapy

Of all those disagreeing with Freud, one man's dissent was powerful enough to bring about the first radical directional shift in the history of modern counselling. J.B. Watson, the founder of behaviourism, instigated the movement that was to become cognitive-behavioural psychotherapy. Watson criticised as unscientific the technique known as introspection, a central pillar of the psychoanalytic edifice. In 1913 he declared: 'Psychology as a behaviorist views it is a purely objective, experimental branch of natural science. Its theoretical goal is the prediction and control of behavior' (cited in Hearnshaw 1989: 216).

This attitude was passionately embraced by Watson's successor and behaviourism's most well-known figure, Burrhus Frederick (B.F.) Skinner. 'We can [read 'must'] follow the path taken by physics and biology by turning directly to the relation between behavior and the environment and neglecting supposed mediating states of mind' wrote Skinner (1976: 20). Here was an explicit rejection of the influence of the unconscious, one of the key platforms of psychoanalytic thought.

Behaviourism examines disturbances between an individual and the surrounding environment. It deals only in 'observables'—behaviours, stimuli and responses—discarding personal and social history. Instead focus was placed on what Skinner called a 'technology of behaviour' (Skinner 1976: 16). The way through one's problems was not via psychoanalytic introspection and catharsis, but through careful observation and clear, intelligent, rational thought.

Behaviourism focuses on learning and learning theory. To radical behaviourists very little of an individual is innate; most is a product of the environment. Behaviourists certainly accept that one can experience internal conflict but make clear that this conflict is learned (Nye 1992). It follows that changing the learning environment is the best way of facilitating change in an individual.

Skinner's enormous contributions to psychotherapy have been reworked and advanced in the cognitive-behavioural therapies developed by Aaron Beck, Albert Ellis and others. Beck's cognitive therapy reinstated the 'invisibles' (in this case, thoughts) into therapy via an understanding that cognitions can affect feelings and behaviours (Beck & Weishaar 1989). Ellis, who founded Rational-Emotive Therapy (RET), believed the attitude taken to one's life largely determines the level of emotional wellbeing. Put directly he claims, 'When you are neurotic, you almost always make yourself that way with illogical and unrealistic thinking' (Ellis 1995: 23). RET seeks to discover, challenge and uproot the irrational thinking that leads to unhappiness.

Like psychoanalysis, cognitive-behavioural therapy has its share of critics. The criticisms of the early behaviourists can still be applied to some modern cognitive-behavioural treatments, in particular the orientation's focus and emphasis on objectivity, thinking and rationality. It is not so much the embracing of these ideas that is potentially problematic but the exclusion of healthy subjectivity, feeling and arationality that limits this orientation.

Humanistic therapy

Just as the impetus to create cognitive behavioural-oriented therapy came from a backlash against the standard (psychodynamic) treatment of the day, so the humanistic orientation in psychotherapy was also founded on a reaction. Humanists felt that the psychotherapy Freud founded was too pessimistic and that behaviourism's rigid scientism omitted too much that was vital to the human condition. Key early figure Abraham Maslow wanted psychotherapy to move away from the 'analytic–dissecting–atomistic–Newtonian approach of the behaviorisms and of Freudian psychoanalysis' (Maslow 1987: xvii) and towards a more holistic therapy. Rather than being consumed by intrapsychic warfare, or dominated by irrational thinking, he saw the human being as an organism that was striving towards optimum potential. Rather than being chased and harassed by demons, humans are seen as naturally moving towards a superior self. The presence of neurosis was seen as a symptom of a failure to actualise as a human organism (Maslow 1978). This actualising tendency is the 'foundational premise on which humanistic therapies are built' (Cain 2002: 6).

Carl Rogers, a major figure in humanistic psychotherapy and founder of person-centred counselling, embraced this idea of actualisation. This natural, organic process could, he believed, be limited or derailed by any number of disruptive processes. The correct therapeutic response was to trust that the energy or drive towards self-actualisation was still present in the client, and encourage this to re-emerge via a particular sort of psychotherapeutic relationship (Rogers 1962). This relationship, nurtured by the counsellor, has three core conditions: empathic understanding, unconditional positive regard (or respect for the client) and congruence or genuineness on the part of the counsellor (Rogers 1980). Rogers claimed the presence of these three conditions were 'necessary and sufficient' to bring about change within the therapeutic relationship (Rogers 1957). He did not interpret, offer advice, challenge 'irrational' belief systems, inquire at length about family relational dynamics or discuss behavioural responses to stimuli. He listened, sought to understand the experiential world of the client and reflect back that understanding. If the counsellor facilitates the core conditions in a counselling relationship and the client is able to experience these qualities in relation to him/herself, then Rogers believed 'change and constructive personality development will *invariably* occur' (1982: 35).

Rogers's idea of therapy has an almost infinite theoretical depth, a fact sometimes obscured by the exquisite simplicity of the structure of the three core conditions. It might sound easy to offer one's client respect and understanding while being genuine in the role of counsellor but there is often some chafing between these conditions in practice. To ensure the emergence of these conditions in the therapeutic relationship, Rogers spoke of a need for the counsellor to 'embody' rather than simply know of these qualities. He spoke of the counsellor necessarily embracing an empathic 'way of being' (Rogers 1980: 137) so as to see the client as a 'person who is in the process of *becoming*' (Rogers 1958: 123). His idea was as profound as it was simple: 'I should expect that in those moments when real change occurred, that it would be because there had been a real meeting of persons in which it was experienced the same from both sides' (Rogers 1960: 53). Person-centred counselling will be addressed further below.

The main criticism of person-centred therapy is that it is not 'enough'. It is not scientific enough say some academics, not directive enough claim the behaviourists and not deep enough protest the psychoanalysts. A more general criticism is that while the three core conditions might be necessary, it can be argued that they fall short of being sufficient for therapeutic change.

Counselling in practice

Counselling can be practised whenever there are discomforting behaviours, ruffled souls or confused minds. The process, regardless of orientation, involves an opening up, an exploration, a questioning of the mystery that surrounds the client's main issue(s). Working with and within this mystery, exploring the who, what, when, where, how and why of the individual's emotional, cognitive, behavioural, spiritual and psychological responses is the purpose of the practice of psychotherapy. This work, unusual in its depth and focus, has the potential to be intimate, challenging and life changing.

Efficacious counselling always operates holistically. Hence, counselling practice (whether formal or informal) must incorporate an awareness of the totality of the client. This entails the practitioner knowing when they are capable of applying the necessary treatments and when it is necessary to work collaboratively with other health professionals. To work otherwise risks severely limiting the effectiveness of treatment and delaying recovery. Tacit or ignorant support of the Cartesian severance of mind and body, as is common in the orthodox biomedical approach to health, may even prolong the symptoms carried by clients. In other words, 'non-psychological' factors can influence the psyche and vice versa. Addressing either element in isolation will limit the ultimate efficacy of treatment.

The emotional and psychological health or all-round 'wellness' of a client may be related to breath, the senses, nutrition and diet, physical movement and exercise, thought patterns, work and play, sex, relationships with others, spiritual practice and the ability to fashion meaning out of existence (Travis & Ryan 1988). A counsellor not only needs to be cognisant of this list, but must hold an awareness of the interplay between our experiences, feelings and body chemistry (Juhan 1987).

Depression, for example, is an experience that demands a holistic response. 'Depression' is a psychological label, and it is accepted that psychotherapy can be an effective treatment. However, depression manifests in many forms and on many levels and can impact on the behavioural, cognitive, attitudinal, affective and somatic (physical) lives of a client (Gotlib & Colby 1987). Treatments for depression vary as widely as the locations of the symptoms and include herbal medicine (Astin 1998), antidepressent drugs (Therapeutic Guidelines Limited 2000), electroconvulsive therapy (Nolen-Hoeksema 2004), homœopathics (Kent 2000), aromatherapy (Worwood 1996), Ayurvedic medicine (Heyn 1987), Bach Flower Remedies (Bach & Wheeler 1979) and exercise (Milkman & Sunderwirth 1993). Note that none of the modalities on this incomplete list are 'psychological', yet all lay claim to assisting in remedying this 'psychological' malaise. Indeed most, if not all, contributors to this book would have treated clients with depression using their particular area of expertise as a primary modality. As all psychological problems impact on areas outside the psyche, holistic practice is essential. A counsellor cannot work in isolation and must be mindful of the personal and medical milieux in which the client exists.

The counselling relationship

Sitting deep within all psychotherapeutic paradigms is an embedded imperative to establish a relationship of difference with the client. This means that the counsellor must be significantly different from parents, partners, friends or workmates so as to be able to view the client from a unique perspective. Some of this difference resides in the necessarily artificial structure of the counselling process. Here the counsellor and the client meet in the same physical space, often at a regular time and day. The dialogue is largely mono-directional, with the client presenting with a 'problem' or 'issue' that they wish to discuss. The counsellor will often charge money for the time spent with the client. The counsellor is bound to hold the contents of each session confidential, while the client can relay any part of the session to whomever they please. The counsellor is bound by a statute of ethical directives aimed at preventing the therapeutic relationship becoming any other sort of relationship (e.g. sexual, platonic) deemed to be harmful to the client. The client is aware of at least some of these structural boundaries which are aimed at providing a unique field or space for the client to explore difficult aspects of their life confidently. While there is difference in the detail, much of the spirit of the above description holds true in informal counselling conducted by health professionals other than 'counsellors' or psychotherapists.

This section will focus on the practice of counselling from Rogers's person-centred point of view for the following reasons:

- **its structural and theoretical simplicity;**
- **its suitability as a stand-alone orientation or as a basis for use with other techniques;**
- **its proximity to the common psychotherapeutic components deemed to be of greatest help to clients (Hubble *et al.* 2000);**
- **its wide applicability outside of traditional counselling-type relationships (Kirschenbaum & Henderson 1989);**
- **its appropriateness to a general healthcare context; and**
- **its holistic values.**

As a prelude to a discussion of person-centred practice, it is helpful to look briefly at the application of microskills before discussing the core conditions for client change. Microskills are the nuts and bolts of therapy, the things that are likely to be found naturally in a good quality conversation and in all types of high-quality healthcare. Appropriate eye contact, comfortable proximity to the other and minimal encouragers (nods, hmms and I see's) are examples of these techniques (Ivey 1988; Egan 1998). The most important of these skills are those of attending and listening.

Attending and listening

Before the core conditions of empathy, respect and congruence can be offered to the client, the counsellor must embody what Egan describes as a 'certain intensity of presence' (1998: 62). To be present and attend to another in this way one must be as 'awake' and 'aware' as possible. The active nature of this sort of attending echoes the etymology of the Latin root *attendere* meaning 'stretch to' (Barnhart 1995). Note too that 'attendant' is the original meaning of 'therapist' (Spinelli 1997).

The etymology of the word 'listen' is also instructive. 'List' has a number of modern meanings including a series of names, the border of a cloth, to lean or incline and a shared linguistic origin with the word 'lust' (*lystan*) (Barnhart 1995). Good listening and good lusting both demand an enormous amount of attention and attending. Compare the 'lean' of listening to the 'stretch to' of attending.

In counselling, hearing is passive whereas listening is active. 'This listening,' claims Kopp, 'is that which will facilitate the patient's telling of his tale, the telling that can set him free' (1976: 5).

What the counsellor hears when listening are words, the lapis, the core, the base material of psychotherapy. Words, spoken and heard, are the counsellor's primary medium when working toward positive therapeutic results (Andrew 2000). Freud recognised that words held 'a magical power' (1916–17: 17). In a therapeutic situation words are quintessential in that the 'soul can be made up on the spot simply through speech' (Hillman 1992a: 217). This is a vital statement. It is too often forgotten that the 'psyche' part of the word psychology is drawn from the ancient Greek word for the soul. Etymologically, psychology is the study of the human soul (Barnhart 1995). If Hillman is right then it is spoken words (rather than dreams as Freud suggested) that form the royal road to the soul, the 'omphalos', or core, of psychology.

Words are not all a counsellor 'listens' for, however. Audible utterances are always combined with silent, non-verbal information (bodily behaviour, facial expressions, somatic responses, physical characteristics and appearance). Sometimes these two streams of information contradict each other. This potential complexity is heightened by the fact that everything the client is expressing emanates from a variety of contexts. These might be social, cultural, gender based, sexual, temporal, economic and political contexts. The counsellor also communicates in verbal and non-verbal ways and from their own collection of contexts. Somehow, from within this semantic soup, human understanding and meaning must emerge.

Underpinning person-centred therapy is a basis of trust in what Rogers calls the 'exquisitely rational' nature of human beings (Raskin & Rogers 1989: 163). From a person-centred orientation humans are fundamentally good and capable of discovering and implementing high-quality solutions to life's concerns. This positive view of human nature has at its core a direction and goal-state called self-actualisation. Rogers believes that humans naturally wish to move towards this state, enticingly described by Maslow as a time or situation where one is 'more integrated . . . more open to experience, more idiosyncratic, more perfectly expressive or spontaneous . . . more creative, more humorous . . . closer to the core of his Being, [and] more fully human' (Maslow 1968: 97). To Rogers (1962) the key to this movement in therapy is a strong relationship between client and therapist. It is here, in this relational space, that healing occurs and *not* in the ideas, directions and interpretations of the 'expert' therapist. When counselling isn't working its failure can often be traced to problems within the therapeutic relationship. This relationship is characterised by three necessary and sufficient conditions of change: empathy, unconditional positive regard and congruence. The counsellor brings these conditions to life in the therapeutic relationship via the attitudes they hold toward the client.

Empathy

Empathy comes from the Greek *pathos*, or suffering, via the German *einfühlung*, which suggests 'in-feeling' (Barnhart 1995). It is related to but different from sympathy, which signifies 'with-feeling'. It has been described as the key to the counselling process 'in which one person so feels into the other as to temporarily lose his or her identity. It is in this profound and somewhat mysterious process of empathy that understanding, influence and the other significant relations between persons take place' (May 1989: 62).

There are two types of empathy, one organic, natural and perhaps innate. The other is the skill of empathy that can be taught and employed in a counselling setting. Both are valuable and have many similarities. Both aim at understanding.

Organic empathy is an innate quality that many counsellors have to some extent. Its presence can be demonstrated by a tendency for others to be drawn to you to talk informally about their problems. The *skill* of empathy 'is not something one is "born with"; rather, it can be learned' (Rogers 1980: 150). It can improve and deepen organic empathy. Both forms of empathy require a keen ear and eye, patience, imagination and the ability to synthesise, reflect on and respond to the content and process of a counselling session.

This 'vicarious introspection' (Kohut, cited in Lee and Martin 1991: 106) is an:

active, immediate, continuous process . . . [in which] the counselor makes a maximum effort to get under the skin of the client, to get within and to *live* the attitudes expressed instead of observing them, to catch every nuance of their changing nature, to absorb him- or herself completely in the attitudes of the other (Rogers 1989: 171).

Empathy is more than understanding alone. A counsellor attending to and listening to a client may understand something of the client's situation. This understanding only becomes empathic understanding when this is directly communicated to the client and when the client receives and acknowledges this communication. Rogers considered empathy as an expression of therapeutic 'relatedness' (Neville 1989: 84). Empathy is often difficult to achieve because underpinning this way of being are qualities such as respect and warmth for the client, concreteness, immediacy, imagination and authenticity.

High-quality empathic understanding is as desired as it is rare. For an individual to be attended to, to be listened to and to have their situation understood on a deep level is profoundly healing. Barrett-Lennard observed that:

the experience of being literally heard and understood deeply, in some personally vital sphere, has its own kind of impact—whether of relief, of something at last making sense, a feeling of inner connection or somehow being less alone, or of some other easing or enhancing quality (Barrett-Lennard 1993: 6).

Unconditional positive regard

The second of Rogers's core conditions is unconditional positive regard, also known as respect, warmth, acceptance, non-possessive caring, prizing and love.

> When the therapist is experiencing a positive, nonjudgmental, acceptant attitude toward whatever the client is at that moment, therapeutic movement or change is more likely. It involves the therapist's willingness for the client to *be* whatever immediate feeling is going on—confusion, resentment, fear, anger, courage, love, or pride . . . When the therapist prizes the client in a total rather than a conditional way, forward movement is likely (Rogers 1986: 198).

Most respect or regard in life is conditional. Love and care are offered under the proviso that certain criteria are accepted, met and adhered to. In short, 'I love you (conditions apply)'. The practice of person-centred therapy aims to create an exception to this situation. The level of unconditional positive regard one is able to offer is largely a reflection of one's personal level of self-regard, self-knowledge, self-acceptance, self-forgiveness and self-love.

Reflecting on his life, Rogers spoke of the effect of replacing a judgemental attitude with one of acceptance. 'I have found it of enormous value when I can permit myself to understand another person' (Rogers 1982: 18). The words 'permit myself to understand' suggest a move away from the safety of habitual judgement or evaluation. One of the reasons we judge in this way is because understanding is risky: 'If I let myself really understand another person, I might be changed by that understanding. And we all fear change' (Rogers 1982: 18). Acceptance spans the positive as well as the negative, differences as well as similarities: '. . . when I can accept another person, which means specifically accepting the feelings and attitudes and beliefs that he [or she] has as a real and vital part of him [or her], then I am assisting him [or her] to become a person . . .' (Rogers 1982: 21).

How far we as a society have to go before we fully embrace unconditional positive regard can be ascertained by a cursory glance through a daily newspaper. Usually the press reports a wide range of stories about misunderstandings, prejudice (subtle and explicit) and adversarial conduct. The news is a chronicle of social disrespect. An attitude of unconditional positive regard in therapy offers both an antithetical position to this human infighting and a fundamentally different way of being with another. As a client, one has no need to defend, justify or advocate one's position or situation. In the freedom of this unconditional expanse one can move, organically, towards actualisation.

Congruence

Congruence, the third of Rogers's core conditions for change, is also known as genuineness or 'realness' (Rogers 1980). It reflects the correspondence between and alignment of the counsellor's thoughts, feelings and behaviours. It involves being there for the client as 'you' within the role of counsellor, rather than being there for the client 'as' the role of counsellor. Congruence is a manifestation of unconditional positive regard for oneself.

Rogers and Sanford regarded congruence as 'the most basic of the attitudinal conditions that foster therapeutic growth . . . [T]he therapist is transparent to the client, openly being the feelings and attitudes that at that moment are flowing within [him or] her' (1989: 1490). This does not mean that the therapist shares their own problems or random thoughts.

> It does mean, however, that the therapist does not deny [himself or] herself the feelings being experienced and that the therapist is willing to express and to *be* any persistent feelings that exist in the relationship. It means avoiding the temptation to hide behind the mask of professionalism . . . (Rogers & Sanford 1989: 1491).

The 'mask' that Rogers warns us about can be seen upon the face of the distant, authoritarian, white-coated expert often found in orthodox medical settings.

Rogers claimed that '[I]n my relationships with persons I have found that it does not help, in the long run, to act as though I am something that I am not' (1982: 16). Nor, he added, has it been helpful '. . . to act in one way on the surface when I am experiencing something quite different underneath' (Rogers 1982: 17). Choosing to be oneself is 'the deepest responsibility' one can assume (Rogers 1982: 110).

Like empathy and unconditional positive regard, congruence in its crystalline form is almost impossible to find. It seems to involve the major life tasks of discovering who you are, accepting yourself and then allowing that acceptance of self to express itself openly in the world. It is not purity that is demanded here, however, rather a movement towards the best human attempt possible to be real, respectful and understanding.

These core conditions are profound teachings and like many such teachings they appear to be simple. On the level of cognitive comprehension they probably are. Activating and practising these conditions in action, in real life, in a relationship with oneself and others, is endlessly complex and difficult. As these ideas interact with each other in therapy, one discovers new depths, contradictions, paradoxes, problems and strengths between them. Each counsellor or health practitioner must work with these ideas with the aim of finding, defining and redefining a personal meaning for each one of these conditions.

In the end it is not microskills, models, theories, core conditions and techniques that make therapeutic practice successful. People, engaged, present and committed, make therapy work. 'Psychotherapy,' said Frankl, 'is more than mere technique in that it is art, and it goes beyond pure science in that it is wisdom. But even wisdom is not the last word . . . Wisdom is lacking without the human touch' (1970: 7, 8).

The evidence

Does psychotherapy work? This broad and generic question is one of the few in counselling that is easy to answer. Yes, it does work: 'psychotherapies, in general, have positive effects' (Lambert *et al.* 1986: 157). This position has been supported by a variety of research designs including single-subject case studies (Yalom 1974; Wedding & Corsini 1989), analysis of the process of the therapy session (Rogers 1942) and meta-analysis and reviews of outcome studies (Lambert *et al.* 1986).

While there is broad agreement among academics and practitioners that counselling in general is effective, this congeniality does not extend to discussions about the efficacy of specific counselling approaches. Echoing the bifurcations that have seen psychotherapy split and resplit into often opposing groupings, research into therapeutic effectiveness has also fallen into factional infighting over what works in therapy. A noisy 'psycho-barracking' has broken out between different orientations, each proclaiming ascendancy and efficacy over the 'opposition's' style of therapy. Psychoanalysts are labelled cold, inefficient and ineffective, behaviourists are called heartless, Orwellian, environmental manipulators, while the humanists are derided as being touchy-feely, unscientific, bleeding hearts. These claims are usually made with more emotional intensity that intellectual rigour.

This inter-orientational antagonism started at the beginning of modern psychology when the first dissenting psychoanalyst parted company with Freud. While rancour still exists, both in the field and in academic writing, recent research has pointed to a way of determining the effectiveness of therapy while bypassing the often petty scraps and arguments of the different theoretical schools. Drawing on earlier research that found no significant difference in the effectiveness of different types of therapy (Luborsky *et al.* 1975; Frank 1977; Lambert *et al.* 1986), a small number of cross-orientational elements or conditions integral to effective counselling practice have emerged. Looking across the vast range of psychotherapeutic orientations, researchers have discovered four conditions or 'common factors' that have been found most directly to influence client change (Hubble *et al.* 2000). To the surprise of many practitioners, the most influential change factor in this quartet was the client and their everyday environment: 'the active efforts of clients are responsible for making psychotherapy work' (Bohart & Tallman 1999: xi). This factor explained 40 per cent of the variance of client change. Researchers found that a strong and respectful client–counsellor relationship was the next most potent portent of change, accounting for 30 per cent of change variance (Miller *et al.* 1997). The client's sense of hope for the future and a belief in the therapeutic process accounted for 15 per cent of change variance, while the final 15 per cent reflected the therapist's theoretical orientation. These researchers stressed that one particular brand or flavour of therapy is not fundamentally superior to any other.

When clients are asked what constitutes effective counselling, their responses reverberate with a fundamental humanity. Drawing on client-generated data, Spinelli (1999) condenses the components of effective psychotherapy down to a very simple, almost atheoretical, tri-pointed equation: the client wants to speak, the client wants what is said to be heard and the client wants the listener to be as human as possible. There are echoes here of Howe's (1993) findings that clients want their counsellors to accept them, understand them and engage in dialogue with them. The elements of effective counselling can also be found in good conversation and strong relationships. It is simple, clear, fundamental and elegant and a powerful human-to-human exchange.

How does one know when counselling is working? This is often difficult for a counsellor to know. Even if clear goals are set, remain relevant through the course of counselling and are largely achieved, a counsellor cannot know if old, dysfunctional patterns might re-emerge after the final session. For a client, success is often easier to gauge. The answer has a visceral origin: one simply knows if life is, or seems to be, better. Perhaps the truest test of therapeutic effectiveness is a never-ending research project run informally, constantly and daily in thousands of consulting rooms around the world. Does psychotherapy work? Ask a client.

The future

What is the future of counselling practice? Undoubtedly, the form of counselling is changing. Psychotherapy is being practised increasingly outside of the psychiatrists' and psychologists' consulting rooms. Health professionals both within and outside the medical mainstream are recognising the power of counselling and are incorporating psychological skills into their practice. Training in counselling skills is being broadened into the mainstream medical and complementary therapies as links between mind and body are being more seriously and widely recognised. Postgraduate courses in counselling that bypass the traditional requirement for an undergraduate degree in psychology are growing in popularity. Additionally, 'integrated practice' is becoming an increasingly common way of working. An integrated practice will feature practitioners of different modalities working together, allowing a practitioner in a non-counselling field to work (via active referrals, case management and direct consultation) with a trained counsellor.

A similar softening of traditional boundaries can be seen in the research literature which reports a mixing together and a possible rapprochement between formerly antagonistic schools within the field of counselling (Norcross 1986). As these rivalries are being reconciled, earlier, pre-scientific material is being returned to and re-evaluated. The work of Hillman (1991) and Moore (1994) is important and influential in this regard. Both men have worked hard to resuscitate and reinstate 'soul' or psyche in psychology and to present these ideas beyond academia. In parallel, the idea of 'spirit' has found its return to counselling via transpersonal psychology (sometimes referred to as the fourth force in counselling). Therapists like Wilber (1993, 1997, 2000) and Grof (1985) have combined post-positivist science, mythology and studies into altered states of consciousness to offer a truly radical restructure of psychotherapeutic reality. As the soul and spirit have long been neglected, so the body has been ignored in most psychotherapies. The work of Kurtz (1990) and Murphy (1992) among others is seeking to right this neglect. The body is also part of Hellinger's (1989) revitalised and radicalised family therapy, which has its origins in an eclectic collection of recent and ancient practices. Similarly, the practical value of psychology's estranged antecedent, philosophy, is being rediscovered by philosophical counsellors who are finding that thousand-year-old truths can assist clients (de Botton 2000; Marinoff 2000). Cognitive therapists are also using fundamental truths in their efforts to empower their clients by instructing them in assertive behaviour (Smith 1988) and in so doing repoliticising the client within the therapeutic process.

A different sort of politics continues to be the major factor in inhibiting change to counselling practice. The 'art versus science' debate continues to inhibit researchers and distract practitioners. While many academics stress the necessity of viewing psychotherapy scientifically (Nathan & Gorman 1998), researchers and writers such as Grof speak of the 'deep crisis' facing psychology due to its adherence to an old scientific paradigm: 'The world view long outdated in modern physics continues to be considered scientific in many other fields [like psychology], to the detriment of future progress' (1985: 17,18). Perhaps this perennial debate needs also to broaden its scope to encompass 'art', 'science' and other ways of viewing the world, perhaps under an umbrella of 'rigour' (rather than dogma) in thought, feeling and practice. One senses the need for psychotherapy to complete the journey through its adolescence and embrace a more mature position. The idea that counselling can genuinely assist individuals and societies is understood. The need to apply this understanding and fulfil its potential has never been greater.

Conclusion

Some aspects of psychotherapy exist independently of time. Writing almost a century ago, in an essay entitled 'New paths in psychology', Carl Jung wrote:

anyone who wants to know the human psyche will learn next to nothing from experimental psychology. He would be better advised to abandon exact science, put away his scholar's gown, bid farewell to his study, and wander with human heart through the world. There, in the horrors of prisons, lunatic asylums and hospitals, in drab suburban pubs, in brothels and gambling-hells, in the salons of the elegant, the Stock Exchanges, Socialist meetings, churches, revivalist gatherings, and ecstatic sects, through love and hate, through the experience of passion in every form in his own body, he would reap richer stores of knowledge than text-books a foot thick could give him, and he will know how to doctor the sick with real knowledge of the human soul. He may be pardoned if his respect for the so-called cornerstones of experimental psychology is no longer excessive. For between what science calls psychology and what the practical needs of everyday life demand from psychology there is a great gulf fixed (Jung 1916: 246–7).

The chasm that Jung identified between counselling theory and daily existence is beginning to close. This chapter has looked at some of the ideas and practices that have made counselling more accessible and helpful to those who seek its benefits. Counselling has become a vital component in holistic healthcare. It has a long history of assisting people whose minds and souls are troubled by inner and outer turmoil. It is a pre-historical form of healing brought into modern western thought by Sigmund Freud and his writings on the unconscious.

Throughout the last century behaviourists, humanists and others have continued the exploration of psychological ideas and counselling practice, broadening and enriching our understanding of the psyche. While countless forms, styles and methods exist, research into the effectiveness of counselling has shown that a number of fundamental, relational factors, particularly the client–practitioner interaction, form the basis of positive psychotherapeutic assistance. For this reason this chapter has focused on the practical application of relationship-based, humanistic, person-centred counselling practice in both formal and informal settings. Special attention has been paid to the core principles of empathic understanding, genuineness in the practitioner and respect and acceptance of the client. Running parallel to these ideas has been the application of counselling theory in allied health and other helping professions, areas that had previously disregarded or failed to acknowledge formally the importance of counselling practice in their work. The discipline continues to expand in a fluid fashion, exploring new ways of engaging in the endless mysteries of the human soul.

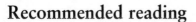

Recommended reading

Grof, Stanislav 1985, *Beyond the Brain*, State University of New York Press, New York.

Yalom, Irvin 1991, *Love's Executioner*, Penguin, Harmondsworth.

McLeod, John 2003, *An Introduction to Counselling*, 3rd edn, Open University Press, Buckingham.

Kirschenbaum, Howard and Henderson, Valerie Land (eds) 1989, *The Carl Rogers Reader*, Houghton Mifflin, Boston.

Moore, Thomas 1994, *Care of the Soul*, HarperPerennial, New York.

9

Flower essences
Bach Flowers/Australian Bush Flower Essences

Bach Flowers
Nicole Heneka

Flower essences have been used as a healing tool for centuries. The modern usage of these essences, however, began in earnest with the Bach Flowers that were developed in the early 1900s by an orthodox medical practitioner who had become disillusioned with the approach of medical science to disease.

Dr Edward Bach studied medicine at Birmingham University and finished his medical training at University College Hospital in 1912. He set up a practice in Harley Street, London, but after treating many patients felt dissatisfied with the results of orthodox treatment, especially in relation to chronic conditions. One of his fundamental beliefs was that a patient's state of mind and personality were the key to the cure of physical disease processes and chronic illness (Bach 1931). Observations of his own patients led Bach to the conclusion that each patient needed to be treated as an individual, not as a set of symptoms relating to a specific disease, and that the 'cure' itself should be gentle and effective without side effects of its own.

The need to develop these ideas fuelled Bach's interest in immunology and through his research at the Immunity School at University College Hospital he discovered that certain intestinal bacteria secreted toxins which caused chronic diseases (Weeks 1973). When these toxins were removed, the chronic conditions also resolved. These conditions ranged from skin complaints and inflammatory conditions to chronic infections.

In 1920, while working as a bacteriologist at the London Homoeopathic Hospital, Bach read Samuel Hahnemann's *Organon*. Hahnemann was also a doctor and the founder of homœopathy (see Chapter 11). Homœopathic medicine focused on the patient's state of mind and characteristics as well as the physical manifestations of a disease. It also worked with minute doses of substances to bring about physical and mental changes to achieve a cure. These homœopathic principles held by Hahnemann were very similar to Bach's in terms of treating the person rather then the disease.

Hahnemann had recognised three 'poisons' which needed to be removed before a chronic condition could resolve. The patient was treated with minute doses of homœopathic medicine which were repeated when the previous dose had stopped working. Bach, using homœopathic methods of preparation, began to develop 'vaccines' from the organisms that he had found to cause intestinal poisoning. The vaccines, or *nosodes*, were administered orally to reduce further any adverse reactions (Weeks 1973). Bach classified the intestinal bacteria into groups based on their fermentation action on sugar. There were seven main groups, each of which promoted a cleansing of the intestinal tract and elimination of the toxins produced by the specific intestinal bacteria. Patients were tested to determine which bacterial group was predominant in the intestine and then given the appropriate nosode (Weeks 1973).

Bach was delighted with the results of the vaccines because they offered a safe and gentle approach to conditions that had previously been considered incurable. Medications and their resulting side effects could also be dramatically reduced or eliminated altogether using these vaccines. At the same time, Bach closely observed the personality picture of the patients being treated with the nosodes (Weeks 1973). Drawing on his knowledge of people, based on years of observation and careful case taking, he began to categorise people according to their emotional states. Bach found that there were twelve major states of mind that affected most people. These included fear, indecision, indifference and impatience. Based on these different states of mind, he developed a theory of personality types. These seven personality types are outlined below, each one corresponding to one of the seven vaccines Bach had developed (Bach 1931).

From his observations, Bach believed that people with similar emotional states did not necessarily suffer from the same diseases, but would *react* to their illnesses in a very similar way. It was this reaction that determined the progression of their illness and so Bach believed that treating the state of mind was crucial to achieving cure. He began prescribing the nosodes based on the patients' personality and emotional symptoms. This method of prescribing was found by Bach to be more effective than just testing for bacterial groups. Bach began diagnosing patients based on their emotional states alone with great success.

The seven oral vaccines, known as the 'Seven Bach Nosodes', were enthusiastically adopted by the medical profession in England, Germany and America. Homœopaths around the world also welcomed this method of treating chronic disease (Weeks 1973). Bach applied himself to further simplifying and *purifying* this method of healing. Just as Hahnemann had developed homœopathic medicines from substances he found in nature, so Bach felt that the vaccines he had developed from bacteria might be replaced with substances based on plants and herbs. He began collecting and testing plants with which he hoped to replace the seven bacterial nosodes.

The remedies

Adhering to his idea of plant-based remedies, Bach developed the first three of his flower essences. He used the flowers of impatiens (for impatience), mimulus (for fear of known things) and clematis (for people living more in the future than the present) and prepared them in the same way he had prepared his vaccines. These remedies were prescribed to patients who fitted the personality picture. Bach had outstanding success with these three remedies. He began treating patients based purely on their personality types and published a paper in *The Homœopathic World* in February 1930 entitled 'Some new remedies and their uses' documenting his cases.

Based on the excellent results he achieved in the treatment of chronic disease, using plant-based remedies and prescribing to a patient's personality state, Bach decided to give up all other methods of treatment and begin developing more flower essences. He knew he had started on the path to a radically different system of medicine from the prevailing medical thought of the time. He handed over his practice and the work on the bacterial nosodes to his colleagues and prepared to start his work over again along very different lines (Weeks 1973).

In 1930 Bach left London and settled in a small village in Wales. At his doorstep were a vast variety of plants that became the foundation of his search for more remedies. He knew that the new remedies had to be gentle in their action, pleasant to take and result in a healing of the mind and the body. Bach spent each day examining and studying the different plants. He noted where and how they grew, the conditions where they grew best and their botanical characteristics. By this time he had become very sensitive to subtle energies and the 'vibrations' of plants. The development of the flower essences was based very much on intuition and what Bach 'felt' when he held a plant in his hands. Sometimes he was intuitively drawn to a plant for certain personality states. At other times he became overwhelmed with the emotion that would be treated by the particular plant (Weeks 1973).

In August and September of 1930 Bach found and prepared six new remedies which he added to the initial three. All, bar one, were wildflowers common to the English countryside. From 1931 to 1932 three more remedies were developed. Bach thoroughly tested each remedy and carefully documented his results. With twelve remedies completed, he wrote and published *The Twelve Healers* (Bach 1933), a book describing each remedy, its indications, preparation and dosage instructions. The next two years saw Bach add another seven remedies.

From March to September in 1935 Bach developed a further nineteen remedies. Unlike the first series of remedies, where he had been intuitively drawn to and able to feel the vibrations of a plant, this second series resulted from him intensely feeling the state of mind that would benefit most from the new remedy. He suffered great mental anguish and accompanying physical symptoms until each new remedy had been discovered.

These 38 remedies became the Bach Flower Remedies we know today. Although each remedy addresses a specific emotional state, Bach categorised the remedies under seven headings, corresponding to the initial seven bacterial nosodes (Bach 1931):

- **fear;**
- **uncertainty;**
- **insufficient interest in present circumstances;**
- **loneliness;**
- **oversensitivity to influences and ideas;**
- **despondency and despair; and**
- **overcare for the welfare of others.**

In addition, a 39th remedy for emergencies was developed and named Rescue Remedy. Probably the best known of the Bach Flower Essences, Rescue Remedy is made up of five individual remedies:

Cherry plum—for the fear of losing control
Clematis—to bring a person back into the present
Rock rose—the emergency remedy when there is extreme fear or terror
Star of Bethlehem—for great distress and shock
Impatiens—for impatience and stress

Rescue Remedy is a good general remedy indicated for any emergency, shock or stress. An accident or injury, receiving bad news, nervousness and anxiety are all instances where Rescue Remedy can be used. It can be taken every few minutes if necessary until the person feels calmer. Rescue Remedy is also incorporated into a cream, which is especially beneficial for children.

Preparing the remedies

Having developed a range of remedies that would address the mind, the other dimension of Bach's work was to develop a method of preparing his remedies that was also in keeping with his philosophy of healing. Walking through a field early one morning, Bach saw the dew on the petals of a flower. He felt that the dew contained the 'vital force' of the flower and it was this energy which would bring about healing. Bach then developed a method for preparing remedies that would enable him to 'capture' the energy of the flower. This was different from the method he had used for the nosodes and the initial remedies (Weeks 1973).

There are three stages in the preparation of the remedies:

1. **the mother tincture: prepared by either the sun or boiling method;**
2. **the stock bottle (practitioner dispenses); and**
3. **the prescription, treatment or medicinal bottle (patient takes).**

The sun method (for flowers and petals) and boiling method (for flowering twigs) were developed to extract the essence of each flower (Weeks & Bullen 1990). Each method utilises the sun and purified water to draw out the essence of the flower.

The sun method

The sun method is used for flowers that bloom in the late spring and summer.

- **Flowers are picked around 9 a.m. as they will have been bathed in some sunshine by then and the blooms will be open.**
- **Picked flowers are placed in a plain glass or crystal bowl filled with pure water and left to sit in direct sunlight for three hours.**
- **The flowers are removed and the water that remains is mixed with equal parts of brandy.**
- **This is the mother tincture.**

The boiling method

The boiling method is used for the flowers and twigs of trees, bushes and plants that bloom in the late winter or early spring before there is significant sunshine.

- **An enamel or stainless steel saucepan is three-quarters filled with the appropriate flowers and twigs.**
- **The twigs are covered with pure water, brought to the boil and boiled, without the lid, for half an hour.**
- **After boiling, the saucepan is left to stand in the sun until cold.**
- **The twigs are removed and the sediment is allowed to settle.**
- **The liquid is poured through filter paper.**
- **Equal parts of brandy are added.**
- **This is the mother tincture.**

Two drops from the mother tincture are then added to a 25 mL bottle containing brandy. This becomes the stock bottle from which the practitioner dispenses. In keeping with Bach's philosophy, this is a very simple method of preparation.

Bach's philosophy of healing

In his book *Heal Thyself* (Bach 1931) Bach detailed his philosophy of healing. He believed that there were fundamental truths which needed to be acknowledged in order to understand the nature of disease. Prime among these is that the soul (or higher self) is the essence of a person. According to Bach, through intuition, the soul guides us so that we can evolve as human beings. Bach describes intuition as the ability to be yourself without being influenced by others. It is about being spontaneous and following your own desires. He felt that when the soul is allowed to guide you then true happiness, spiritual and physical health is found. True happiness, Bach believed, brings with it qualities of courage, wisdom, strength and love.

Conversely, disease is seen as a result of conflict between the soul and personality, which leads you away from your optimal path in life. When a person is swayed by the influence of others or stops following their inner convictions it causes an inner conflict. This leads to feelings of unhappiness which in turn attract the qualities that are the antithesis of happiness: greed, cruelty, self-absorption, ignorance, pride and hate. These states of mind interfere with the normal and harmonious functioning of a person. Over time, these 'negative' emotions effect physical changes in the body which result in disease (Bach 1931).

Bach saw the mind as the controller of the mental and physical aspects of a person. If the mind is disturbed, for example through fear, depression or worry, the sense of inner joy and harmony is lost. This is communicated to the rest of the body resulting in physical symptoms and, eventually, disease.

Bach assessed his patients based on their individual emotional signs and symptoms. He treated the patient at this level because that was where the clearest indication of conflict between soul and personality could be found. According to Bach, if the mind regained the lost sense of happiness, for example through the use of the flower essences, the body would be restored to its previous state of health and harmony. The Bach Flowers work by energetically helping a person reconnect with that fundamental sense of happiness that comes with letting the soul guide one's life. In the flower essences Bach had remedies that targeted what he believed to be the true cause of illness, the underlying emotional state which had led to an imbalance of the system. Through the energy of the flower essences, a person could be guided back to spiritual health and, therefore, emotional and physical health (Bach 1931).

The Bach Flowers in practice

In complementary medicine there is an emphasis on the treatment of the person as a whole rather than as a collection of symptoms. This extends to addressing the emotional state because there is such a strong relationship between the physical body and a person's state of mind. There is plenty of evidence that emotions will affect the body in a tangible and physical way. A good example of this is nervousness. On a physical level nervousness can manifest as trembling, nausea, perspiration and diarrhoea. Each of these symptoms can be treated, but the cause of the nervousness has not been addressed. Even a prescription that addresses all of these symptoms will not 'cure' the person experiencing them. A person feeling nervous may be thinking 'what if I make a mistake?' or 'everybody will be looking at me'. It is these thoughts that are causing the physical symptoms. Going a level deeper might determine that it is the 'fear' of making a mistake or a lack of self-confidence that is causing the thought process. So, although the physical symptoms of nervousness can be similar for many people, the underlying thoughts can be very different.

The physical manifestations of these thoughts over a period of time will affect the body on a physiological level. In the case of nervousness, adrenalin is responsible for many of the physical symptoms. This 'stress' response can develop into a number of chronic conditions. Treating only the physical signs and symptoms will not cure the condition. This is where the Bach Flowers become an important part of clinical practice. As a modality, the Bach Flowers address a wide variety of emotional states that can, and do, manifest as physical symptoms. Using the Bach Flowers, the practitioner has a specific tool with which to address these underlying states. This enables a truly holistic approach to the treatment of the patient.

To appreciate this it is helpful to consider how one of the Bach Flower remedies may be prescribed using a hypothetical case. A female patient presents with insomnia and headaches. This has been happening for three weeks. She is very tired, finds it difficult to concentrate and is becoming very short tempered. Initially there are several remedies that could be indicated:

- **Olive: for tiredness**
- **Walnut: to help ground and focus**
- **Holly: for anger**

After questioning the patient, it is revealed that three weeks ago she found out she would have to attend a court hearing on a matter she thought had been resolved. Since then the patient has worried almost continuously about the upcoming court appearance. She goes over and over the different scenarios in her head to the point where she can't sleep. The patient cannot get the worrying thoughts out of her head.

So although there were three remedies which could have been considered appropriate initially, further questioning led to the *cause* of her current symptoms, that is, the worrying thoughts about the court case. The remedy that is indicated in this case is White Chestnut. This remedy is for persistent worrying thoughts that a person just cannot get out of their head. A person might become fixated on an idea or go over and over an argument or an unpleasant situation. Taking White Chestnut will help to break the cycle of worry and help the person come back to a state of mental peace.

Dispensing the remedies

In practice, the Bach Flower Essences come as a kit of the 38 individual remedies plus Rescue Remedy. Two drops from these stock bottles are added to a 25 mL dropper bottle which contains three parts pure water and one part brandy (as a preservative). Glycerine or vinegar can be used for people who are sensitive to alcohol or the remedies can be applied to pulse points on the wrists, ankles, temples, neck and behind the knee.

As a general rule, up to five remedies can be combined in one bottle. Rescue Remedy counts as one remedy even though it is made up of five remedies itself. For all remedies the patient takes four drops four times a day either under the tongue or in some water. The remedy can be taken more often if required—this is especially beneficial in acute cases. A 25 mL dosage bottle usually lasts about three weeks. This period is a good time to review the patient's progress and change the remedy if necessary. Bach Flowers can also be added to herbal medicine mixtures or creams and ointments.

Since the Bach Flowers are an energetic medicine, the patient cannot overdose. They are safe to use in pregnancy, for infants and children of all ages. The Bach Flowers do not interfere with any other medications the person may be taking. Animals, and even plants, also respond well to the Bach Flowers. There are no side effects but because they address the emotions directly it is important to monitor a patient's emotional wellbeing while they are taking Bach Flowers. The prescription may need to be changed over time as certain states resolve and new ones emerge. This is because the emotions can be seen to be like layers of an onion and as each layer is removed another one takes its place until the core is reached.

In contemporary practice, the Bach Flowers give the practitioner an avenue to treat the mind as well as the body. The changes and improvements in a patient's condition can be remarkable. However, it is very important to appreciate the limitations of these remedies. In adhering to naturopathic principles, the patient as a whole needs to be treated. Physical signs and symptoms also need to be addressed. By supporting the body and the mind, a far more effective treatment can be given for any condition.

Support on an emotional level may need to extend to counselling or psychotherapy. Referral is essential in these cases as the needs of the patient may go beyond what the complementary therapist has been trained to provide. Under no circumstances should a patient be advised to give up orthodox prescriptions and rely solely on the Bach Flowers. This applies to both medications for physiological and emotional conditions. Bach Flowers can be given in conjunction with any orthodox medication. It is then up to the patient and their doctor to discuss any revisions of their prescription.

Conclusion

There is a lot of literature available on the Bach Flowers and on Bach himself, as well as other resources like repertories and pictorial cards. These references give the modern practitioner access to a gentle and effective system of medicine and prescription. Bach's vision of a simple and gentle method of healing that is available to all people has been realised. Used correctly, and in conjunction with other modalities, the Bach Flower Essences are a valuable addition to modern medical practice.

Recommended reading

Bach, E. 1931, *Heal Thyself*, C.W. Daniel, Saffron Waldon.

Bach, E. 1933, *The Twelve Healers*, C.W. Daniel, Saffron Waldon.

Weeks, N. 1973, *The Medical Discoveries of Edward Bach, Physician*, Keats Publishing, Connecticut.

Weeks, N. and Bullen, V. 1990, *The Bach Flower Remedies: Illustrations and Preparations*, C.W. Daniel, Saffron Waldon.

Australian Bush Flower Essences
Ian White

The concept of healing that was shared by such great healers as Hippocrates, Paracelsus, Hahneman and Steiner was a simple one. They all believed that good health was the result of emotional, spiritual and mental harmony and found that when they treated their patients' psychological imbalances their diseases were cured. This belief is embodied in the philosophy of the healing modality of flower essences.

The Australian Bush Flower Essences work on the mind and spirit but predominantly work on the emotional level, harmonising negative feelings and belief patterns held in the subconscious mind, and are very specific in the issues and emotions which they address. They are obtained by extracting the healing vibrational quality from the highest evolved part of the plant, the flowers.

The history of flower essences

Ancient records show that over 3000 years ago the Egyptians were collecting the dew from flowers to treat emotional imbalances. The Australian Aborigines have also long used flowers to heal emotional imbalances. They would also collect the dew or else eat the whole flower to obtain the vibrational healing aspect of the plant. The early settlers reported that when the local Aboriginals fell ill they would treat themselves by floating waratahs in water for a number of hours and then drinking the water (Nixon 1987).

The earliest written European records of flower essence usage dates back to Abbess Hildegard von Bingen in the twelfth century and Paracelsus, the famous Swiss medical professor, alchemist and herbalist of the sixteenth century. Both prepared remedies from the dew of flowers in order to treat their patients' emotional problems and physical ailments. Flower essences have also been widely used in Asia, the Indian subcontinent and South America.

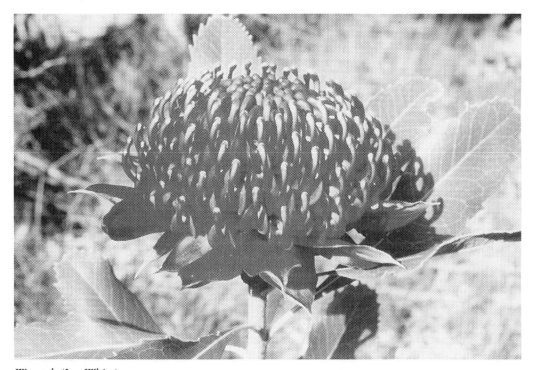

Waratah (Ian White)

Up until the mid-nineteenth century the majority of people in many countries were familiar with the emotional healing qualities of the plants and flowers growing around them. This is evident, for example, in Europe with the numerous books published in the eighteenth and nineteenth centuries on the subject of the 'language of flowers' wherein the emotions associated with each specific flower were listed (Greenaway 1978; McIntre 1996). Today we still see the remnants of this system in that people associate roses with love and rosemary with remembrance.

As detailed earlier in this chapter, the flower essences were further developed in the 1930s by Edward Bach (1886–1936) and since the 1980s there has been a great resurgence of flower essence development around the globe. There have been seven International Flower Essence conferences held in different countries since the inaugural conference in France in 1990. The Australian Bush Flower Essences carry on this very long healing tradition of flower essences.

Development of the Australian Bush Flower Essences

My family and I have been practising herbal medicine in Australia for five genera-tions. My great-grandmother and grandmother were among the first white people to study seriously the medicinal properties of our Australian plants. I grew up living next door to my grandmother in the bush at Terrey Hills in New South Wales. As a young boy I spent as much time as possible helping her prepare herbal extracts and tinctures as well as accompanying her on regular bushwalks where she would point out specific plants and trees and discuss their healing qualities with me. It was during this time that I developed a deep appreciation of the immense healing qualities of the Australian plants. I initially studied psychology at university but during my first summer vacation I developed a debilitating case of dysentery while travelling in India. On returning home I rebuilt my health by using herbs, yoga, meditation and natural medicine. For the rest of my degree I attempted to combine psychology with natural healing. However, by graduation I realised that all the things I was interested in were addressed by natural therapies and immediately commenced my naturopathic degree. This is where I came across the concept of flower essences. Their simplicity, afford-ability and the fact anyone can use them excited me but in the late 1970s the only system available was the English one. It struck me as strange that no one was researching Australian flowers, especially given the powerful healing properties of the Australian flora. This led me to start investigating Australian plants through research into their Doctrine of Signatures (see Chapter 10), Aboriginal practices, intuitive methods and kinesiology. I was carrying on the family tradition but focusing rather on the emotional and spiritual healing properties of our Australian flora.

For two years I was a driven man. On waking each morning I would feel the urgency to head off into the bush to research and develop what came to be known as the Australian Bush Flower Essences. During that period three other naturopathic colleagues and I trialled them on our patients to determine if my findings were accurate and could be verified. At the end of this time I was exceptionally satisfied and excitedly started to publish my research and make the Bush Essences available. The first thing that I noticed with the Bush Essences was how quickly they worked. Instead of prescribing them four times a day for a month, the essences needed only to be taken morning and night for a two-week period. The results were spectacular. Patients were certainly aware of the beneficial changes when they were prescribed the Australian Bush Flower Essences and I also noticed very profound and quick allevia- tion of physical symptoms. Soon people from all around the world were working with the Australian Bush Essences. Currently there are 65 individual Bush Flower Essences and from these I have developed fourteen combination remedies, five creams and five mists.

The Bush Essences very much address the unique and new needs of society in the twenty-first century. As the needs of society change new essences come through to help meet those needs. The Bush Essences address such contemporary issues as learning difficulties (e.g. dyslexia, Attention Deficit Disorder, Attention Deficit Hyperactivity Disorder), communication skills, creativity and protection from electro- magnetic radiation and solar radiation. There are also specific Bush Essences that address issues of sexuality, learning, toxic environments, spirituality, communication and relationships. These essences address such basic emotions as fear, grief and anger together with the major personality archetypes.

Australia has the highest number of flowering plants in the world. According to the geologists, it was the first continent to experience erosion and thus the first with soil. Consequently, botanists claim that the first flowering plants occurred in Australia. Today the Australian flora displays striking colour with a predominance of red and purple along with unique ancient forms. Australia is one of the most physically and psychically unpolluted countries and metaphysically has an ancient, powerful energy. This energy, combined with the strength and purity of the country, manifests itself in the flora and is encapsulated in the flower essences made from those plants. This is why the Australian Bush Flower Essences have a worldwide reputation for being incredibly quick acting and for having profound healing abilities even on the physical body.

Flower Essences and vibrational healing

As alluded to at the beginning of this chapter, the philosophy of flower essences views physical symptoms as merely the manifestation of emotional and spiritual imbal- ances. Recently there has emerged a heightened understanding that all living things have a unique energetic vibration, and keeping that energy in balance is essential for their wellbeing. Flower essences, being a form of vibrational therapy, can be a very effective healing tool to bring all aspects of any imbalances into alignment.

If the attitudes, thoughts, emotions and physical body are aligned and working harmoniously, then good health and wellbeing are assured. Richard Gerber, the author of *Vibrational Medicine for the 21st Century* (Gerber 1988), states that vibrational medicines, which are high-frequency subtle energies, are able to act on the subtle energy bodies at the emotional, mental and spiritual levels. There is then a flow-on from the subtle bodies into the physical.

Gerber states that the term 'vibration' is a synonym for frequency, and that the only difference between dense matter such as a piece of wood and subtle matter such as a flower essence is the frequency at which they vibrate. Subtle matter vibrates at exceedingly fast speeds. The vibrational medicines that contain high-frequency subtle energies are able to act on the subtle-energy bodies and at the level of the emotional, mental and spiritual body.

Gurudas, the author of the book *Flower Essences* (Gurudas 1983), postulates that when an essence is ingested or absorbed through the skin, it is initially assimilated into the bloodstream. Then it settles midway between the circulatory and nervous systems. There, an electromagnetic current is created by the polarity of the two systems. The essence then moves directly to the meridians, which are vital mechanisms of interface between the subtle bodies and the physical body (see also Chapter 5, 'Acupuncture'). From the meridians the flower essence is thought to be amplified by silica in connective tissue out to the chakras and various subtle bodies and then back again to the physical body.

According to Gurudas, of the three major forms of vibrational remedies (flower essences, homœopathic remedies and gem elixirs) flower essences are the most effective modality to reach and treat the subtle-energy bodies, along with the meridians and physical body.

Preparation and administration

All of the Bush Essences are prepared by the sunshine method, a technique that was originally developed by Edward Bach to simulate nature's production of dew (see 'Bach Flowers', above). Under ideal environmental conditions, flowers growing in the wild, far away from pollution, roads or power lines, are collected, placed into a bowl of pure water and left in sunlight for approximately two hours. Under the action of the sun the healing quality of the flowers is released into the bowl of water. The flowers are then removed from the bowl. This remaining flower water is then added to an equal amount of brandy, the latter acting as a preservative. This resulting compound is referred to as the mother tincture. The mother tincture is further diluted to what is known as stock. Practitioners prepare dosage bottles for their clients from their stock bottle. Several essences can be combined in the one dosage bottle but there is rarely a need to work with more than five.

The standard Bush Essence dose is to take seven drops from the dosage bottle, under the tongue, on rising and retiring. These are powerful periods for the psyche and at the same time it is very easy to remember to take them and affords high patient compliance. To address an emotional imbalance the remedy is normally taken for two weeks, whereas to address a physical problem the remedy will normally need to be taken for a least a month. There is no harm in taking the remedy for longer periods.

Contraindications

One of the most positive aspects of the Bush Essences is that they are self-adjusting, totally safe and without side effects. Since prescribing is predominantly for emotional states and the essences are safe, anyone can prescribe them. However, someone who does possess counselling or diagnostic skills could incorporate the Bush Essences at an even deeper level.

The only time to hesitate in prescribing the Australian Bush Flower Essences would be if the person were unable to take alcohol, whether for religious, social or health reasons. In such cases vegetable glycerine can be substituted for the brandy.

Working with other modalities

The Bush Essences are unique in that they can be and are easily incorporated with all healing modalities.

Many acupuncturists put the drops onto the needles once they have been placed in the patients. Emergency Essence is sprayed in intensive care wards and Emergency Essence drops are used in obstetrics wards to assist in childbirth and can be given to patients to help them recover from the trauma of surgery. Emergency Essence is a combination of seven essences and is used to ease distress, fear, panic and trauma. It is the first-aid remedy of the Bush Essences.

Slender Rice Flower is also used after surgery to enhance scar healing and lessen the incidence and effects of adhesions and scar tissue. Mulla Mulla is successfully employed on patients undergoing radiation therapy where it reduces the amount of burning as well as enhancing the healing of any such burns and at the same time easing the emotional trauma some people experience during this treatment. She Oak has been successfully used as an alternative treatment for hormone replacement therapy. It helps to hydrate the cells in the body, helping to slow the ageing process and maintaining vaginal lubrication. It also helps the body to utilise oestrogen precursors in food such as soy and yams. She Oak helps women maintain their optimum level of sex hormones even during menopause. Many psychiatrists around the world incorporate the Bush Essences as a major part of their treatment with patients. One has also found that the Emergency Essence with added Dog Rose and Dog Rose of the Wild has proved more effective for treating people who have panic attacks than any orthodox drug (*The Essence* 1999).

Reiki and hands-on healers often place specific Bush Essences either on their hands or directly on that part of the client's body to which they intend to direct healing energy.

Massage therapists and body workers can rub Emergency Essence cream directly into any painful areas their clients have and can add specific Bush Essences to their massage oil. Flannel Flower, for example, is used for clients who are uncomfortable with physical touch or intimacy.

Veterinarians widely prescribe the Bush Essences for all manner of emotional and physical symptoms. Animals respond extremely quickly to the essences, as do children. Red Helmet, for example, produces excellent results for animals with behavioural problems such as aggressive dogs and stubborn, rebellious horses. Pituitary tumours, quite common in dogs, are treated with brilliant results using

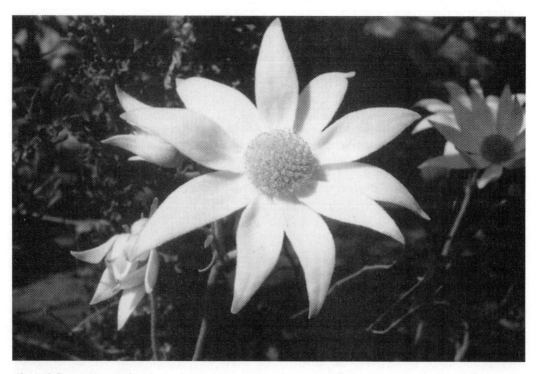

Flannel flowers (Ian White)

Yellow Cowslip Orchid. I know of one veterinary clinic in which a bottle of Emergency Essence is always on the operating tray. Many wildlife agencies involved in animal rescue also use the Bush Essences, especially Emergency Essence.

Naturopaths frequently search for the emotional causes behind physical symptoms and, once determined, the Bush Essences are ideal for addressing these issues. Both my books contain a listing of the Bush Essences that cover the main emotional states and beliefs that frequently create specific physical symptoms. There is also a chapter on iridology in *Australian Bush Flower Healing* (White 1999) that discusses major markings in the eye and indicates which Bush Essences would be the most appropriate for the health conditions that these markings underlie.

Any practitioner, no matter what their modality, would benefit from taking Alpine Mint Bush, which can help prevent practitioner burn-out. They would also benefit from spraying their treatment room at the end of the day with Space Clearing Mist to help remove the psychic residue left when patients release strong emotions. Space Clearing Mist purifies and cleanses all environments of negative emotion, mental and psychic energies.

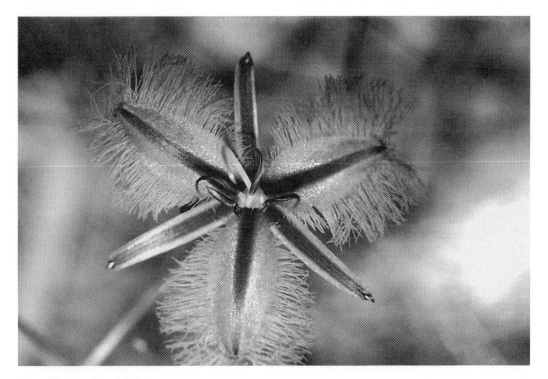

Fringed violet (Ian White)

Case histories

The following few brief anecdotes and case histories illustrate the scope and potential of the Australian Bush Flower Essences.

One woman was in so much pain from arthritis that she was unable to sit down in the chair. The joints of her fingers were swollen, gnarled and deformed. Her condition had commenced four years earlier when her husband had left her for another woman. I prescribed Sturt Desert Pea for her, an essence for grief. After five days she rang back to say that all she had done was cry in that time but also that she was free of pain and the deformity in her hands had gone! Rheumatologists would declare this either as impossible or a miracle.

A young woman in her early twenties wanted a prescription of Bush Essences to help her recover from her impending surgery for cervical cancer. After further discussion she confided that when she was fifteen years old she had been raped. Feeling that this was a likely trigger as to why she developed such a serious illness so early in life, I prescribed Flannel Flower, Fringed Violet and Wisteria to treat the emotional and physical shock and trauma of that event. After a few days she developed a burning sensation in the cervix, but she thought that this was part of the healing process and continued to take the Bush Essences. Three weeks later at the pre-operative check by her gynaecologist, he told her in a somewhat dumbfounded manner that he couldn't detect any signs of her cancer. She also reported feeling comfortable sexually for the first time since the rape. In both of these case histories, I wasn't treating the physical symptoms but rather the emotional incidents that I felt were the causative factors in the client's diseases. Once the emotions are balanced and harmonised the body can then heal itself and often in a very profound way.

The Australian Bush Flower Essences are also being used in orphanages in Brazil with the kitchen staff being instructed to add essences to the food while it is being cooked. In the first orphanage where this treatment program began, each child on average experienced 5.7 cases of bronchitis a year and the annual medical cost to the government per child was 67 reales. Bronchitis is connected to grief, an emotion that one would expect abandoned children to experience deeply. After one year of using Bush Essences in the orphanage the frequency of bronchitis dropped to under one case per child and annual health expenditure went down from 67 to 7 reales.

The Bush Essence combination Purifying Essence is used to help cleanse the body of both emotional and physical toxicity. One woman, a previously heavy smoker who had not smoked for fifteen years, experienced on taking this blend nicotine stains coming out on the fingers she used previously to hold her cigarette. Other patients have even smelt old anaesthetics coming out of their skin after taking this essence.

She Oak harmonises the ovaries and is prescribed for women experiencing infertility or having any hormonal imbalances including pre-menstrual syndrome or menopausal symptoms. A woman aged 41 had been trying to become pregnant for eight years and had tried every available gynaecological therapy. She took She Oak and immediately her gynaecologist discovered to his surprise that her hormones rose to a normal level and she developed a regular menstrual cycle and ovulation. This went on for three months and then she became pregnant. To her doctors this was astounding. While on She Oak her menstrual cycle and ovulation were normal; however, when she was on hormones there was very little measurable hormonal activity. One Sydney doctor claims to have over a 90 per cent success rate treating infertility solely with She Oak.

A doctor who works with the Bush Essences in a Brazilian hospital provided an amazing case history with before and after CAT scan images, showing how she had successfully treated a woman with an ovarian tumour, using only She Oak. The patient had a complete remission and no surgery was necessary.

Bush Essences can help a broad range of learning, emotional and behavioural areas. A most amazing case was a six-year-old boy who had been diagnosed as having Attention Deficit Disorder with hyperactivity, Asperger's Syndrome, eating disorders and learning and speech problems. His behaviour was outrageous. He had slept only three or four hours out of every 24 from the time he was a baby and he had put his younger brother in hospital several times. He had been assessed at school as being at mid-preschool standard and he had no social skills. He would not go out of the house unless forced and fought violently with any children he played with. He made life hell for everyone. On the sixth day after starting to take a mix of Fringed Violet, Sundew, Bush Fuchsia, Crowea, Dog Rose, Kangaroo Paw and Macrocarpa there was a marked improvement. He willingly went to visit his grandmother and allowed her to give him a hug, something he had never done before. On the same day his speech teacher commented that for the first time since she had been working with him he was actually listening and responding. He continued to take the essences, with some changes to the combination, for several months and by the time the next school year had started he was reassessed and found to be middle of the range for his age at reading and comprehension. His new teacher didn't even know he had any problems until his mother told her. His mother said to me, 'I feel that for the first time since he was born I have a normal child'.

These case histories are indicative of the wonderful results being achieved worldwide with the Australian Bush Flower Essences. As a modern and relevant part of the flower essence pantheon, the Bush Essences represent a powerful, safe and easy-to-use system of medicine that works to bring about health and wellbeing by addressing and resolving the causative factors of disease, rather than merely treating the symptoms.

Recommended reading

Gerber, Richard 2001, *Vibrational Medicine for the 21st Century*, Piatkus, London.

Oschman, James 2000, *Energy Medicine*, Harcourt, New Hampshire.

White, Ian 1991, *Australian Bush Flower Essences*, Bantam Books, Sydney.

White, Ian 1996, *Australian Bush Flower Remedies*, revised edition, Australian Bush Flower Essences (ABFE), Sydney.

White, Ian 1999, *Australian Bush Flower Healing*, Bantam Books, Sydney.

10

Herbal medicine
Hans Wohlmuth

Herbal medicine is the use of plants as medicines. Herbal medicine is also known as phytotherapy (especially in Europe; from Greek *phyton* meaning plant), botanical medicine, medical herbalism and herbology (USA). More specifically, the term herbal medicine refers to the therapeutic use of relatively crude and therefore chemically complex plant extracts, or simply the herb in its dried form. In this way herbal medicines are distinct from plant-derived pharmaceutical drugs, which contain single chemical compounds extracted from plants in their pure form.

All human societies of which we have any knowledge have availed themselves of plants for use as medicines. Herbal medicine in the widest sense is therefore a global form of medicine, which exists in a vast (albeit declining) diversity, forming a dynamic part of the rich cultural tapestry of our planet. Some of the most successful and sophisticated systems of herbal medicine prevailing today are Chinese Herbal Medicine (an integral part of Traditional Chinese Medicine) and the herbal medicine that forms part of the Ayurveda, the traditional system of medicine/health from India. These systems are treated elsewhere in this book.

This chapter is concerned with the type of herbal medicine that is prevalent in industrialised, western societies (in particular English-speaking countries), as distinct from both Chinese and Ayurvedic herbal medicine. Often referred to as 'western herbal medicine' (for want of a better term), this form of herbal medicine can best be defined as the therapeutic use of medicinal plants within a holistic context. Apart from being practised as a stand-alone therapeutic modality, it also forms part of the practice of naturopathy in English-speaking countries. Western herbal medicine is, as will be outlined below, essentially European in origin with significant influences from herbal traditions from other parts of the world, most notably North America and Asia (Wohlmuth *et al.* 2002).

It is important to be aware that the word 'herb' means different things to different people. To a botanist a herb is a herbaceous, that is, non-woody, plant, in contrast to shrubs and trees, both of which have woody stems. At the grocery store the term 'herb' is likely to be interpreted as meaning a culinary additive such as chives, parsley or dill. In herbal medicine, however, 'herb' is synonymous with 'medicinal plant' or, to be specific, the medicinal part(s) of a medicinal plant species, regardless of whether the plant is woody or not. The herb cascara is thus the bark (medicinal part) of *Frangula purshiana*, which happens to be a tree, just as the herb lemon balm consists of the above-ground parts of the herbaceous (non-woody) plant *Melissa officinalis*.

Origin of herbal medicine

Our hunter-gatherer ancestors had access to a large variety of plants in their environment. Many of these were eaten as foods, others were avoided due to their toxicity. At some point our ancestors started using certain plants not as foods but as medicines. We do not know when this occurred but it is likely to have been early in hominoid history, probably long before our own species, *Homo sapiens*, evolved some 300 000–500 000 years ago.

In 1960 the grave of a Neanderthal was discovered in the Shanidar Cave, in the northern parts of present-day Iraq (Solecki 1975). Neanderthals were hominids but are considered to have belonged to a species different from our own, the now extinct *Homo neanderthalensis*. An intriguing feature of this burial site, dated at 60 000 BCE, was the discovery that the dead seemingly had been laid to rest with bunches of flowers that would have grown in the area at the time. Analysis of conserved pollen from the flowers in the grave allowed the identification of eight different plants, seven of which are known to possess medicinal properties. Among these were a species of yarrow (genus *Achillea*), a species of *Ephedra* (source of the alkaloid ephedrine) and a species of mallow (genus *Althaea*). There is no way of knowing why these particular plants were chosen to accompany the dead Neanderthal on his final journey. They may well have been chosen simply because they grow locally and were flowering at the time. But it is also possible they were chosen because of their medicinal qualities, as a medicine kit for the journey into the great unknown.

It seems perfectly plausible that other, now extinct, hominids should have used plants as medicines when one considers that other mammals are known to do exactly that. The best-known examples of this come from some of our closest living relatives, the African great apes, which appear to use several plants for strictly therapeutic purposes (Huffman *et al.* 1998).

There is no doubt, however, that humans make use of plants specifically for medicinal purposes on a scale that exceeds use by any other mammal. The ethno-botanist Timothy Johns has advanced the hypothesis that the extensive use of medicinal substances by humans coincided with the transition from hunter-gatherer to agricultural society (Johns 1990). Hunter-gatherers had a richly varied plant diet and consumed on a daily basis a very wide range of biologically active phytochemicals, the types of compounds that are the pharmacologically active ones in medicinal plants. A high dietary intake of these phytochemicals would have maintained a high degree of health, so the argument goes. The advent of agriculture brought a sedentary lifestyle and a dramatic change in diet, from the highly diverse plant intake of hunter-gatherers to the reliance on often a single staple crop for survival. While agriculture allowed for population concentrations and urbanisation, it also led to many new health problems, as a result of a change in lifestyle and an impoverished diet lacking the variety of phytochemicals. The suggestion is that it was this situation that necessitated the introduction of specific sources of health-giving phytochemicals, namely herbal medicines.

The question of just how humans were able to identify plants with specific therapeutic qualities from local floras comprising many hundreds and sometimes thousands of species, many of them toxic, remains a mystery. The conventional view is that it occurred primarily through trial and error, possibly aided by the careful observation of animals. If this is true, large numbers of people through the ages must have suffered the toxic and sometimes fatal effects of plant toxins as a result of such experimentation. A somewhat more esoteric explanation, but nevertheless one that possibly should not be discounted, suggests that certain individuals throughout the history of humankind, usually tribal healers, have possessed a particular ability or 'dowsing instinct' allowing them to identify plants with specific medicinal qualities with far greater accuracy than would be achievable by simple trial and error (Griggs 1997).

Possibly the most important explanation for the ability of humans to identify therapeutic plants is an evolutionary one. The evolution of the human species has probably provided us with a certain degree of inherited phytochemical knowledge, enabling the recognition of, for example, the antimicrobial properties of aromatic essential plant oils or the toxic but also potentially pain-relieving properties of bitter alkaloids. This, coupled with the highly developed ability of humans to learn and pass on detailed information, and the thousands of human generations, may have resulted in the human species' sophisticated knowledge about medicinal plants and their uses.

A brief history of western herbal medicine

The history of herbal medicine is rich and fascinating and is, of course, to a large extent the history of medicine itself. For an engaging and comprehensive account readers are referred to Barbara Griggs's *New Green Pharmacy—The Story of Western Herbal Medicine* (Griggs 1997), from where much of the present information has been sourced.

The oldest written reference to medicinal plants and their use is the Chinese *Pen Ts'ao*, written about 4800 years ago and listing more than 360 species of herbs.

Another ancient manuscript, the Ebers Papyrus from Egypt, dates from about 1500 BCE and mentions a large number of plant and animal remedies. It also contains recipes for many specific formulae as well as magical chants (Mann 1992).

Hippocrates (c.460–377 BCE) of Greece is often referred to as 'the father of medicine'. He could equally be regarded as one of the founders of holistic herbal medicine. He prescribed individualised treatments for his patients, recommended exercise and dietary regimens and selected his herbal treatments from more than 400 species of plants. Hippocrates was also an exponent of humoral medicine and viewed disease as an imbalance of the four humours (black bile, blood, yellow bile and phlegm), which were derived from the concept of the four elements: earth, fire, air and water. Accordingly, Hippocratic treatment aimed at restoring the balance of the four humours.

Diocles, a student of Aristotle, wrote the oldest Greek herbal, the *Rhizotomika*, in the fourth century BCE. It was a Roman army surgeon by the name of Dioscorides (c. 40–80 CE), however, who wrote the most influential early European manual of medicinal plants, *De Materia Medica*, in the first century CE. This comprehensive work included illustrations and descriptions of about 600 plant species, along with text detailing their uses, doses and potential toxic effects.

Galen (c. 129–199 CE), like Hippocrates, practised humoral medicine but his approach to therapy was rigid, quite unlike the flexible and individualised approach of Hippocrates. Galen introduced a complex herbal classification system based on the humoral properties of each plant. According to this system each plant was assigned a 'temperament' (hot, cold, moist, dry or temperate) and a grading (first, second, third or fourth degree). For example, herbs that were deemed to be strongly heating (e.g. ginger and chillies) were said to be 'hot in the third degree' (Mills 1991).

The works of Galen were translated into Arabic and later Latin, and it is an astounding fact that his ideas had a stranglehold on European medical thought for about 1500 years.

One person who challenged Galenic medical authority was the Swiss-German doctor Philippus Theophrastus Bombastus von Hohenheim (1493–1541), better known as Paracelsus. He had a keen interest in alchemy and introduced the use of chemicals and metals such as mercury into medical practice. He is also credited with being the first to search for 'active principles' in plants. Despite his seemingly more modern views on some aspects of medicine, Paracelsus still believed in the Doctrine of Signatures, which states that plants carry 'labels' (or signatures) which indicate what they can be used for. Although the Doctrine of Signatures has been part of many different cultures, there is clearly no rational biological explanation for this concept, which is consistent only with creationist or supernatural cosmologies where humans are seen as being provided with (labelled) medicinal plants by a creating power. Numerous examples were cited as 'evidence' of the Doctrine of Signatures: plants with yellow flowers such as greater celandine (*Chelidonium majus*) for jaundice; plants with small tuberous storage roots such as pilewort (*Ranunculus ficaria*) for haemorrhoids; and plants that appear to carry leaves with fine holes in them (in fact translucent oil storage cells) such as St John's wort (*Hypericum perforatum*) for stab wounds. Despite some correlations, this kind of argument does not stand up to scrutiny and is akin to, say, an idea that the first letter of a plant name should indicate what it might be used for—hence cascara for constipation and foxglove for fibrillations.

In England, John Gerard's famous *Herbal or General Historie of Plantes* was published in 1597, and in 1649 the apothecary Nicholas Culpeper (1616–54) translated the *London Pharmacopoeia* from Latin into English, much to the consternation of the medical establishment, who saw this as a threat to their exclusive medical knowledge. Culpeper also wrote several original herbal works, none more famous than *The English Physician* (1653), in which he presented herbal medicine in an astrological framework.

Across the Atlantic Samuel Thomson (1769–1843) also encountered the ire of the medical establishment. Having been successfully treated with herbs as a child, Thomson was appalled by the bloodletting and heroic medicines of the day, which he believed were counterproductive and dangerous. Having no formal medical training, Thomson was self-taught and his simple but effective herbal medicine practice was dismissed by the medical profession as quackery. Thomson's theory on medicine was simple and vitalistic: he held that all disease was caused by cold (resulting from obstructions to the flow of vital energy) and accordingly treatment should be heating and aim to restore the flow of vital energy. Thomson's system of medicine was brought to England by Albert Coffin in 1838, where it became established in the north of the country. After Thomson's death in 1843 his system of medicine developed into what became known as physiomedicalism.

It was not only lay people like Samuel Thomson who were concerned about the horrors of heroic medicine. Dr Wooster Beach (1794–1868) started a movement of American medical doctors that became known as the eclectics. Eclectic medicine included many herbal medicines and promoted treatments that acted 'in harmony with physiological laws'. Followers of Thomson, physiomedicalists and eclectics alike used European herbs as well as native North American plants, the use of which was mostly learnt from Native American peoples.

Twentieth-century western herbal medicine arose from the physiomedical and eclectic traditions but was also influenced by European folk medicine, especially from Germany. Over the last couple of decades increasing amounts of scientific information about many herbal medicines has become available, and science is increasingly shaping the practice and future of contemporary herbal medicine. Figure 10.1 illustrates the major influences on western herbal medicine.

Figure 10.1   Major influences on western herbal medicine pre- and post-1900

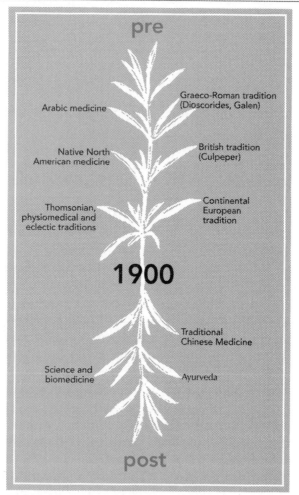

It should be emphasised that medical knowledge has been exchanged and medicinal plants traded for many centuries, and this type of cross-pollination has influenced all the major schools of medical thought through the ages. Hence medicinal plants from distant parts of the world have been used in western herbal medicine for centuries. The last twenty years, however, have seen an increasing number of Asian medicinal plants in particular incorporated into the western *materia medica* (literally 'medicinal materials' and refers to the medicinal substances used in a given system of medicine). Most of these plants have a long history of use in traditional medical systems such as Traditional Chinese Medicine and Ayurveda.

Theoretical foundations of western herbal medicine

The roots of western herbal medicine are ancient, yet at the start of the twenty-first century the modality finds itself vying for a place in mainstream healthcare in industrialised countries. At the same time, herbal medicine is becoming increasingly science based and as a result the theoretical foundations of the discipline are to some extent in a state of flux. Today's practitioners of western herbal medicine occupy a broad spectrum as far as theoretical foundations are concerned.

At one end of the spectrum are the traditionalists with strong philosophical allegiance to Thomsonian and physiomedical traditions and their vitalistic approach. At the other end of the spectrum are those who accept the biomedical model but see real value in the holistic approach to health and disease and the therapeutic qualities of herbal medicines. In this context it may be worth pointing out that it is entirely possible to use herbal medicines in a non-holistic, reductionist manner. Doing so, herbal practitioners would argue, does not amount to true herbal medicine but rather to allopathic medicine practised with plant-based medicines. Thus, the holistic approach is central to the practice of contemporary western herbal medicine. In a holistic framework, the emphasis is on treating the patient rather than their disease. The patient is viewed as comprising a physical body, with mental, emotional and spiritual aspects, all of which potentially influence the individual's state of health. In addition, the patient is viewed in the wider context of personal relationships, community and environment, and it is recognised that each of these could play a role in the person's health.

Vitalism in herbal medicine

Vitalism can be described as 'a doctrine that ascribes the functions of a living organism to a vital principle distinct from chemical and other forces' (Delbridge 1990). As such, vitalism is a doctrine that requires the invocation of the spiritual or supernatural and can be viewed as the antithesis to reductionism.

Vitalism was central to the medical philosophy of Samuel Thomson and the physiomedicalists, who saw the 'vital force' as controlling the body. Consequently, manifestations of health and disease were seen as the attempts of the 'vital force' to maintain the functional integrity of the organism (Priest & Priest 1982). Vitalistic concepts, especially the idea of 'supporting the vital force' as a treatment objective, are still common among practitioners of herbal medicine in the English-speaking world, although the concept is poorly articulated and little has been written about vitalism in contemporary herbal medicine literature. Vitalism plays a central role in many traditional systems of medicine such as Ayurveda and Traditional Chinese Medicine, where the concept of the 'vital force' is manifest as *prana* and *Qi*, respectively.

While a thorough discussion of vitalism is beyond the scope of this chapter, a brief overview might prove useful. Vitalism in the western world dates back to Hippocrates, Plato (427–347 BCE) and Aristotle (384–322 BCE) (Seaman 1999). Aristotle regarded living beings as consisting of the physical body and the soul, although these two elements were seen as inseparable. Aristotle's philosophy, which also included the view that in living beings everything spontaneously tends towards an appropriate aim, came to have an enormous influence on medical and biological thought, mostly through the work of Galen, whose influence remained dominant until the sixteenth century (Federspil & Sicolo 1994).

The first major challenge to vitalism came with René Descartes (1596–1650), whose view that only humans possessed a soul meant that the bodies of living organisms, including humans, were essentially machines, albeit very complex ones, and that their workings were guided only by the laws of physics. Descartes's mechanistic doctrine represents the origin of modern reductionism (Federspil & Sicolo 1994). In the seventeenth century, a 'new vitalism' emerged, which departed radically from the classic vitalistic doctrine. Whereas Aristotle and Galen had viewed the soul as inseparable from the matter in the living body, G.E. Stahl (1659–1734) and his followers saw the soul as a separate entity to the physical body.

Vitalists of the nineteenth century asserted that life does not develop as a result of physical and chemical phenomena but rather in spite of them, as a result of a (vital) force that is unlike any physical force. This view was articulated clearly by the Italian physician and vitalist G.A. Giacomini (1796–1849), who stated that 'The living being is controlled by a power in opposition to the physicochemical laws' and 'It is nature that cures disease. And by the term "nature" we mean an activity, a force within the living organism' (Federspil & Sicolo 1994).

The French physiologist Claude Bernard (1813–78) took a more moderate view and became an exponent of what has been termed 'moderate vitalism'. As a physiologist, Bernard realised that living organisms could not adequately be described by simply the sum of their constituent parts, as strict reductionism would suggest. Bernard wrote that 'the [physiologic] elements, although different and independent, do not simply associate with one another, but their unification expresses something more than the simple addition of their separate properties' (Federspil & Sicolo 1994). Bernard was, however, strongly opposed to vitalistic views incorporating the supernatural and stated, 'I would agree with vitalists only if they limited themselves to admitting that living beings present manifestations absent in the inanimate world and, for this reason, constitute a peculiar character of it' (Federspil & Sicolo 1994).

It is against this historical backdrop that vitalism in Thomsonian and physiomedical herbal medicine should be seen. The place of vitalism in modern herbal medicine is controversial. Many proponents of traditional herbal medicine argue that vitalism and its concept of a 'vital force' are fundamental parts of the theoretical and philosophical framework of herbal practice. In contrast many others, who view herbal medicine as an essentially scientific practice employing medicinal plant preparations as pharmacologically active therapeutic agents, see vitalistic concepts as irrelevant, antiquated and unhelpful to the promotion of herbal medicine as a valuable part of contemporary healthcare.

While the concept of a life force may provide a meaningful philosophical framework for some practitioners, there is clearly no scientific basis for the existence of an external force of this kind.

Herbal medicines

Herbal medicines are medicines made from plants. A survey of some 259 of the most widely used plants in western herbal medicine in Australia found that the vast majority are flowering plants (angiosperms). Approximately one-third of the species belong to just five botanical families: the daisy family (Asteraceae), mint family (Lamiaceae), rose family (Rosaceae), carrot family (Apiaceae) and legume family (Fabaceae) (Wohlmuth 2002). The study also surveyed the biogeographical origin of medicinal species and the morphological plant parts used for medicinal purposes. These results are shown in Table 10.1 and Table 10.2 respectively.

Table 10.1   Biogeographical origin of 259 species used in western herbal medicine (after Wohlmuth 2002)

Europe/Europe and parts of Asia	37.4%
Asia	19.3%
Africa	3.0%
North America	21.6%
South America	3.5%
Pacific (incl. Australia)	1.2%
Native to several continents	14.0%

Table 10.2   Morphological plant part used for medicine (after Wohlmuth 2002)

Plant part used	
Aerial parts	37.8%
Underground parts	27.8%
Fruit/seed	13.9%
Bark	8.5%
Flower	4.6%

Herbal medicines are relatively crude extracts of medicinal plants and are characterised by containing a range of chemical constituents, several of which may contribute to the pharmacological effects of the medicine. This contrasts with

Table 10.3 Chemical constituents of herbal medicines and pharmaceutical drugs

Therapeutic agents	Chemical constituent(s)
Herbal medicines	
Meadowsweet (*Filipendula ulmaria*), flowers and leaf	Flavonoids (incl. different glycosides of quercetin and kaempferol); phenolic glycosides (incl. salicylaldehyde primveroside and methyl salicylate primveroside); essential oil (incl. salicylaldehyde, phenylethyl alcohol, methyl salicylate); tannins (incl. rugosin-D); and others (Mills and Bone 2000)
Licorice (*Glycyrrhiza glabra*), root	Triterpenoid saponins (incl. glycyrrhizin); glycyrrhetinic acid; flavonoids (incl. flavanones, chalcones and isoflavonoids); sterols (Mills and Bone 2000)
Plant-derived pharmaceutical drugs	
Lanoxin®	Digoxin
Oncovin®	Vincristine sulphate
Synthetic pharmaceutical drugs	
Telfast®	Fexofenadine
Zocor®	Simvastatin

plant-derived and synthetic pharmaceutical drugs, which typically contain a single, purified active compound, as shown in Table 10.3.

Plants as sources of pharmacologically active compounds

It has been known for centuries that many plants contain compounds with powerful pharmacological effects. Most pharmacologically active plant constituents are so-called secondary metabolites, such as alkaloids, saponins and coumarins. These secondary metabolites are compounds that do not appear to be essential to the short-term survival of a plant, in contrast to primary metabolites such as carbohydrates, lipids, proteins and nucleic acids. The first secondary metabolites to be isolated from plants in the early nineteenth century were all alkaloids with powerful pharmacological effects: morphine (1816), strychnine (1817), atropine (1819) and quinine (1820) (Mann 1992). In the twentieth century many pharmaceutical drugs were based on plant compounds. In 1985 it was estimated that 25 per cent of pharmaceutical drugs dispensed in the USA between 1959 and 1980 were based on active principles from plants (Farnsworth *et al.* 1985).

Compounds extracted from plants are still being used in pharmaceutical drugs. Well-known examples are the analgesic alkaloid morphine, extracted from the opium poppy (*Papaver somniferum*), and the cardiac glycoside digoxin, extracted from the Grecian foxglove (*Digitalis lanata*). Many other pharmaceutical drugs are derived from plant compounds, either by chemical modification of a plant compound or by having their synthetic structure modelled on plant compounds. The steroidal drugs are an example of the former, being produced semi-synthetically from steroidal plant precursors, mostly from soybeans (*Glycine max*) or yams (*Dioscorea* spp.). The world's most successful pharmaceutical drug, acetylsalicylic acid (Aspirin®), was developed from naturally occurring plant salicylates. It was first marketed in 1899 by the German pharmaceutical company Bayer.

Pharmacologically active plant compounds are typically small molecules which, like other drugs, can interact with protein targets called receptors in the human body. The main way in which a herbal medicine differs from a plant-derived pharmaceutical drug is that it contains multiple chemical compounds, many of which may contribute to the effect of the remedy. In contrast, pharmaceutical drugs (plant derived or not) normally consist of a single, purified chemical compound which will interact with one specific receptor. For example, a tincture of peppermint is a herbal medicine, whereas morphine, a pure plant compound, is a pharmaceutical drug. Table 10.4 lists some characteristic differences between herbal medicines and pharmaceutical drugs.

Table 10.4   Differences between herbal medicines and pharmaceutical drugs

Herbal medicines	Pharmaceutical drugs
Relatively crude plant extracts	Synthetic or highly purified
Multiple active compounds	Single active compound
Potentially multiple targets of action	Single target of action

Types of herbal medicines

Herbal medicines are used topically and orally and come in a variety of forms. The simplest form of herbal medicine is a herbal tea made from the dried herb. Teas may be prepared either as infusions, where the herb is steeped in freshly boiled water, or as decoctions, where the herb is simmered in boiling water. Which is the more appropriate method depends on the constituents and the nature of the plant material. The therapeutic effects of medicinal teas should not be underestimated provided good-quality herb is used in an appropriate strength and dose.

Apart from dried herbs, the majority of retail preparations are in solid dosage forms such as tablets or capsules, whereas preparations for practitioner dispensing are more commonly liquid extracts. These extracts are made by extraction of the plant material using a mixture of ethanol and water as solvent. More dilute forms of liquid extracts are often called tinctures. Another type of liquid extract uses a glycerol–water mixture as the extraction medium; the resultant extracts are called glycerol extracts or 'glycetracts' and have the advantages of being alcohol free and sweet tasting. Glycerol is not, however, a good universal solvent for most plant constituents and in most cases a glycerol extract will be inferior to an equivalent ethanol–water extract. Fresh juices of a variety of medicinal plants are also available in bottled form in some countries.

Tablets and capsules may contain powdered dried herb, but increasingly solid or semi-solid extracts are used for these dosage forms. Such extracts are often prepared by drying liquid extracts. In recent years an increasing number of highly concentrated extracts have become available. Some of these have high raw material (herb) to extract ratios. The widely used ginkgo leaf extract, for example, has an average herb to extract ratio of 50 to 1, that is, 50 kg of ginkgo leaf is used to produce 1 kg of extract. It is obvious that in the case of highly concentrated preparations, the extraction must be highly selective. In the example of the ginkgo leaf extract only 2 per cent of the raw material ends up in the extract; the rest is discarded. Concentrated extracts are often prepared by way of sophisticated extraction methods such as supercritical fluid extraction or the use of repeated extraction with multiple solvents. What defines these extracts as still being herbal and not pharmaceutical drugs is the fact that they retain a high degree of chemical complexity.

Most of these concentrated extracts are also *standardised*, which means that standardised extraction and manufacturing processes have been employed in their production. In the case of standardised extracts of high quality, the process of standardisation includes agronomic practices such as seed selection and cultivation, as well as the application of quality assurance systems that effectively monitor all steps of production, from the growing plant to the finished extract. Standardised extracts are also characterised by containing quantified levels of one or more *marker compounds*. The level of a marker compound is usually given as a minimum content or as a range. Undesirable constituents may also be specified by way of a maximum level (e.g. ginkgolic acids in ginkgo leaf extract). Marker compounds may be compounds with known pharmacological activity or may be compounds that are characteristic of the particular plant species.

Essential (or volatile) oils are chemically complex constituents of many medicinal plants. They can be selectively extracted by steam distillation. The use of pure essential oils in herbal medicine is very limited, but examples of oils that are used therapeutically are peppermint oil and tea tree oil (the steam-distilled oils of *Mentha* x *piperita* and *Melaleuca alternifolia*, respectively).

Quality issues in herbal medicine

There are numerous quality issues pertinent to herbal medicines. These range from basic issues of correct botanical identification, harvest, drying and storage methods, to issues of good manufacturing practice and stability (see Table 10.5). The most obvious limiting factor to the quality of a product is the quality of the raw material from which it is made. Most herbal medicines are made from dried plant material and the timing and methods of harvest, as well as the drying and storage conditions, are critical.

It is fair to say that there is enormous variation in the quality of herbal medicines currently on the market in most countries. It is also evident that regulating authorities as well as responsible sectors of the industry are making concerted efforts towards improving quality standards of herbal medicines.

Table 10.5   Parameters that impact on the quality of herbal medicines and measures taken to control them

Parameter	Measure
Botanical identity of raw material	Correct botanical identification
Correct medicinal part(s) of plant	Correct morphological identification
Quality of raw material	Good agricultural practice; correct harvest and post-harvest handling; tests for marker compounds, contaminants (heavy metals, micro-organisms, pesticide residues)
Extraction and manufacturing	Good manufacturing practice; use of appropriate methodology; test for marker compounds
Stability	Stability testing on extract/product
Quality use	Appropriate packaging and labelling (indications, dosage, warnings)

Evidence for western herbal medicine

Evidence for efficacy and safety is a cardinal issue in all forms of natural and complementary medicine, as indeed it is also in mainstream medicine. Herbal medicine and other forms of natural medicine frequently stand accused of being supported by little or no evidence. In the case of western herbal medicine this can be comprehensively refuted as considerable evidence exists for its efficacy and safety. The issue of evidence is rather more complicated, and individual herbal medicines can claim different levels of evidence for their efficacy. Likewise, their use is associated with different levels of risk.

When assessed on the available evidence, western herbal medicine seems to be generally effective as well as safe. In terms of evidence in support of the efficacy of herbal medicine, it should be recognised that many different types of evidence may contribute to the overall picture. When assessing the evidence for a particular herbal medicine it is the totality of the different types of available evidence that

Table 10.6   Types of evidence relevant to the therapeutic use of medicinal plants

Clinical evidence	Non-clinical evidence
Empirical data from traditional use (e.g. pharmacopoeial monograph)	Data from *in vitro* (test tube) studies
Published case studies	Data from animal studies
Uncontrolled trials	
Randomised controlled trials	
Systematic reviews of randomised controlled trials	

should form the basis of the assessment. Different types of evidence relevant to the assessment of herbal medicines are listed in Table 10.6.

A documented history of traditional use is an important type of evidence for many herbal medicines. Traditional use refers to the continuous use, over hundreds or sometimes thousands of years, of a remedy for a specific health problem. Traditional use normally occurs within a traditional medical system (such as western herbal medicine or Traditional Chinese Medicine) or an indigenous group. With few exceptions, all herbal medicines used in western herbal medicine are supported by evidence from traditional use. In cases where the same plant has been used in several traditional systems of medicine or by separate indigenous groups for the same ailment, the evidence of traditional use carries more weight.

In addition to traditional use many herbal medicines are now also supported by different types of clinical or scientific evidence, ranging from *in vitro* (test tube) investigations of biological activity to systematic reviews of randomised controlled trials. *In vitro* data can provide valuable information about the pharmacology and toxicology of herbal medicines, but cannot be extrapolated directly to use in humans. Important determinants of the clinical effects such as bioavailability and metabolism cannot be assessed in test tubes. However, data from *in vitro* studies are valuable when combined with information about traditional use or other clinical data. Table 10.7 gives examples of herbal medicines supported by different levels of evidence.

The practice of western herbal medicine

The initial visit to a practitioner of western herbal medicine (be it a herbalist or a naturopath) is likely to last for at least an hour. The practitioner will take a comprehensive case history and may carry out a physical examination as appropriate. The case history will include the patient's presenting complaint, medical history and

Table 10.7   Types of evidence supporting the therapeutic uses of some herbal medicines

	In vitro data	Traditional use	Randomised controlled trial (RCT)	Systematic review of RCTs
Burdock (*Arctium lappa*) in chronic skin disease		•		
Echinacea (*Echinacea* spp.) in the common cold	•	•	•	
St John's wort (*Hypericum perforatum*) in mild–moderate depression	•	•	•	•
Ginkgo (*Ginkgo biloba*) leaf in peripheral arterial occlusive disease and cognitive deficit	•		•	•

family history, diet, lifestyle, social situation, emotional wellbeing, use of pharmaceutical drugs and supplements and so on. If biomedical diagnostic tests are required, the practitioner will refer the patient to a general practitioner. Well-trained practitioners will base their clinical diagnosis on biomedical diagnostics, while some may also use unproven diagnostic tools such as iridology.

Once a diagnosis has been made, the practitioner will provide the patient with dietary and lifestyle advice and determine the appropriate herbal treatment. The treatment may be aimed at different therapeutic outcomes. Part of the treatment may aim to provide symptomatic relief and make the patient feel better in the short term, while another aspect of the treatment may address the perceived causes of the problem (thus honouring the fundamental principle of 'treat the cause, not just the symptoms').

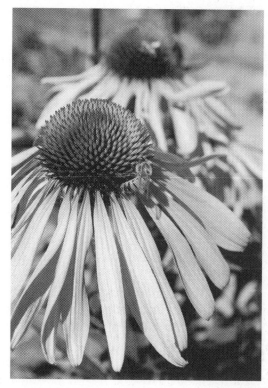

Echinacea purpurea (Echinacea) (Hans Wohlmuth)

Yet another part of the treatment may be constitutional in nature, that is, aimed at treating underlying weaknesses (acquired or inherited). Treatment aimed at providing symptomatic relief should not be undervalued. After all, the patient's most immediate concern is usually to feel better, and short-term improvement is the most effective way of ensuring that the patient returns for follow-up consultations, where underlying issues and causative factors can be addressed.

A second visit will normally take place one or two weeks after the first and will nearly always be shorter in duration. Herbal treatment can vary from days to years, depending on the nature of the patient's health problems. As in other holistic health-care modalities, there is an emphasis on actively involving the patient in their treatment and healing process, rather than being a passive recipient of a treatment prescribed by the practitioner. The practitioner's role as educator and motivator is important in encouraging the patient to take responsibility for their own health. This approach is a core tenet of the therapeutic relationship in holistic medicine, and it contrasts with the rather more paternalistic relationship between doctor and patient that traditionally has prevailed in conventional western medicine. Another characteristic of holistic medicine is the emphasis on prevention, and this approach is incorporated into herbal practice whenever possible.

The herbal treatment

Herbal treatment is characterised by the fact that it is tailored to the specific needs of the individual patient. Therefore, two patients with the same medical diagnosis would rarely be given identical herbal treatments. For example, two patients may present with osteoarthritis; one may also suffer from frequent digestive upsets while the other is experiencing bouts of anxiety. Although the herbal medicines aimed at treating the osteoarthritis may be the same for both patients, the holistic herbal prescriptions would differ. This emphasis on individualised treatment is often expressed in the maxim 'treat the patient, not the disease'.

In accordance with traditional principles herbal treatment is often supportive and normalising in nature. The body's eliminative functions and the digestive system (including liver function) tend to receive particular attention, reflecting the importance placed on healthy digestion.

A western herbal medicine practitioner will generally prescribe medicines based on their actions rather than their indications. The term 'action' refers to a pharmacological or physiological property (e.g. sedative, diaphoretic or anti-inflammatory), whereas the term 'indication' refers to a condition or disease state for which the medicine can be used (e.g. insomnia, the common cold or tendonitis). This mode of prescribing facilitates a holistic treatment of the patient rather than an exclusive focus on the treatment of their disease.

Herbal medicines are dispensed in a variety of ways. When dispensed by a practitioner the medicine commonly contains extracts of several different herbs. For this reason practitioners tend to favour the use of liquid extracts, which allow for the convenient blending of individualised formulations from single-herb stock extracts in the practitioner's dispensary. In recent years the use of standardised botanical extracts in capsule or tablet form has become increasingly common. These preparations have the advantages of a consistent chemical composition and being easy and convenient to take, although they do not allow the practitioner to make up an individualised formula for the patient. Most western herbal medicine practitioners have a dispensary in their clinic from where the prescription will be made up and dispensed. Dietary advice is also a common part of herbal treatment.

Compliance

Patient compliance is an important issue in herbal therapy, as it is in any other kind of therapy. If the patient does not take the prescribed medicine and follow other recommendations provided, a successful treatment outcome cannot be expected. The use of liquid herbal extracts presents particular challenges in terms of compliance, especially owing to their taste. Patients who are not familiar with herbal medicines may find the strong taste (exacerbated by the alcohol content) a major barrier to compliance. This problem can often be overcome by taking the extract in a little fruit juice. The inconvenience of the medicine being in liquid form can also compromise compliance, especially if the patient is required to take the medicine in the middle of the day. Prescribing a medicine to be taken twice daily (morning and evening) rather than three times daily tends to result in better compliance. The key to good patient compliance is motivation and the setting of attainable goals for the patient. Asking a patient to make drastic and immediate changes to diet and lifestyle is far less likely to succeed than a more long-term plan that involves gradual change. Encouraging the patient to take responsibility and gain control of their own health is also an important strategy to obtain good compliance.

The scope of herbal medicine

The majority of the world's population has access only to traditional, mostly herbal, medicine, so it could be argued that any ailment or disease could be treated with herbal medicine. Some people living in rich industrialised societies, however, have the luxury of being able to choose herbal treatment from a palette of healthcare options which include orthodox modern medicine. In this scenario the different healthcare modalities are complementary to each other, and the selection of one over another is often a matter of personal choice. Without doubt, orthodox medicine is superior for the treatment of many acute and life-threatening conditions. Herbal medicine, however, has much to offer in the treatment and management of a wide range of conditions that do not constitute medical emergencies.

Many common acute illnesses, such as the common cold, influenza, sinusitis, digestive upsets, insomnia, urinary tract infections and menstrual pain, to mention but a few, can be treated successfully by herbal therapy. It is often in the management of chronic conditions, however, that herbal medicine comes into its own. Herbal medicines are generally well tolerated and associated with only minor side effects. This makes them suitable for use in chronic conditions, where long-term treatment is required. In terms of chronic disease it should be emphasised that herbal medicine is unlikely to cure where conventional medicine has failed, but herbal medicine is often highly successful in managing the symptoms of chronic conditions, resulting in improved quality of life for the patient. The holistic approach to health and disease and the focus on individualised treatment makes herbal medicine an excellent option for the management of chronic disease such as elevated cholesterol levels, problems associated with poor circulation, osteoarthritis, non-insulin-dependent (type 2) diabetes, chronic hepatitis, asthma, anxiety, mild to moderate depression, pre-menstrual syndrome, benign prostatic hyperplasia and chronic skin conditions.

The role of herbal medicine in serious or life-threatening conditions is supportive and complementary to conventional medicine. Herbal medicine cannot substitute for insulin in diabetes, anti-viral drugs in HIV/AIDS or chemotherapy in cancer. What herbal medicine can offer in these conditions is improved quality of life through amelioration of secondary symptoms and side effects of pharmaceutical drugs. Needless to say, only experienced practitioners should treat patients with these conditions, and wherever possible it should be done in concert with the patient's medical practitioner.

Herbal therapy, like any other kind of therapy, has its limits and a well-trained and experienced practitioner is aware of when these limits are being reached. Referral to another health professional may be required, be it a naturopath, counsellor, psychologist, osteopath or medical practitioner. Herbal medicine complements a wide range of other therapeutic interventions, in particular nutritional therapy. In the hands of a skilled practitioner herbal medicine can also be successfully combined with conventional medical treatment, with due attention to the potential for drug interactions between herbal medicines and pharmaceutical drugs. As with any case of patient co-management, a superior treatment outcome can be achieved if all practitioners involved are willing to communicate and cooperate.

Safety issues in herbal medicine

The view held by some that herbal medicines are inherently safe because they are 'natural' is of course false. Nature abounds with very poisonous plants; one only needs to think of a plant like hemlock (*Conium maculatum*), the 'state poison' used for executions in ancient Greece, to be reminded of the power of plant poisons. While many poisonous plants were used in conventional medicine in days gone by, contemporary western herbal medicine does not employ the use of plants with significant toxic potential. In most countries legislation prevents the use of highly toxic plants in herbal medicine.

The safety issue in herbal medicine has a scope that extends far beyond poisonous plants. It includes side effects and other types of adverse reactions, interactions with pharmaceutical drugs, the use of herbal medicines in pregnancy and lactation and a range of issues arising from inadequate quality assurance.

Available evidence suggests that western herbal medicine is very safe. Safety data obtained from clinical trials consistently show that herbal medicines are safe and associated with only mild side effects compared with pharmaceutical drugs (Carraro *et al*. 1996; Woelk 2000). When the number of serious adverse events arising from the use of herbal medicines is related to the number of people in the community using these preparations one can only conclude that the risk associated with herbal medicines is minimal (Barrett *et al*. 1999). Given that adverse reactions arising from herbal medicines are less likely to be reported than adverse reactions to pharmaceutical drugs (Barnes *et al*. 1998), the evidence still suggests that herbal medicines are generally safe. Serious but very rare adverse reactions to herbal medicines may be liver toxicity or severe allergic reactions, but most reported adverse events are mild and transient in nature.

Many cases of adverse reactions to herbal medicine arise from a lack of good manufacturing practice rather than as a result of plant toxicity (Drew & Myers 1997). Failure of good manufacturing practice may involve botanical misidentification, substitution, adulteration, contamination (e.g. with micro-organisms or heavy metals), incorrect preparation or incorrect recommended dosage.

Herb–drug interactions

Herbal medicines have the potential to interact with pharmaceutical drugs and modify their pharmacological effects in the body. The opposite is of course equally true: drugs can interact with herbal medicines. Interactions can compromise treatment and can in some cases put the patient at serious risk.

Based on knowledge of the chemical constituents in medicinal plants it is possible to hypothesise about a vast number of potential herb–drug interactions.

The clinical experience suggests, however, that such interactions present less of a problem than could be expected. For this reason it is important to differentiate between *hypothetical interactions*, of which there are many, and *documented interactions*, of which there are relatively few.

Knowledge of herb–drug interactions is still in its infancy and there is no doubt that more cases will be documented in the future. Increased knowledge and documentation of interactions is a positive development for western herbal medicine as it provides for safer and more effective practice. Recent years have seen a marked increase in our understanding of herb–drug interactions, and clinical trials are now being conducted with the specific purpose of investigating potential interactions between herbal medicines and drugs. Currently, the most detailed information about interactions pertains to St John's wort (*Hypericum perforatum*). Extracts of this plant can interact with pharmaceutical drugs through several mechanisms. One of these involves stimulation of drug-metabolising enzymes, resulting in reduced bioavailability and efficacy of certain drugs, when these are co-administered with St John's wort (Johne *et al.* 2002).

Herbal medicine in pregnancy, lactation and childhood

In pregnancy, especially during the first three months, the intake of any medicine, be it herbal or conventional, should be minimised as information about the effects on the human foetus is limited. For herbal medicines the knowledge about the safety (or lack thereof) of herbal medicines comes from traditional use, sometimes supplemented with data from animal studies.

The most widely used herbal medicine in pregnancy is probably raspberry (*Rubus idaeus*) leaf, which is considered a facilitator of labour and commonly taken as a tea during the last trimester of pregnancy. While its efficacy remains to be conclusively proven there is nothing to suggest that this use is unsafe.

Morning sickness is a common problem in early pregnancy and herbal medicines such as ginger (*Zingiber officinale*), German chamomile (*Matricaria recutita*) and fennel (*Foeniculum vulgare*) tea have been safely employed to provide relief for centuries.

Many medicinal plants are regarded as unsafe in pregnancy and their use is avoided. Included in this category are plants that present a risk of inducing spontaneous abortion, such as pennyroyal (*Mentha pulegium*) and juniper (*Juniperus communis*). Despite many herbs having been assigned 'abortifacient' properties in the past, no herbal medicine can be used safely and effectively to induce abortion.

In breastfeeding it should be considered that most compounds absorbed by the mother will end up in the breast milk and therefore be ingested by the baby, albeit in lowered concentrations. This is particularly important in newborns, whose ability to

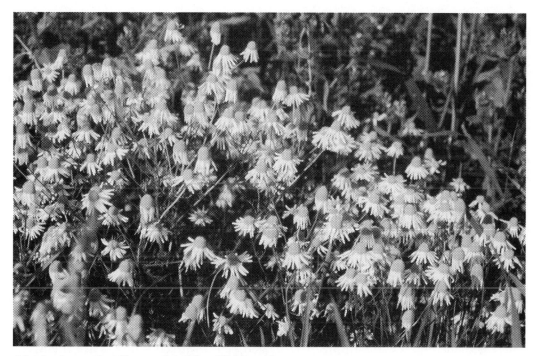

Matricaria recutita (Chamomile) (Hans Wohlmuth)

metabolise and excrete foreign compounds is incompletely developed (Bryant *et al.* 2003). In general, western herbal medicine is well suited to the treatment of children. Qualified practitioners select mild-acting herbs dispensed in appropriate doses, to which children tend to respond extremely well.

Conclusion

Contemporary western herbal medicine has evolved from an ancient system of traditional medicine dating back more than 2000 years, to the time of Hippocrates. As the discipline evolved, it benefited from numerous influences. Major early influences were Greek and Roman medicine followed by Central European and British herbal traditions. The eighteenth and nineteenth centuries saw the incorporation of many medicinal plants of North American origin, knowledge of which was mostly gleaned from North American indigenous peoples.

During the latter part of the twentieth century science played an increasing role in the development of the major herbal traditions, including western herbal medicine. Although this has led to concerns about the future of herbal medicine in some sections of the herbal profession, it also promises to make the practice of herbal medicine increasingly evidence-based in terms of both safety and efficacy. This, combined with the persistent demand for a range of natural healthcare options by a large section of the community, has seen herbal medicine move towards becoming an accepted part of mainstream healthcare in many western countries in recent years.

This move towards the mainstream brings with it new challenges. Preserving a holistic approach to health and disease is paramount if herbal medicine is to survive as a distinct medical system. The increasingly scientific approach must be employed in a way that prevents the herbal medicine of the future from becoming conventional medicine practised with plant-based pharmaceuticals. Science has immense potential to further the use and acceptance of herbal medicine, but it must be applied in a manner that respects the holistic philosophy so crucial to the successful practice of herbal medicine.

Quality control is another area that presents itself as a challenge for the future. Complex natural products such as herbal medicines pose inherent problems in terms of quality and safety, and the herbal medicine industry must successfully address these problems if herbal medicine is to become a viable part of mainstream healthcare in the future.

The continuing development of herbal medicine relies heavily on research. Research is expensive, and it is more difficult to protect intellectual property relating to herbal medicines than pharmaceutical drugs. This in turn makes it harder for the herbal industry to recuperate its investments in research and development, and adequate funding for future herbal medicine research will require financial commitments from both industry and governments.

Herbal medicine is already responding to these new challenges, and the resurgent interest in plants as medicines from the public, healthcare professionals and scientists leaves little doubt that herbal medicine will take its rightful place in the medicine of the future.

Recommended reading

Chevalier, A. 1996, *Encyclopedia of Medicinal Plants*, Dorling Kindersley Ltd, London.

Eldin, S. and Dunford, A. 1999, *Herbal Medicine in Primary Care*, Butterworth-Heinemann, Oxford.

Ernst, E. (ed.) 2000, *Herbal Medicine—A Concise Overview for Professionals*, Butterworth-Heinemann, Oxford.

Griggs, B. 1997, *New Green Pharmacy—The Story of Western Herbal Medicine*, Vermillion, London.

Mills, S. and Bone, K. 2000, *Principles and Practice of Phytotherapy*, Churchill Livingstone, Edinburgh.

11

Homœopathy
Ian Howden

Homœopathy presents a major challenge to conventional science and medicine. It is almost diametrically positioned in relation to contemporary wisdom as it uses as medicine solutions that are diluted to a point beyond that which is measurable by normal scientific means. Even though conventional science cannot explain homœopathic principles in theoretical terms, the practical evidence of its efficacy is manifestly present. Homœopathy numbers among the most popular therapeutic systems in the world, owing largely to a long homœopathic tradition in India. Although scientific and medical research cannot adequately account for the success of homœopathy, there is a large body of clinically based evidence in support of this therapeutic approach.

As at 2003 there have been more than 240 clinical trials conducted in a range of countries to substantiate homœopathy's clinical effects (Linde & Melchart 1988; Kleijnen *et al.* 1991; Reilly *et al.* 1994; Linde *et al.* 1997; Jacobs 2002). Furthermore homœopathy is today an integral part of natural and complementary medicine as it is practised traditionally in Australia and much of Europe and North America. Consequently, homœopathy is now institutionalised in tertiary settings in Australia and many other countries. Homœopathy is therefore a rich field, not only for scientists, who may well yet find scientific explanations for the 'minimum' dose, but also for the medical profession in general.

Homœopathy is a distinct approach to therapeutics that stands apart from all other modalities in terms of its depth and breadth. It offers a rational, holistic, vitalistic and safe alternative based on simple principles and a very clear methodology. This chapter presents an introductory overview of homœopathy. It reviews the field of homœopathy—its history, philosophy and practice—and describes the fundamental importance of homœopathic principles in the development and practice of western medicine today.

Early history

From Hippocrates to Hahnemann

Homœopathy is based on a principle that has underpinned the western medical tradition for as long as that tradition has existed. It is centred around the principle that 'like cures like'—first found in the works of Hippocrates (Hippocrates 1952) around 400 BCE. This principle has often re-emerged in the development of western medical tradition since that time, particularly in the work of Galen (Hippocrates 1952) and Paracelsus (Hartmann 1973), and most particularly in the writings of Samuel Hahnemann at the end of the eighteenth century (Hahnemann 1880, 1896, 1990, 1996).

Samuel Hahnemann (1755–1843) was an eminent German physician, academic and linguist before he abandoned his medical practice and developed his new therapeutic method which he called homœopathy. The name was derived from the Greek *homoios* (like) and *patheia* (suffering)—therefore 'similar suffering'—and was based on this same principle that 'like cures like'.

Hahnemann interpreted this law of 'similars' to mean that a substance can cure those conditions it is capable of causing, and he devoted a large proportion of his life to 'proving' substances of nature. By 'proving' is meant that Hahnemann devised a carefully controlled set of protocols to enable the 'symptoms' of a substance to be deduced from their toxicological effects when ingested by healthy subjects. For example, when the plant deadly nightshade (*Belladonna atropa*) is ingested in sufficient quantity the symptoms produced will always be violent, including the intensity of its fever, its thirst and its hallucinations. And this same *Belladonna* is capable of curing similarly violent symptoms when it is administered in a homœopathically appropriate dose.

Hahnemann documented the causative properties of a range of substances, some of which were previously unknown to therapeutics. These 'provings', when published in his homœopathic *Materia Medica* (Hahnemann 1880), formed the basis for the development of homœopathic materia medica, a development that has continued unabated to this day.

The time of the development of homœopathy coincided with the period that is often referred to as 'the Enlightenment'. This period in the late eighteenth century was a time when reason and scientific rigour had become more culturally widespread and was applied to all manner of pursuits. Hahnemann, too, was concerned to document his methodology as an expression of reason and scientific rigour, and so it is strange that homœopathy is sometimes characterised as 'unscientific'. It is quite clear that Hahnemann's prime motivation in developing his new art was to develop a system of medicine that was rationally based (see Hahnemann 1990), in sharp contrast to the *ad hoc* therapeutic approaches being used in the medicine of his day. He felt that bloodletting, leaching and crude forms of surgery were unsatisfactory forms of therapy and he was intent on developing a methodology to enable the safe and effective application of the principle that 'like cures like'.

Provings

Hahnemann was particularly interested in the work of Dr William Cullen (1712–90) that centred on the use of Peruvian bark (*Cinchona officinalis*) in the treatment of malarial fever. Cullen had suggested that the herb's value lay in its bitter yellow juice which, in the light of the ancient Doctrine of Signatures, he understood to resemble bile. Hahnemann was keen to distance himself from the Doctrine of Signatures and to embrace the new scientific methods in his development of a rational system of medicine. He suspected a relationship between medicine and cure that was to prove even more groundbreaking. Accordingly, he abandoned his practice of the conventional medicine of the times and embarked upon a time of careful experimentation on himself using the juice of the Peruvian bark. The results of these experiments proved seminal in the development of modern homœopathy.

As a result of his experimentation, Hahnemann found that the ingestion of sufficient quantities of this Peruvian bark juice produced in him symptoms very similar to those of the malarial fever for which it was known to be of great therapeutic benefit. And so began his series of planned 'provings' using a range of substances (some of which were new to therapeutics) which he began using on close colleagues, friends and family. His endeavour was to develop a methodology to test his newly discovered hypothesis that like can be cured by like—*similia similibus curentur*.

Until recently homœopathy has relied almost entirely on information collected from 'provings' along with limited reports of toxicological data and data from accidental poisonings for the development of its materia medica. Since the closing years of the twentieth century, however, the homœopathic journals indicate an increasing awareness of the potential shortcomings of 'provings' as the sole means available to determine the curative potential of homœopathic preparations. In developing an understanding of homœopathic materia medica the modern homœopath is encouraged to look in all possible directions, including towards natural science, to find more about the 'peculiar features' of substances.

Decimal and centesimal potencies

In order to limit the possible iatrogenic effects of his medicines, Hahnemann developed a method called *potentisation* (Hahnemann 1996) by which a substance is serially diluted by taking one part of a given solution and adding it to a water and/or alcohol solution. Concentrations of 1:10 are simply referred to as decimal potencies (denoted by the letter X) and concentrations of 1:100 as centesimal potencies (denoted by the letter C). Between each step of dilution the container holding the substance is struck firmly (succussed) against a solid but 'giving' object (often a leather bound book) to release the energy of the substance into the diluted mixture. Hahnemann claimed that this process of succussion had the effect of increasing the 'potency' of the substance despite the increased dilution. He used this process to make potencies up to 30C (equivalent to one part of the therapeutic substance to 10^{60} parts of water) or even 200C (equivalent to one part of the therapeutic substance to 10^{400} parts of water).

With substances which are insoluble in water or alcohol Hahnemann advised that the mixture should be ground with pure lactose in a porcelain mortar and pestle until it reaches a concentration of 1:1 000 000 (i.e. $1:10^6$), by which time, he hypothesised, all substances are soluble in water. The process of dilution and succussion is then continued as required.

Hahnemann developed this methodology through six editions of his *Organon of the Medical Art* (Hahnemann 1990) and two editions of his *Chronic Diseases* (Hahnemann 1896), spanning some 27 years. Over that time his general approach changed radically, particularly in relation to all aspects of posology, that is, in relation to issues of potency, dosage and frequency. However, through all his struggles to develop a simple and replicable approach he always remained firm as to the absolute centrality of the principle that 'like cures like' to sound therapeutics. In this Hahnemann continued an established tradition going back at least to Hippocrates.

Indications for homœopathy

Hahnemann placed all disease within the therapeutic reaches of homœopathy. Whether diseases are acute or chronic, including those diseases resulting from the inherited effects of what he called the chronic 'miasms' (explained later in this chapter), homœopathy can deal with them. The only condition for the use of Hahnemannian homœopathy is that it must be possible to match the dominant disease symptoms of the patient, as they are manifested via the physical, mental and emotional signs and symptoms of the patient (often called a 'diagnosis'), with a range of carefully documented toxicological effects of an appropriate elemental, plant or animal substance (often called a 'proving').

The legacy of James Tyler Kent

By the fifth edition of the *Organon* in 1833 Hahnemann had expounded the fundamental principles and tenets on which the philosophy and practice of homœopathy could be developed. His therapeutic approach is best described as 'watch and wait' and his preference was for low to medium centesimal potencies administered in water. It was this fifth edition of the *Organon* (Hahnemann 1996) that found its way to Dr James Tyler Kent in America later in the nineteenth century. It was thus on this philosophical base that North American homœopathy developed and became quite different from the system developed in Europe by Hahnemann.

The first way the theoretical approaches of Hahnemann and Kent differed is in terms of what has since been referred to as 'constitutional' prescribing. To

Hahnemann's 'acute' and 'chronic' diseases Kent added a 'constitutional' picture of the patient. He suggested that the remedy being sought should be appropriate to a disease picture which encompasses the patient's disease history as well as their known predispositions and allergies, the pattern of their life disease and particularly the broad emotional and mental patterns that are often evident in a person's life (Kent 1995). It was Kent who first directed homœopathy towards archetypal patterns found in all of nature. It is to Kent's notion of constitutional type that we can trace the range of theoretical approaches to materia medica and case taking which have arisen in homœopathy particularly since the 1970s. The more recent influences of contemporary homœopaths such as Sankaran, Scholten, Vermeulen and Whitmont have been revolutionary in the development of western homœopathy, but even greater was the influence of James Tyler Kent in the 1850s in introducing this concept of constitutional archetypes.

The other way in which Hahnemann and Kent differed was in their experimental approaches to the use of ultra-high potencies. Whereas Hahnemann had assumed a therapeutic limit to the effective action of the higher homœopathic potencies (particularly 200C and above), Kent was willing and eager to experiment well beyond the 30th and 200th centesimal potencies predominantly used by Hahnemann. Kent recognised the power of the highest potencies (Kent 1995) and wrote of the dangers of the homœopathic aggravation: 'I'd rather be in a room with a dozen [people] slashing with razors than in the hands of an incompetent prescriber of high potencies' (Kent 1975: 526).

On the other side of the Atlantic Hahnemann had also experimented with the power of different potencies. Hahnemann's response to the dilemma posed by the potential aggravation resulting from repeated dosing, particularly with the higher potencies, was to develop the milder 50 millesimal potencies which are discussed later in this chapter.

The fundamental principles of homœopathy

Hahnemann isolated three major principles on which he based his new therapeutic system. These principles, which he developed during the writing of the six editions of his *Organon of the Medical Art* (Hahnemann 1990) between the years 1806 and 1823, are discussed below.

The law of similars—like cures like—*similia similibus curantur*

The implication of this 'law of similars' is that a substance is capable of 'curing' precisely those conditions that it is also capable of causing. This principle, which is much older than homœopathy, has also been recognised well beyond the bounds set by homœopathy. For example, Nicholas Culpeper, a founding father of modern herbal medicine, wrote in the seventeenth century:

> Neither is there any better remedy under the sun for the bite of a viper . . . than the head of the viper that bit you, bruised and applied to the place, and the flesh eaten, you need not eat more than a dram at a time . . . Neither any comparable to the stinging of bees and wasps etc. than the same that stung you, bruised and applied to the place (Culpeper 1995: 356).

This is indeed a well-worn principle.

The law of the minimum dose—potentising

Hahnemann was aware that even when toxic substances are used for therapeutic purposes they will inevitably leave drug residues in the body. These residues, which are known in orthodox western medicine as the 'iatrogenic' effects of a substance, are themselves capable of altering the health of the patient. They are still today recognised as being responsible for a large number of the diseases treated in modern hospitals. Hahnemann was keen to reduce these drug-related side effects while retaining the curative (causative) effects of the substance. To this end he developed potentisation, the process of serial dilution and succussion, so that a minimum dose of a medicine was possible.

Science continues to struggle to either verify or disprove the efficacy of this process of dilution, succussion and trituration. Avogadro's number suggests that there are unlikely to be any molecules of the original substance beyond a dilution of $1:10^{23}$—equivalent to the twelfth centesimal potency (12C) or the 24th decimal potency (24X) (Baker 2002). Since homœopathic preparations are frequently used in the 30th (30C which represents a dilution of $1:10^{60}$), 200th (200C—$1:10^{400}$) and 1000th (M—$1:10^{2000}$) centesimal potencies and beyond, the dilutions might not be expected to register any atoms of the diluted substance. Something has been transmitted nonetheless as evidenced in the numerous clinical trials referred to earlier. The size of the dilutions achieved from the serial dilution and succussion process involved in the manufacture of homœopathic preparations are so minute that it is still impossible to scientifically verify their existence, let alone their efficacy. As spectrometers and even nuclear magnetic resonance machines are only capable of measuring matter at much lower dilutions, these machines are incapable of proving or disproving the presence of 'energy' in extreme dilutions. It is not yet possible to see or measure the latent power that is apparent when an appropriate homœopathic preparation is administered according to sound homœopathic principles.

As mentioned, Hahnemann is reported to have mainly used therapeutic substances at dilutions of up to the 30C potency although some accounts suggest that he may have experimented up to the 200C potency (Haehl 1985). Certainly he intimated that, in his opinion, the increase in therapeutic power that he postulated occurs with increasing potency must at some point come to an end (Hahnemann 1896). In North America James Tyler Kent experimented with much higher potencies and found that not only did they work but they also often overstimulated the system and caused considerable aggravation of the condition. By 'aggravation' is meant any exacerbation of the patient's condition that can be directly attributed to the administration of a therapeutic substance. These differences in opinion over the effects of different potencies remain unresolved.

A general principle of homœopathy suggests that the 'finer' diseases (particularly those affecting the mind and the emotions) will respond well to higher homœopathic potencies. Higher potencies would generally be understood to include the 200C potency and above. This must of course be weighed against the further observation that the highest potencies may well result in stronger aggravations as the remedy 'takes hold', particularly when administered to those of sensitive disposition. It was due to the severity of some aggravations from even the lower potencies that Hahnemann developed the '50 millesimal potencies'—his 'new perfected' potencies, which he introduced in the sixth edition of the *Organon* (Hahnemann 1990: 219). This radically different and 'perfected' approach to potency enables high levels of dilution of the therapeutic material but with far fewer successions—and therefore far less 'energising'.

The 50 millesimal potencies require serial dilution and trituration only to the $1:10^6$ dilution, followed by a one-off dilution and succussion, essentially of 1 part to 50 000. Hahnemann instructed that this mixture (LM1) be taken as required in water, with the medicine bottle being succussed between doses. These potencies could be taken up to the LM30. By this means Hahnemann was attempting to retain the 'curative' properties of the substance while limiting the unpleasant (and potentially dangerous) aggravations. It is evident that Hahnemann intended the 50 millesimal potencies (which were not available to Kent) as a replacement for the decimal and centesimal potencies of the earlier editions of the *Organon*. However, the sixth edition, in which they were introduced, was not published in English until 90 years after his death and was not verified as to its authenticity until late in the twentieth century (Schmidt 1994). It remains to be seen whether this work will change the basis of current practice.

Even 'classical' homœopaths of the early twenty-first century are therefore faced with a range of legitimate approaches to posology. Whether the substance becomes stronger or weaker at sub-Avogadro levels of dilution and succussion continues to be a subject of research, but homœopathic clinical practice adequately confirms that therapeutic action occurs when remedies are administered according to Hahnemannian guidelines, even in the tiniest doses. Although different philosophical 'streams' of homœopaths will disagree as to the efficacy of ultra-high and ultra-low potencies, the safety of homœopathic preparations when they are administered with care is acknowledged generally.

The law of the single remedy

Hahnemann taught the value of using single homœopathic substances for the treatment of sick human beings. Such substances are called *simplex* remedies and are each manufactured from a single substance which has been 'proved' on healthy human beings in order to identify its therapeutic uses (e.g. *Belladonna* 30, *Belladonna* 200, *Sulphur* M). A *complex* remedy, on the other hand, is made from a number of substances combined in a single dose (such as the many homœopathic flu or teething combination remedies that are often available from health food stores and pharmacies). Each constituent of a complex remedy is selected because of the symptoms it exhibits when proved separately. But only the sequential matching of substance to symptoms that is made possible with a simplex remedy enables a truly safe and maximally therapeutic effect.

Hering's law of direction of cure

Constantine Hering was another key figure in the developmental stage of homœopathy. Although his 'law of the direction of cure' is really not the exclusive property of homœopathy, it is homœopathy that has particularly emphasised its therapeutic value. This 'law' states that cure takes place:

- **from within outwards;**
- **from above downwards;**
- **from the more important organs to the less important organs; and**
- **that symptoms disappear in the reverse order of their appearance.**

It is interesting that although this 'law' is named after Constantine Hering, the primary source for it seems to be nowhere to be found in his collected writings. Although this is a set of guidelines rather than of rigid rules, it provides valuable signposts after the administration of a homœopathic potency which enable the practitioner to trace changes in disease symptoms. It also enables the homœopath to check the progress of the disease to determine whether or not apparent changes are due to the operation of the remedy or because the disease is continuing unabated. The guidelines provided by Hering often give the homœopath the confidence to leave an illness largely unmedicated.

Diagnosis and 'repertorising'

Miasmatic theory

Much chronic disease is at least partly dependent on the inherited predispositions of the patient. The homoeopathic theory relating to inheritance is called 'miasmatic theory', although on this subject not all homœopaths share a common understanding. J.H. Allen usefully defined a miasm as any force that is engrafted upon a patient making them more liable to every disease that comes along. He suggested that in treating disease, understanding miasms enables an intelligent approach to the problem (Allen, J.H. 1910).

Samuel Hahnemann recognised three main inherited miasms that he named the Sycotic miasm (characterised by over-absorption), the Leuetic miasm (characterised by under-absorption) and Psora (broadly characterised by skin diseases and distorted function). Hahnemann alluded to a possible fourth, the tubercular, or pseudo-psoric, miasm, and this was confirmed by H.C. Allen in *The Materia Medica of the Nosodes* (Allen, H.C. 1910). More recently Leon Vannier (1955) has suggested a fifth, the oncotic or canceric miasm.

Many contemporary homœopaths speculate about other miasms resulting, for example, from the residues from petrochemical products or from the wide range of rays to which human beings are nowadays exposed (e.g. radio, TV, microwave, X-ray, electricity). Yet others suggest further possible 'taints' resulting even from the recent genetic manipulation of food, animals and people.

Case taking

Hahnemann documented a step-by-step approach to the accurate collection of the details of the disease. Although he was particularly detailed in his instructions as to how to take a case his intention was clear. He was in search of an accurate picture of the patient that would enable comparison with the information documented in provings. In Aphorism 83 of the *Organon* Hahnemann concluded that: 'this individualising examination of a case of disease . . . demands of the [practitioner] only impartiality, sound senses, attentive observation, and faithfulness in recording the disease picture' (Hahnemann 1990: 130). His methodology required that the practitioner ask undirected questions to enable the patient to tell their story in their own words, only prompting when absolutely necessary. The twentieth century has added many valuable resources to supplement the invaluable guidelines provided by Hahnemann in taking an accurate case (e.g. Kaplan 2001).

Hahnemann summarised his approach to case taking in Aphorism 104 where he stated that 'once the totality of the symptoms that principally determine and distinguish the disease case—in other words the image of the disease—has been exactly recorded, the most difficult work is done' (Hahnemann 1990: 141). By this he meant that once the pattern of disease has been accurately mapped, all that remains is to match that disease picture to a remedy picture found in a homœopathic materia medica.

Repertorising

The 'symptoms' of each homœopathic preparation as they are identified in the provings are recorded in homœopathic repertories. Each symptom, called a rubric when it is recorded in a repertory, is listed according to the part of the body it affects or the nature of the pain it causes. Over 110 repertories are now available, ranging from the first one developed by Benninghausen (Boger 1983) to the most recent, Prisma (Vermeulen 2002), and the many computerised versions continuing to enter the market.

The painstaking task of finding each symptom in the repertory is a mechanical process to narrow down the range of possible remedies from which to make a choice of 'similimum' for each patient. The similimum is the homœopathic substance whose symptoms as manifested in the provings best reflect the symptoms of the disease as manifested in the patient. In acute disease this process is somewhat simplified. The homœopath is interested to find a 'four-legged stool', that is, a remedy which has at least four major symptoms in its provings which match four major symptoms of the patient's acute disease symptoms. In more chronic and constitutionally based pre-scribing, however, the process is more complex, requiring a wider range of symptoms to be sought and matched, and it will often require the assistance of some form of repertorising.

Repertorising does not, in itself, determine the homœopathic preparation to be administered. At its best, repertorising is a very valuable quantitative procedure to narrow down the range of possible therapeutic substances indicated for the treatment of any disease condition. The mechanical nature of this process lends itself well to computerisation and the early twenty-first century has witnessed the development of a number of user-friendly and comprehensive computer programs to assist in the mechanical task of repertorising.

Once a case has been repertorised the homœopath must decide between the major indicated remedies. This choice can only be made by a person who is skilled in case taking and the homœopathic materia medica. To this person, the professional homœopath, falls the task of choosing an appropriate remedy, potency and frequency from the plethora of information about both person and remedy.

Homœopathy in the twentieth century and beyond

It was not until the latter part of the twentieth century that medical science began to realise that the destruction of viruses and bacteria is only one possible way to respond to the germ theory. Holistic therapies such as homœopathy have emerged in response to the demand for a therapeutic approach that best enables the treatment of the 'whole' human being. With the emergence of the germ theory of disease in the early twentieth century and the subsequent development of antibiotics and penicillin and their promise to 'stop disease in its tracks', disciplines such as homœopathy with its concentration on 'holism' and its acknowledgement of a 'vital force' soon lost favour in the fast industrialising West. By using drugs to kill the invading bacteria (later they were also repetitively used by many doctors to try to treat viruses), orthodox medicine hoped and expected that the accompanying 'disease' would also recede. Unfortunately the theory did not take account of the iatrogenic effects of these new drugs themselves or of the possible inadequacies of purely symptomatic prescribing, and today homœopathy is again considered by many to be an effective treatment in a wide range of disease.

The story of western homœopathy between the time of James Tyler Kent and the resurgence of interest in homœopathy in the latter half of the twentieth century is so rich with famous British, European, North American and Indian names that it is possible to single out only a few for special mention. To the outsider much of this period may appear to be a latent stage of homœopathic development. In fact an enormous amount of important work, particularly in the understanding of homœopathic materia medica, occurred during this time. Many new provings were conducted and a great deal of information was added to the growing store of homœopathic knowledge. The books by homœopathic historian Julian Winston (1999, 2001) provide an invaluable guide to the depth of homœopathic philosophy and literature in the period from 1810 to the Second World War. This was a time when the foundations were laid to enable the demand for this sound, rational therapeutic system to grow exponentially in the period from the Second World War to the early twenty-first century.

After the Second World War there was a gradual resurgence in interest in the homœopathic principle. In this environment, where increasing numbers of the public realised that disease and health are integral parts of an holistic concept, homœopathy blossomed. George Vithoulkas made perhaps the most valuable contribution to this re-emergence by explaining the logic of homœopathy to a mass audience and by highlighting the importance of the mental and emotional realms in understanding the evidence base of any therapeutic approach (Vithoulkas 1989). Once Vithoulkas published *The Science of Homœopathy* in 1973, the way was opened for a number of authors in a wide range of disciplines to add their weight to the growing body of scientific evidence that was accumulating in support of the homœopathic principles. Contemporary homœopathy is premised on the idea that a person is an integrated being arising from an interrelationship between body, mind, soul and spirit. The success of homœopathy depends on the ability of natural practitioners to recognise the interconnectedness between all aspects of a person. This translates into a principle of treating the 'whole' person.

In the early twenty-first century a variety of applications of the law of similars are being trialled throughout the world in search of boundaries to the therapeutic possibilities of the homœopathic principle. For example, Jan Scholten, a contemporary Dutch chemist and homœopath, has explored ways to understand the curative properties of metals, minerals, compounds and salts by understanding their place in the Atomic Table of Numbers (Scholten 1993, 1997). More recently he has turned his attention to exploring the homœopathicity of many herbs by understanding the botanical family to which they belong. Scholten (and a range of other contemporary homœopaths) are exploring archetypal patterns which manifest in the mineral, plant and animal kingdoms, particularly through provings, since these patterns also manifest in human beings as disease.

The sources of remedies

Samuel Hahnemann documented a method by which a homœopathic preparation can be manufactured from a very wide range of natural products (Hahnemann 1990). For example, the source may be a herbal tincture, for example *Belladonna* (deadly nightshade), *Pulsatilla* (pasque flower) or *Viscum album* (mistletoe); an element or compound like sulphur (pure flowers of sulpha), mercury (soluble mercury) or calcium carbonate (pure lime); an animal product, for example *Apis* (honey-bee), Lac caninum (dog's milk) or Ambra grisea (secretion of the whale); or even from lesser understood substances such as X-rays, diamond or uranium. In fact any substance of the natural world may yield a remedy.

More recently the type of remedy called nosodes has been prepared from diseased human tissue or its by-product (e.g. Morbilinum is made from the secretions of the measles pustule while Parotidinum is made from the secretion of the parotid gland in mumps). Although Hahnemann identified the miasms and their effects on the human being in chronic disease, he in fact counselled against the use of human disease products themselves in the treatment of human beings (Hahnemann 1990: 99—footnote).

Some homœopaths also use sarcodes, remedies manufactured from healthy tissue purportedly to strengthen similar diseased tissue, while others use remedies called 'tautopathic' preparations, often manufactured from orthodox pharmaceutical drugs (e.g. penicillin, the oral contraceptive pill or aspirin), to treat allergic reactions to those drugs. Remedies manufactured from substances known for their allergenic effects on sensitive human beings (e.g. house dust, mould), called 'isopathic' preparations, are used by some homœopaths to treat allergic reactions to those substances, although Hahnemann suggested the use of a *similar* substance rather than the allergen itself to treat such conditions. All of these preparations are capable of manufacture to dilutions unverifiable by the most sensitive modern scientific equipment.

Clinical trials and research

The need to provide scientific legitimacy for homœopathy and the resultant search for 'mechanism' have seen a dramatic rise in the conduct of clinical trials in the past 30 years, often comparing the use of a homœopathic potency against a placebo. Many of these trials have been designed to test the efficacy of the law of similars, while many others seek to understand further the action of the higher centesimal potencies. In order to satisfy the requirements of natural science, the majority of these trials have also been double blind, with cross-over design and placebo controls. Many homœopaths are not satisfied that the clinical trial provides an adequate format to test effectively the outcomes of homœopathic therapy, with its extended consultations and individualised prescriptions.

Since the early 1970s there have been over 240 clinical trials undertaken to test the efficacy of homœopathic preparations. Although many of these trials have been published in peer-reviewed medical journals, few have been the subject of statistically significant independent replication. Of the three major meta-analyses undertaken to date, one published in the *British Medical Journal* in 1991 (Kleijnen *et al.* 1991) and the other two in *The Lancet* (Linde & Melchart 1988; Linde *et al.* 1997), all concluded that, although many of the trials conducted have been of low methodological quality, the results are generally positive when comparing the results from administering a homœopathic preparation and a placebo. Reilly's study of random controlled trials published in *The Lancet* came to very similar conclusions (Reilly *et al.* 1994).

Clearly there is a need for more rigorous research to test the clinical relevance of the homœopathic principles. The race is on to independently replicate previous trials, in full realisation that once a statistically significant replication has been achieved, the way is then clear for further studies to proceed to test mechanism, various potencies and frequency of dose.

Among other methods being trialled for research into the efficacy of homœopathic practice are '*n* at 1' trials, whereby a large number of single-patient trials are compared. Similarly, whole-practice research concentrates on the results from the entire therapeutic experience rather than isolating the effects of the remedy for particular scrutiny. These methods hold particular promise at this point and, in this regard, contemporary homœopaths may also stand to benefit more broadly from the social sciences and other empirically based studies of human behaviour. A major stumbling block for homœopathy in the twenty-first century is that high-quality research is very expensive to undertake. Although some moves are underway to patent individual homœopathic potencies it is unlikely that research into homœopathy will generate any significant profits in the foreseeable future.

Radionics and other black boxes

Since the early nineteenth century when Korsakov proposed a means of potentisation that enabled the same bottle to be used through all potencies, various technological innovations have been developed to enhance the manufacture of homœopathic potencies, to assist in the diagnosis of the patient or the disease and to simplify the process of repertorising. Perhaps the most contentious technologies have been in the field of electronic diagnosis, where information from a range of sources can be used to diagnose and to determine a supposedly 'appropriate' remedy, and in radionics, whereby many practitioners now 'manufacture' their homœopathic potencies by means of an electronic box. Such technologies have flourished since the 1970s and are not confined to homœopathic application.

While no definitive opinion can be proffered regarding the effects of radionically prepared remedies or electronic diagnosis, the methods do not satisfy Hahnemann's criteria nor have they been accepted by any of the classical figures through homœopathic history. They cannot therefore be legitimately seated under the banner of homœopathy.

Homœopathy and the medical community

Naturopathy

Naturopathic philosophy as it is practised in the western world in the twenty-first century centres on principles such as vitalism, first do no harm, removal of the cause and holism. No naturopathic modality is better placed than homœopathy to address each of these principles.

Vitalism is that principle whereby practitioners endeavour to draw upon the 'vital energy' of the being in order to effect cure, rather than concentrate on the mere removal of individual symptoms. Central to Hahnemann's treatise was an understanding of what, since the work of Stahl in 1707, has been called the 'vital force' (Steiner 1985: 113), a term which aligns homœopathy with the tradition of vitalism that is as old as history.

Similarly the 'minimum doses' resulting from Hahnemann's process of potentisation were developed by Hahnemann and then later by Kent, to address the issues of safety that are also central to naturopathy.

Orthodox medicine

Western orthodox medicine is regularly confronted, in its own practice, by the 'scientific' application of the law of similars. Orthodox vaccinations, oncology, desensitisation therapies, hormesis—all have brought this principle into legitimate mainstream contention. The formal relationship between homœopathic practice and orthodox medicine varies radically between countries. In some countries (e.g. much of Europe) the homœopathic principle is integral to many orthodox medical practices while in other countries the relationship is often more tenuous.

In North America, for example, the right to use homœopathic potencies is enshrined in the US Constitution. Yet the history of the American Medical Association has been closely connected with many attempts to limit the popularity of homœopathy (Coulter 1994). In many Asian countries (particularly India) the relative cheapness of homœopathic potencies makes this form of therapy predominant. In Australia, although non-medical homœopathy predominates, the demands of the marketplace of the twenty-first century are requiring that more medical and pharmaceutical practitioners undertake professional homœopathic training. Dentistry and veterinary science are also experiencing a resurgence in the demand for a therapeutic approach to disease and therapy which is based on sound homœopathic principles.

Limitations of treatment and the need for referral

Theoretically the limitations presented by a homœopathic approach to disease are defined only by the skill of the practitioner. If a substance of nature is available which is capable of causing the totality of the disease symptoms being experienced by the patient, homœopathic philosophy would predict that a potency prepared from that substance would be capable of strengthening the body's opposition to that disease. In practice, however, the modern homœopath is often confronted by a confusing array of symptoms sometimes based on inherited predisposition, cause and suppression, not to mention a minefield of legal requirements that change from country to country and often from state to state. Referral is often necessary, either because of the complexity of the case or because of the limited experience of the practitioner, even in cases where there are no obvious legal or therapeutic impediments to treatment.

Classical homœopaths strive to treat the patient with a single therapeutic substance. They are also generally unwilling to use any therapeutic modality other than homœopathy. Little research has been conducted on the possible pharmacological interactions between homœopathic preparations and, for example, herbal medicines, acupuncture or even orthodox medical drugs. It is inadvisable to combine any therapeutic modalities unless the possible interactions between the modalities are well understood.

Conclusion

Hahnemann developed an entirely new methodology in the early nineteenth century, with its novel approaches, particularly in relation to case taking, remedy preparation, the proving of therapeutic substances and his development of a theory of the miasmic nature of chronic disease. The principle on which this new therapy was based—that like cures like—has been central to human philosophies throughout antiquity. The legacy of Hahnemann to medical science has been to provide a new detailed methodology following rational, holistic, vitalistic, safe and replicable lines to test this age-old principle of disease and its cure.

Although the jury is still out on the mechanisms by which homœopathic substances exert their action, this discipline has proved itself to be capable of withstanding rigorous and intensive scrutiny and research. The works of many great homœopaths in the latter part of the twentieth and early twenty-first centuries, such as Whitmont, Scholten, Vermeulen and Sankaran, and researchers such as Eskinazi, Schwarz and Russek, Linde *et al.*, Kleijnen *et al.*, Reilly and Jacobs have all helped to ensure that homœopathy continues to grow into the twenty-first century both in its interpretation and in its practice.

Recommended reading

Coulter, H.L. 1994, *Divided Legacy: A History of the Schism in Medical Thought*, 2 vols, Centre for Empirical Medicine, Washington DC.

Hahnemann, S. 1990, *Organon of the Medical Art*, edited and annotated by Wenda Brewster O'Reilly, based on a translation by Steven Decker, Birdcage Books, Redmond, Washington.

Hahnemann, S. 1896, *The Chronic Diseases—Their Peculiar Nature and Homœopathic Cure*, vol. 1, B. Jain, New Delhi.

Kaplan, B. 2001, *The Homœopathic Conversation. The Art of Taking the Case*, Natural Medicine Press, London.

Kent, J.T. 1995, *Lectures on Homœopathic Philosophy*, B. Jain, New Delhi.

Winston, J. 1999, *The Faces of Homœopathy*, Great Auk Publishing, Wellington, New Zealand.

12

Massage therapy
Vicki M. Tuchtan

The art and science of massage therapy is today enjoying a rediscovery. Massage was practised centuries ago by an array of ancient civilisations and physicians and included in ancient shamanic rituals. Nowadays massage therapy is used by many as a pleasurable way to relieve the stresses of modern living and is holding its own in the face of increasing scientific investigation into its worth. This chapter investigates the development of massage therapy throughout the years, defines the modern practice of massage therapy, discusses the effects of and indications for massage therapy and describes some of the research findings surrounding the practice of massage therapy.

> The touch of massage is not simply an ordinary touch or contact of the hand with the body, but is a skilled or professional touch. It is a touch applied with intelligence, with control, with a purpose; and simple as it is, is capable of producing decided physiological effects (J.H. Kellogg 1895).

Massage therapy through the ages

The practice of massage therapy is an ancient healing art that dates back many thousands of years. In ancient times it was believed that demons or evil spirits were often the cause of disease states. Folklore suggests that shamanic healers used magical powers to cleanse the body of such forces and massage often formed a part of many rituals (Calvert 2002). According to Kellogg (1895) an ancient Chinese text, believed to be written around 2700 BCE and describing the system of Kung fu, was probably the foundation stone for today's modern system of massage therapy. Another relevant ancient Chinese text is *The Yellow Emperor's Classic of Internal Medicine*. Believed to date from around the fifth to third centuries BCE, the text was translated into English in 1949 by Ilza Veith. In this translation Veith refers to massage of the skin and flesh as part of the treatment approach for complete paralysis and chills and fever.

Other ancient civilisations believed to have employed massage therapy include the

Egyptians, Indians, Greeks and Romans. Used in conjunction with bathing, the Greeks and Romans enjoyed the luxury and therapeutic worth of massage therapy. The renowned Greek physician Hippocrates, known today as the 'father of medicine', was a significant proponent of massage. He made famous the term rubbing, or *anatripsis*, which he deemed a necessary skill for all physicians of the time (Calvert 2002). Another Greek physician, Asclepiades, completely rejected the medicines of his time and relied solely on the practice of massage in his treatments, believing that massage restored the flow of fluids in the body. In his practice of massage, Asclepiades discovered that through gentle stroking sleep could be induced (Kellogg 1895). Asclepiades went on to establish his own school and was known by his followers as the father of physical medicine (Kamenetz 1980).

Another celebrated physician, Galen, was a prolific writer on the topics of exercise and massage (*c.*130–201 CE). According to Kamenetz (1980) Galen classified the three qualities and quantities of massage as 'firm, moderate and gentle' and 'much, moderate and little' respectively. By combining the qualities with the quantities, Galen described nine different forms of massage therapy, each for different conditions. Having been a student of Hippocrates, Galen was appointed physician to the gladiators of Rome at the age of 28 (Calvert 2002). He was significant in the development of massage therapy during this period; Calvert (2002: 56) comments that 'his writings, as they relate to massage, can be considered as representing five centuries of Greco-Roman anatripsis theory and practice'.

With the fall of the Roman empire the practice of massage therapy was significantly diminished as 'Christianity gradually became a permeating influence, and to reinforce its authority, knowledge that was considered to be heretical or non-Christian was suppressed' (Callaway 2002). Throughout the Middle Ages in Europe, people once again believed that disease states resulted from the invasion of an evil spirit or were the consequence of one's evil thoughts or actions.

Despite what was occurring in Europe, the Arabs continued the practices of the Greeks and Romans. An important text of the time, the *Canon Medicinae*, written by the Arab physician Avicenna (980–1037 CE), promoted the benefits of massage, hydrotherapy and exercise (Calvert 2002; Callaway 2002).

The renaissance of science and medicine in Europe during the fifteenth century saw the resurgence of massage therapy. Late in the fifteenth century a man by the name of Gazius published the work *Florida Corona*, which included a culmination of the ancient writings on massage therapy by authors such as Hippocrates, Galen and Avicenna (Kamenetz 1980). In 1569 the Italian-born Mercurialis (1530–1606) published *De Arte Gymnastica*, described by Kamenetz (1980: 18) as 'the most important book of the century on exercise by a physician'. Although focused largely on exercise, the book does include details of massage therapy based on the work of Galen (Calvert 2002).

Paré (1510–90) was another physician who expounded the positive attributes of physical therapy. He used the terminology described by Galen for the various forms of massage therapy, and applied such techniques for the recovery of surgical patients. Paré is said to have 'recommended vigorous rubbing of the scalp . . . for the treatment of alopecia' (Kamenetz 1980: 19). Over the next 200 years or so physicians advocated the practice of massage therapy for all manners of complaints despite little writing on the practice of massage and even less evidence for the use of massage therapy in such conditions being available. Glisson detailed massage and exercise for the management of rickets, Quellmalz recommended massage for chronic constipation, Tissot advocated friction massage for sprains, Shaw promoted massage for scoliosis and Bonnet prescribed massage for chronic rheumatic disease (Kamenetz 1980).

Modern massage

Kamenetz (1980: 24) states that 'many people date the era of modern massage from the appearance of Estradère's doctoral thesis on the subject' in 1886. Estradère systematically reviewed the literature to date on massage therapy, and described the uses of massage therapy according to the body systems. He provided a classification for the strokes used in the practice of massage therapy, which included frictions, pressure, percussion and other passive, eccentric and concentric movements. Aside from the work of Estradère, significant contributions to modern massage therapy were made by Ling and Mezger (Kamenetz 1980).

Per (Peter) Henrik Ling was born in Sweden in 1776. A man with a talent for poetry, he was a doctor and educator who also had a passion for advocating the rights of the people, including those of women and children. He had a keen interest in physical activity and took up fencing to learn more about human motion. Working with two other Frenchmen, Ling established the Swedish system of exercise, referred to as 'Svenska Gymnastikens' or Swedish Gymnastics (Maanum 1985).

Over the years Ling developed his system further and dedicated himself to teaching it to the masses throughout Sweden. According to Pyves (2001: 175) 'in modern parlance, Ling's original system was a health enhancement program that used massage alongside of exercise and stretching to promote hygiene and prevent illness'. The modern western massage system is based on the Swedish system of wellness developed by Ling. In fact the basic western method of massage is referred to as Swedish massage therapy.

The Dutch physician Johanne Mezger (1839–1909) was a follower of the Swedish system of massage therapy and employed Ling's massage system in his practice. Today the massage therapy strokes utilised for therapeutic intervention are most often classified according to French terminology and it is Mezger who is credited as first using such terms. The major Swedish massage therapy strokes described by Mezger include effleurage, petrissage and tapotement. The descriptions of friction and vibration, as used in massage prior to this time, were also added resulting in the culmination of the five major Swedish massage therapy strokes used today. During the nineteenth and twentieth centuries 'these five core techniques became the foundation of almost every massage and bodywork training throughout the world' (Pyves 2001: 176). The methods pertaining to these core techniques are outlined later in the chapter.

Massage therapy defined

There is no single philosophical basis to massage therapy as each form of massage has its own philosophical principles that underpin practice. Nevertheless, there are unifying beliefs within the massage community. The majority of massage practitioners adopt an approach to treatment that is holistic, one that seeks to address the whole person, taking into consideration the body, mind and soul. This may be reflected in the environment that is created for massage. For example, aromatherapy oils and appropriate music might be employed by the massage therapist to establish an emotionally and spiritually soothing context for the physical work on the tissues of the body.

Intrinsic to most massage treatments is the idea that the client should be proactive in their healing process. Accordingly, and in proportion to their own training, massage therapists will provide information with the aim of empowering the client to take responsibility for their own health. This may simply involve referral to another practitioner. If the massage therapist is trained in corrective exercise prescription, for example, guidance as to a corrective exercise program that may strengthen or stretch appropriate muscles may be provided. Whatever the disposition of the individual therapist, however, a massage treatment will leave the client feeling physically and mentally nurtured. Yet at its most fundamental level massage is a physical therapy.

In 1952, after reviewing the available literature on the subject of massage, Beard (1952) defined massage therapy as that

> used to designate certain manipulations of the soft tissues of the body which are most effectively performed with the hands and are administered for the purpose of producing effects on the nervous and muscular systems, and the local and general circulation of the blood and lymph (Beard 1952: 614).

Since then, massage therapy has been described as the therapeutic manipulation of the muscles and associated soft tissue of the body (Clews 1988) and the manipulation of soft tissue 'with rhythmical pressure and stroking for the purpose of promoting health and well-being' (Cafarelli & Flint 1993: 61). Matuszewski (1985) describes massage as the use of rubbing, kneading, stroking and tapping to improve circulation, enhance muscle tone and relax the recipient. According to Stelfox (2002: 3), massage therapy 'may be defined as the use of (predominantly) the hands to physically manipulate the body's soft tissues (skin, fascia, muscles, tendons and ligaments) for the purpose of effecting a desirable change in the individual'.

Modern massage techniques

The practice of massage, 'or systematic rubbing and manipulation of the tissues of the body, is probably one of the oldest of all means used for relief of bodily infirmities' (Kellogg 1895). Massage techniques have been refined over the centuries and the most practised style of massage therapy used today in the West is the Swedish system, with Swedish massage techniques featuring in many styles of massage available. Generally speaking in the western world, when most people think of massage therapy they will think of Swedish massage, also referred to as 'classical' or 'relaxation' massage. However, there are many different and varied systems of massage currently in use that may be classified under the broad umbrella of massage therapy. Some of these systems are described in Table 12.1.

Table 12.1   Common systems of massage therapy

System	Description
Relaxation massage	Also referred to as Swedish massage, usually applied to the major areas of the body, including the face and feet
Remedial massage	Remedial massage serves to assess and treat areas of soft tissue dysfunction, and employs a broad array of soft tissue techniques in treatment and management such as trigger point therapy, muscle energy technique and corrective exercise
Sports massage	Sports massage is the application of generalised massage therapy in the sporting arena. Sports massage involves the application of massage and related techniques to enhance performance of recreational and professional athletes
Manual lymphatic drainage massage	A light technique that targets the lymphatic system and aims to reduce oedema and expel toxins from the body
Shiatsu massage	A technique traditionally administered through clothing, involving the application of pressure (acupressure) techniques to acupoints of the body
An Mo Tui Na	Also referred to as oriental massage or Traditional Chinese Medicine (TCM) remedial massage, it is a technique considered more vigorous than shiatsu and is based on TCM practices
Aromatherapy massage	Incorporates Swedish strokes, manual lymphatic drainage and acupressure and serves as the technique used to apply essential oils to the body via the skin
Reflexology	Involves the application of pressure to meridian-based points on the feet, hands and ears to improve function and restore balance in the body

Table 12.2   The five major Swedish massage therapy strokes

Name of stroke	Type of movement	Therapeutic outcome
Effleurage	Gliding	• Promotes relaxation
Petrissage	Kneading	• Stimulates blood and lymph circulation • Promotes relaxation
Tapotement	Striking	• Stimulates circulatory and nervous systems
Friction	Compressing	• Produces vasodilation • Mobilises soft tissue
Vibration	Shaking	• Stimulates circulation • Promotes relaxation

Source: Adapted from Tappan and Benjamin (1998).

Table 12.2 shows the five major strokes employed, together with the desired outcomes. The term 'effleurage' comes from the French verb meaning to touch lightly. Effleurage strokes are usually applied as long gliding movements that flow distally to proximally on the body. Effleurage techniques can be performed with varying degrees of pressure. Light pressure has a general relaxing effect on the body and engages the superficial lymph vessels thereby encouraging lymphatic movement, whereas deeper pressure tends to affect blood vessels, encouraging venous return. Still deeper pressure may have a direct effect on muscle tissue.

Petrissage comes from the French verb meaning to knead. Petrissage involves lifting, rolling, squeezing, stretching and compressing strokes which affect the underlying tissues. Petrissage techniques are said to increase local circulation, reduce tone in hypertonic (or 'tight') muscle and stretch superficial fascia.

Tapotement, from another French verb meaning to tap, is also referred to as percussion. Tapotement strokes are normally performed with alternate hands striking the tissues followed by a quick rebound. Such strokes are generally used to stimulate the client. Like petrissage, tapotement may increase local blood flow and reduce hypertonic muscle tone. Tapotement techniques are used in manual chest physiotherapy to help clear mucus in certain respiratory conditions.

Frictions are generally stationary, non-gliding strokes applied to muscle, tendons or ligaments. These are performed by the therapist applying pressure using the hand, fingers or elbow with a small-magnitude transverse or circular motion. Frictions are used to assist in aligning scar tissue in the latter stages of the healing process and to promote dense connective tissue remodelling. Friction techniques have been shown to increase a joint's range of motion, most likely through an increase of muscle extensibility.

The term vibration is used to describe a range of massage techniques that involve vibration, rocking, shaking and jostling. Typically vibrations involve using a flat hand to apply pressure on the tissues while performing fine or course shaking movements with the hand, much like when one shivers from the cold. It is believed that vibrations have a wide range of effects including normalising hypertonic muscle and relieving pain locally.

A traditional Swedish massage might include all five strokes, although tapotement and vibrations are commonly omitted from the sequence. A relaxation massage targeting the psychological condition might comprise effleurage and petrissage alone as these strokes aim to induce relaxation. To effect physiological changes to the musculoskeletal system a massage might comprise effleurage, petrissage, tapotement and friction, to enhance circulation and mobilise the affected region. Such a practice might be typical of a remedial massage therapist or a sports massage therapist. Additionally, in modern massage practice the basic five Swedish strokes have been developed and advanced beyond the traditional methods. The various forms of massage therapy now may encompass other more specialised techniques, including but not limited to trigger point therapy, myofascial release techniques, acupressure and manual lymphatic drainage techniques. Such techniques would require additional training beyond the level of a relaxation massage therapist.

Effects of massage therapy

Emotional effects

Touch is an instinctive form of communication essential to the survival of all animal species. One of the five major senses, touch is a type of social interaction that occurs naturally between people and is a form of connection that can elicit many and varied responses. When a baby is born touch plays a major part in bringing about the bonding that occurs between a mother and child as the mother nurses her baby for the first time. When nursed and caressed, the baby feels loved, secure and calm, and is known to thrive when exposed to a regular and caring touch. As the child grows to a toddler, their fears and pain are soothed away when a parent places a reassuring hand on their forehead to ease a fever or rubs a knee that has been knocked. As a teenager, a slap on the back or a clasped hand from a peer can yield a sense of belonging. As the teen becomes an adult the instinctive knowledge of the healing power of touch persists. The individual may massage their stomach with a flat hand to soothe an abdominal pain or gently caress the brow of a partner or friend who has a headache. In a more formalised sense adults might enjoy the benefits of a regular massage treatment, to allow themselves time out from their busy schedule. A massage treatment may leave them feeling calm, nurtured, relaxed and dreamy or perhaps energised, enlivened and ready to take on the world, depending on the type of massage undertaken.

Today, many westerners are finding themselves deprived of physical contact, living in an era where unnecessary touch is avoided and physical intimacy is often a challenge. In such instances massage therapy has an important role to play in fulfilling the 'touch' needs of society. Many people seek massage therapy simply as a form of touch therapy and as a sensual experience that makes them aware of their body, stimulates their senses and soothes and cares for their body, mind and soul.

This subjectively nourishing quality of massage is one that will be well known to anyone who has experienced a massage treatment. In an age where evidence-based medicine is pre-eminent, however, clinical trials are being undertaken to show scientifically that massage does indeed positively impact the emotions. In a non-randomised investigation into the effects of massage on mood, Weinberg *et al.* (1988) recruited 183 university students. To determine the relationship between massage, exercise and positive mood enhancement, subjects were required to perform 30 minutes of moderate-intensity exercise, receive a 30-minute full-body relaxation massage ($n = 40$) or rest/read for 30 minutes ($n = 56$). Prior to and immediately after participation subjects had to complete three psychological instruments: the Profile of Mood States (POMS), the Thayer activation checklist and the Spielberger anxiety inventory. Massage resulted in improvements on all six of the POMS subscales—confusion, tension, depression, anger, fatigue and vigour—of which all were significant with the exception of vigour. The authors concluded that in terms of positive mood enhancement, massage and running were the only groups to benefit consistently. Although subjects did not show unusually high baseline scores for the psychological instruments used, this study does suggest that massage may be useful in elevating mood.

Another study validating the ability of massage to affect the emotional state positively actually began as an investigation of the effects of pre-performance massage on stride frequency in sprinters (Harmer 1991). Although no significant increase in stride frequency was noted, subjects did report positive feelings about massage, stating they felt relaxed and refreshed after massage treatment. Some subjects stated a carry-over effect, believing that massage allowed them to perform better in their training sessions up to five days post-massage, suggesting that enhancement of mood elevates performance.

Despite subjects reporting feelings of wellbeing post-massage, it is difficult to quantify the emotional benefits of massage. A study by Fraser and Kerr (1993) investigated the effects of massage on anxiety. The study involved 21 elderly subjects in care, assigned to one of three groups: a five-minute massage with conversation, conversation only and no intervention. Results were obtained pre- and post-test and involved a questionnaire and quantitative measures of electromyography, heart rate and blood pressure. Although physiological improvements consistent with reduced anxiety were observed, these were not statistically significant. It should be noted though that subjective qualitative data collected from the study does support the use of massage for relaxation.

A 1993 study investigated the effects of massage on the behaviour and physiology of children and adolescent psychiatric patients (Field *et al.* 1993). The study involved 72 children and adolescents (32 females) hospitalised with either depression or adjustment disorder. Collectively, the results suggested a reduction in anxiety in both the short and long term for the depressed children and adolescents in the massage group. The nursing observations suggested that massage therapy may have a positive effect on children and adolescents hospitalised with either depression or adjustment disorder, while results from the sleep video showed an increase in the percentage of time sleep occurred while in bed over the five-day period. Despite having a control group, a limitation of this study was that massage therapy was not compared to another form of relaxation therapy.

Field *et al.* (1996) conducted a study to compare the effects of massage and relaxation therapies on anxiety and depression in a group of depressed adolescent mothers recruited from a hospital maternity ward. Thirty-two mothers were randomly assigned to either a massage group (*n* = 16) or a relaxation therapy group (*n* = 16) that consisted of yoga and progressive muscle relaxation. All treatments lasted for 30 minutes and were administered twice a week over a five-week period. The results of this study showed that anxiety reduced on the first day for both groups, and on the last day of treatment for the massage group. The massage group also exhibited lower depression scores on the first and last days of treatment and less anxiety after their sessions. It is important to note that only the massage group experienced a reduction in stress levels, as measured by a decrease in the levels of cortisol in the urine across the course of the treatment.

Another study illustrating the psychological impact of massage investigated the effects of massage therapy on depression, anxiety and immune function in adolescents diagnosed with HIV/AIDS (Diego *et al.* 2001). Twenty-four seropositive patients received either massage therapy or relaxation therapy involving progressive muscle relaxation. After treatment on the first and last days, both the massage and the relaxation groups showed an immediate reduction in anxiety post-treatment, while only the massage group reported a reduction in depression. Those receiving massage also showed evidence of heightened immune function. The authors believe the positive effects of massage therapy may be explained by the ability of massage to reduce stress and anxiety, which in turn lowers cortisol levels and leads to improved immune function.

Many people can attest to the calming and relaxing sensations they experience after receiving a massage therapy treatment. Such claims are backed up by research findings which suggest massage therapy can improve emotional states, reduce anxiety levels, assist with depression and relieve stress. With improved mood comes the benefit of enhanced immune function. Such reflex effects (see below) of massage are of prime interest to researchers; the findings outlined above have the potential for wide application across a vast array of conditions and age groups.

Physical effects

While the nurturing and psychological aspects of human touch are central to the therapeutic value of massage there are also objective physical benefits to be acknowledged. On the physical level when performing any massage therapy stroke, the therapist is endeavouring to elicit one of two possible effects. These effects of treatment, as first described by Mennell (c. 1917), are referred to as reflex and mechanical effects.

A reflex effect may be described as an involuntary response and is an indirect effect of the massage treatment. The downward shift of blood pressure that is observed with massage is an example of an indirect, or reflex, response, brought about by dilation of blood vessels as a result of the application of deep effleurage movements (Salvo 1999). Reflex effects commonly result in neural and endocrine changes and are thought to be a significant factor in the overall benefits of massage therapy.

On the other hand, mechanical effects are direct effects and include the direct influence that the manual therapy has on the soft tissues of the body. Such mechanical effects also influence the fluid environments of the body and affect the motility of the intestines and their contents (Mennell c. 1917; Cassar 1999; Fritz 2000). A direct effect implies that a mechanical response has occurred because of the application of direct force or pressure when administering massage. Such a direct effect may include the resolution of oedema through the use of effleurage, which promotes lymph and venous return (De Domenico & Wood 1997). It should be noted that these actions are interrelated and interdependent. As such, the direct and indirect effects of massage should not be thought of as isolated entities.

There are many claims made throughout the literature about the benefits of massage, yet few have been substantiated through rigorous investigation. It has been said that massage reduces pain (Trevelyan 1993; Tappan & Benjamin 1998), increases metabolism, stimulates the lymphatic and circulatory systems and makes for rapid healing (Beck 1988). According to Tappan and Benjamin (1998) massage can also induce relaxation, reduce oedema, improve a joint's range of motion and enhance the confidence of the recipient. Recommended as an aid for recovery from exercise (Smith et al. 1994), it is claimed that massage is useful for stress management (Matuszewski 1985) and can soften scar tissue and loosen adhesions (Ortolani 1978).

De Domenico and Wood (1997) describe the physiological benefits of massage as being improved blood and lymph circulation, improved flow of nutrients, increased removal of metabolic wastes, resolution of oedema, pain reduction, enhanced joint mobility and improved muscular function, as well as stimulation of autonomic and visceral functions. Listed as psychological benefits are physical relaxation, relief from tension, pain and anxiety and improved 'wellness'. Elton (1995: 84) states that 'while much has been written about the theory of massage, there is still much room for research, to separate the physical from the physiological and psychological effects'. To appreciate fully the effects of massage it is illuminating to examine the research that pertains to each condition.

Pain

Pain reduction is a physiological benefit of therapeutic massage described by many authors (Trevelyan 1993; De Domenico & Wood 1997; Tappan & Benjamin 1998) yet little is known about the exact mechanism behind the analgesic action of this therapy. Is the perception of pain altered through purely physiological pathways or can massage positively affect the emotional state of the recipient thereby psycho-logically blocking the pain experience?

According to the gate-control theory of pain established by Melzack and Wall in 1965, sensory input of pain is transmitted to the spinal cord and the brain. Once nerve cells in these areas are sufficiently excited, a theoretical gate opens and allows transmission of pain signals to the brain, where they are processed. The brain is able to close the gate and alter pain perception, through psychological input such as feelings of wellness. Thus, if a person's mood is positive the pain signals to the brain may be blocked. Hence, a person's thoughts and emotions can directly influence the pain experience and the subjective pleasure of massage may thus yield pain relief. Another way to alter pain perception is to confuse the input of sensory information arriving at the lower centres of the central nervous system by application of a different stimulus, such as the application of massage.

In the clinical domain Davis et al. (1990) investigated the pain management tech-niques tried by 82 people with rheumatic disease. Fifty-nine per cent of young adults and 25 per cent of old adults had used massage as a technique to manage their pain. Both groups found massage more helpful in managing pain than non-prescription medicine and electrical stimulation. Old adults found massage more beneficial than relaxation techniques, exercise, bracing and conversation for pain management. It is interesting to note that the percentage of massage users was significantly greater in the young adults than the old adults; perhaps this is consistent with the current turn toward complementary therapies such as massage and the awareness among young adults of such avenues of health management.

One study conducted over a 30-day period (Field et al. 1997) investigated the effects of daily massage on anxiety, pain and functional ability in children aged between four and sixteen years with mild to moderate juvenile rheumatoid arthritis (RA). Although not statistically significant, the results of this study show a reduction in anxiety, in both the children receiving the massage and the parent performing the massage. Salivary cortisol levels were reduced post-massage and level of pain, as measured through self-report, parental and physician assessments, was also lowered. Despite a small sample size the researchers recommend further investigation in the area of pain, anxiety and functional ability in RA populations, stating that 'massage seems to be a cost-effective therapy' (Field *et al*. 1997: 617).

Nixon *et al*. (1997) investigated the effect of relaxation massage on pain perception and usage of analgesia medication after abdominal surgery. Patients who received massage post-operatively perceived less pain than patients in the control group yet did not exhibit a reduction in analgesia medication use. One incidental finding of this study is that the massage therapy intervention was particularly effective for pain reduction in the older patients.

Another study (Field *et al*. 2003) investigated the effects of combined massage and movement therapy on the pain associated with fibromyalgia. Forty subjects diagnosed with fibromyalgia were randomly assigned to either a control group ($n = 20$) to undergo relaxation via the use of progressive muscle relaxation or a massage/ movement group ($n = 20$). The authors noted that both the control and the massage/movement groups showed a decrease in anxiety and pain after the first and/or last sessions. However, results for the massage/movement group also showed improvements in mood, a reduction in anxiety and lower levels of pain across the three-week study period. Further investigations are required to determine the longer lasting effects of massage/movement for chronic pain conditions such as fibromyalgia.

It is evident that many sufferers of chronically painful conditions such as fibromyalgia tend to seek out a wide variety of options to assist in relieving their pain. As massage therapy becomes more widely used in the clinical realm more and more patients experiencing pain will choose to receive massage therapy to assist with their condition. As shown above, evidence exists to validate the use of massage therapy for its immediate effects in reducing pain perception but further investigation is required to determine the longer-term effects of massage therapy for pain and the exact mechanism behind its effect.

Circulation

There is an assumption that massage has a significant impact on the cardiovascular and lymphatic systems and there is clinical data to support this. Ernst *et al*. (1987) investigated the effects of whole-body massage on blood fluidity in patients with ankylosing spondylitis. The results of this study showed that twenty minutes of massage produced both acute and long-term declines in haematocrit, which is the percentage of blood composed of red blood cells. Declines in blood and plasma viscosities (thickness or stickiness of solution) were also observed. The investigators concluded that such changes were the result of increased fluid movement or perfusion into blood, indicative of enhanced circulation post-massage, suggesting massage to be of benefit for muscular disorders such as ankylosing spondylitis.

In another study that spanned a ten-year period, 655 patients, primarily experiencing post-mastectomy oedema, were recruited for participation in a longitudinal study investigating massage for oedema (Yamazaki *et al.* 1988). Each participant received a series of pneumatic (mechanical) massage treatments for peripheral lymphoedema (oedema of the arm). Findings suggest that massage applied with undulatory (changing) pressure may be beneficial in improving both lymphatic and blood flow. Yamazaki *et al.* (1988) concluded that such massage is useful to relieve peripheral lymphoedema as it encourages venous and lymphatic return.

Research also suggests that massage may be useful for high blood pressure (hypertension) and related symptoms of anxiety, stress, hostility and depression. A study conducted by Hernandez-Reif *et al.* (2000) investigated the effects of a course of ten 30-minute massage sessions over a five-week period in 30 hypertensive subjects. A control group received instruction on progressive muscle relaxation. Decreases in both sitting and reclining blood pressure (diastolic) measurements were recorded in those receiving massage. Despite both the experimental and control groups reporting less anxiety, only the experimental group (which received massage) reported reductions in hostility and depression. Measurements of salivary and urinary cortisol (a stress hormone) were also reduced in the massage group, indicating a reduction in stress.

When one rubs or massages the skin it becomes reddened after a short period of time, which is indicative of enhanced circulation to the area. During a massage therapy treatment the recipient experiences improved circulation. Such a change in circulatory function is an immediate mechanical effect of massage therapy. The extent to which this mechanical change induces reflex responses is unclear at present and warrants further investigation.

Training in massage therapy

There are an increasing number of training providers delivering courses in massage therapy in both the private and public sectors of the western medical community. The massage profession in Britain, Australia and New Zealand is self-regulating, and a certificate-level award is a common entry point to massage therapy practice. Depending on the training institution a certificate-level award typically involves one year of full-time study.

Quite a different situation exists in the education of massage therapists in the United States. Extensive regulation of the massage profession exists in both the United States and Canada. In the United States almost 30 states license or regulate the industry, and most states require a minimum of 500 hours of training to become a massage therapist (Rich 2002). In contrast, legislation in some parts of Canada requires a massage therapist to undergo over 2000 hours of training and in

British Columbia as much as 3000 hours of training. Whether the massage profession is regulated or not is largely dependent on the government of the day and its directions in policy development.

Massage therapy in practice

The place

Once trained it is relatively easy for a massage therapist to establish their business. The required 'tools of the trade' are minimal. A massage therapist requires little more than a room conducive to treatment, a massage table, linen and lubricant (such as a cold-pressed vegetable oil like sweet almond oil) for massage. Some therapists may choose to enhance the ambience of the massage environment to promote the relaxation effects by using vaporised essential oils, subdued lighting, soft music and warmed towels. Chapter 6 deals in detail with aromatherapy, but massage therapists, depending on their training, may choose to use essential oils as part of their treatments to induce not only emotional but also physical effects.

As the application of massage involves removal of some or even all clothing on the part of the client, the issue of modesty and privacy forms a part of all massage training. Through the use of modest and appropriate draping, the therapist ensures that the personal boundaries of the client relating to undress are not breached, and the treatment is applied in a discreet and professional manner.

A massage therapist can work from home or establish a practice in a multidisciplinary clinic with other complementary medicine practitioners. Leisure centres and spa complexes are two modern environments in which massage practice is particularly appropriate. Another alternative is to have a mobile practice that visits clients in their homes, hotels or the workplace. As a professional healthcare provider, the massage therapist should also be a member of a professional association and maintain adequate insurance cover. In an environment of variable training levels professional memberships can be an indication to a client that the practitioner is adequately qualified to provide a professional service.

Massage and the medical community

Massage therapy is generally considered a safe and effective form of therapy for a vast array of medical complaints, and as such is indicated for a multitude of different situations. When consulting with a client for the first time a relaxation massage therapist takes a detailed case history of the client to ascertain their needs and develop a detailed profile of their current health status. Armed with this case history, the therapist is able to select the most effective treatment strategy to suit the client. When administering massage therapies other than Swedish massage, such as remedial massage, a more detailed case history may be sought and an objective musculoskeletal assessment undertaken.

Factors that a massage therapist would take into consideration when formulating a treatment strategy include any pre-existing diseases or syndromes the client may have and any medications they may currently be taking. Certain conditions or situations may render the application of massage therapy unsuitable and contraindications to treatment are listed in Table 12.3. A massage therapist would refer the client to their primary care practitioner or nearest emergency department for treatment where warranted. In the case of a client who has a past history of a contraindicated condition a therapist may choose to go ahead and treat the client, after first seeking a written clearance from a primary care practitioner. Common medications that may prompt a massage therapist to take caution and modify a treatment include analgesic, anti-inflammatory and anti-hypertensive drugs. Analgesic and anti-inflammatory medications may reduce sensitivity and mask pain, thus clients may not be able to give adequate feedback on treatment techniques being applied. One of the side effects of anti-hypertensive medications is postural (or orthostatic) hypotension, which involves a downward shift in blood pressure when one moves from a reclining to seated position or seated to standing position. As a result the therapist would ensure the client makes a gradual transition to a standing posture post-massage (Tuchtan & Tuchtan 2002).

Table 12.3   Contraindications to massage therapy

- Acute accidents and emergencies (including appendicitis, bronchial asthma, cerebrovascular accident, heart failure, myocardial ischaemia, shock)
- Acute inflammatory conditions
- Acute psychosis
- Aneurism
- Embolism
- Fever
- Abnormal bleeding conditions (including haemophilia)
- Infections (including encephalitis, meningitis)
- Infectious skin conditions
- Kidney failure
- Leukaemia
- Malignant tumours
- Tuberculosis

Perhaps the true place of massage in the medical community is as a form of preventive medicine. This is not to say that massage offers no remedial effects for existing ailments. As the research above illustrates, massage can address physical, emotional and possibly even spiritual issues. There is no doubt, however, that the diversity of effects of massage combine to make it an invaluable tool for maintaining overall wellbeing. Regular massage can ease the mind and soothe the body and can benefit the healthy as much as the unwell. Consequently, the massage therapist is a frontline agent in maintaining the health of the general community. Equally, unless otherwise qualified, the massage therapist is not in a position to be a primary care physician for the acutely or chronically unwell. Armed with a full knowledge of the capacities of their modality, however, the massage therapist functions variously as a health maintainer, a point of referral or a conjunct therapist to help and nurture the client while they are undergoing other more arduous therapies.

Conclusion

Massage therapy is an ancient healing art that dates back centuries. The way in which massage affects the physiological functioning of the body or brings about a change in one's psychological state is yet to be fully understood although advances are being made in this area. Despite the fact that the full benefits of massage as a therapy are yet to be definitively established, there exists the foundations of solid research findings validating the efficacy of massage therapy, particularly in the areas of pain, anxiety, depression and immune function. Massage therapy is non-addictive, readily available and pleasurable. A therapy that is suitable for all ages, massage has a vast array of applications and a multitude of benefits and serves as a powerful tool that plays a vital role in the modern holistic approach to health and wellbeing.

Recommended reading

Cassar, M. 1999, *Handbook of Massage Therapy: A Complete Guide for the Student and Professional Massage Therapist*, Butterworth Heinemann, Oxford.

De Domenico, G. and Wood, E.C. 1997, *Beard's Massage*, 4th edn, W.B. Saunders Co., Philadelphia.

Field, T. 2000, *Touch Therapy*, Churchill Livingstone, London.

Rich, G.J. 2002, *Massage Therapy: The Evidence for Practice*, Mosby, London.

Tuchtan, C.C., Tuchtan, V.M. and Stelfox, D.P. in press, *Foundations for Massage*, 2nd edn, Churchill Livingstone, Sydney.

13

Nutrition
Karen E. Bridgman

Complementary medicine is the 'science' of health and is a healing practice that looks at small changes in a person's physiology at the functional level. The diagnosis is not just disease based and the treatments involve correcting dysfunction and rebalancing the body, ideally before major biochemical changes (such as disease or pathology) take place. Practitioners therefore look for smaller changes in the body, attempting to diagnose functional problems early, and the therapies they use, such as nutrition, work best as a lifestyle shift and are part of long-term, lifetime processes of regulating health.

A history of 'nutrition'

Food (and water) is inseparable from the history and the development of the human race. Without it we would not exist. The search for food and water has been (and is) the crucial factor in our survival and therefore in the development of humanity from very earliest times. As human history began (between ten and four million years ago), the pursuit of food and how we have managed this has given us the leisure time to pursue the arts and develop rituals, cultures and differing ways of being in this world.

Human beings have been on this planet and adapting to its conditions for approximately four million years (Eaton 1989; Horrobin 2001). This translates to about 100 000 generations of humans as hunter-gatherers, eating a varied diet of seasonal foods. Modern humans are creating new problems for their health, partly because of increasing numbers, partly because of the use of technology for food production. This can confer great benefits but can also be damaging to health when technology is used in a way that humans have not had time to adapt to genetically.

Evolutionary traits that have been responsible for human survival in the past may not confer the same advantages today. For example, the hunger drive encourages us to eat when food is available (to build up supplies for shortage), the desire for 'sugars' and fats provides a quick source of energy in difficult conditions and salts provide often poorly available minerals and electrolytes. Unlike today, these foods were often in short supply in a traditional diet and obtaining them conferred a survival advantage. Today these 'desires' are not as useful because in the West there is generally too much food, and too much sugar, fat and salt are added in the processing of foods. Excess consumption of these 'survival' foods now predisposes humans to chronic illness such as diabetes, cancer and heart disease. The western diet with its long term nutrient imbalances drives these 'diseases of western society', the degenerative conditions, that are largely based on excesses of inflammation, oxidation and chemical overload.

Table 13.1   Palaeolithic versus modern American diet charts

	Late Palaeolithic	American	Recommended today
Dietary energy (%)			
Protein	33	12	12
Carbohydrate	46	46	58
Fat	21	42	30
Alcohol	<1	7–10	—
P:S ratio[a]	1.41	0.44	1
Cholesterol (mg)	520	300–500	300
Fibre (g)	100–150	19.7	30–60
Na (mg)	690	2300–6900	1000–3300
Ca (mg)	1500–2000	740	800–1500
Ascorbic acid (mg)	440	90	60

Note: [a]Abbreviations: P:S ratio is the polyunsaturated to saturated fat ratio; Na—sodium, Ca—calcium, ascorbic acid—vitamin C.
Source: Modified from Eaton and Konner (1985).

A comparison of the Palaeolithic and standard American diet is instructive (see Table 13.1). Notice the change in the ratios of the macronutrients: carbohydrates (including fibre), proteins and fats. Also notice the change in the proportions of the micronutrients: sodium (a possible determinant of blood pressure in many people), calcium (a blood buffer and major component of bone) and vitamin C (ascorbic acid), a nutrient known to positively affect the immune system, the cardiovascular system, the skin, the brain and the liver.

Food preservation/food processing

Apart from the local freshly available foods, humans have always had need to preserve foods. From seasons of plenty to seasons of famine, or for travelling long distances over inhospitable lands, preserving foods for provisioning was necessary. Traditional ways of preserving foods were salting, drying in the sun or freezing, fermentation, pickling in a variety of spices, preserving in honey or brine, sealing in airtight packages or containers such as amber or alcohol or burying in cool, wet bogs full of boracic or other acids. All of these methods reflect the ingenuity of humans in their fight for survival and to be fed adequately. These methods not only preserve food but some of them, like fermentation, also increase nutrient density, for instance fermentation increases the B vitamin content of food.

Food preservation made it possible for human ancestors to travel to explore unknown places and for the evolution of social and cultural complexities that developed when humans had enough food to tide them over long periods of enforced leisure, for example during harsh winters. Over the last three or four thousand years food preservation has had positive and negative consequences. It has allowed for the great expeditions, the great navigations and the creation of the trade routes along which knowledge and culture were exchanged. On the other hand, it has also made possible the great armies, the endemic warfare and the colonisation of distant lands (Shephard 2000).

Food technology businesses today make use of many of these techniques to increase shelf life of foods. Originally based on the need to reduce the risk of food poisoning and to allow a consistent and reliable food supply, today's food preservation is unfortunately increasingly based on economics and not on the understanding we now have of nutrition. Many of our processed foods today bear little resemblance to their original product in nutrient density. Foods are refined to the extent that they have an almost indefinite shelf life but this process removes many of the vitamins and minerals needed for health. For example, in the refining of flour between 40 and 80 per cent of the B vitamins are removed (up to 80 per cent of vitamin B1, which is essential for the metabolism of the carbohydrate, and up to 95 per cent of vitamin B6, which has a role in many metabolic functions). Between 50 and 90 per cent of the major minerals such as zinc, iron, calcium, magnesium, potassium and chromium are also removed (Wahlqvist 1981; Briggs 1983; Wardlaw & Insel 1990).

The need for food

Food, water and oxygen are the substances upon which life on this planet is based. Food provides us with both the energy and the nutrients required to build, maintain and repair all our body cells. The study of nutrition is the study of these foods and their nutrients, what they consist of, how the human body digests, absorbs and utilises them and what they do to support life and health.

The nutrients in food are divided into several categories. The macronutrients are the components of foods we require in larger amounts and which are present in foods in large amounts. They include carbohydrates, protein and lipids (fats and oils). Micronutrients are the vitamins, minerals, flavonoids and other components in foods that we require in small amounts only, but which are just as important as their larger-volume components. A single nutrient deficiency, whether it be a macronutrient or a micronutrient, can be equally as devastating for human health.

The macronutrients in food supply energy for our bodies to function, mainly from carbohydrates and fats (lipids). Proteins supply energy if necessary but this is an inefficient process by comparison; carbohydrates and fats having about a 95 per cent energy conversion and proteins about 65 per cent. Glucose (a simple carbohydrate) is the primary fuel for brain and central nervous system function and is very important for energy production in the liver and muscles.

Food also supplies the base substances for all our hormones. Cholesterol (a lipid) is the basis of many hormones, including the hormones responsible for sexuality and reproduction (oestrogen, progesterone, testosterone), for a major anti-inflammatory hormone (cortisol) and for vitamin D (cholecalciferol) production from our skin (vital in calcium and bone metabolism). Lipids are also vital structural and functional components of the brain. The essential fatty acids particularly are crucial for both the development of our brain and for its correct function, as well as being major regulators of inflammation.

Proteins (and fats) in food form the structural components of our bodies and during periods of growth it is important to increase the protein in the diet in proportion to body weight; for example, in children and teenagers. As people age and growth slows, they often need less protein since it is mainly used for repair of body structures that are damaged. Proteins also form hormones such as adrenalin and noradrenalin for stress management and insulin for blood sugar management and energy production. Neurotransmitters are largely made of proteins and these govern mood and behaviour.

The micronutrients (vitamins, minerals, amino acids, flavonoids, etc.) do not provide calories (energy) but are vital for metabolism to take place. They have an enormous number of roles to play in the maintenance of life and in the health of the body; for example, vitamin B6, zinc and magnesium are largely responsible for the activity of thousands of enzyme systems from digestion, hormonal regulation, central nervous system activity and much more. It is vital for us to obtain the required balance of all these micronutrients in critical amounts for survival, and in higher but less critical amounts for optimal health.

Nutrition as healing

Nutrition forms the basis of complementary medical practice and there are two major approaches to the study of nutrition (Bland 1999):

1. **The traditional focus of modern nutrition, which is the deficiency and negative outcomes approach and problem avoidance. For example,**

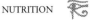

elimination of high oxalate foods to prevent kidney stones; reducing fats in the diet to lower cholesterol; avoiding sugars to manage dysglycaemia.

2. The functional approach, which looks beyond just redressing deficiency and problem avoidance and focuses instead on the alteration in function that could generate these problems. Using the same examples, a practitioner of functional nutrition would:
   - increase elimination of oxalates and add probiotics to the diet to regulate oxalate metabolism and reduce kidney stones;
   - improve liver function, reduce sugars and balance gastrointestinal absorption of specific types of fats to regulate cholesterol; and
   - improve sugar metabolism and steroid hormone balance and manage stress, along with decreased sugar intake to regulate blood sugars and manage dysglycaemia.

Both the traditional and the functional approaches have their uses and can work together, but the functional approach is more positive and has greater potential for improving the overall health of the system. The functional perspective recognises nutrient deficiency as a basis for intervention but increases the effectiveness of clinical nutrition as a modality by determining why the metabolic pattern that has created the deficiency has changed, and intervening to correct this. It looks more holistically at the relationships that create health and disease.

Dietary measures

Nutritional therapies can be used in many ways. At one end of the spectrum are dietary therapies such as water or juice fasting, using foods as therapies (such as vegetable juices for extra antioxidants in the management of cancer, especially beetroot/carrot), or altering dietary patterns (eliminating certain foods) to reduce allergies or intolerances. There is also a range of diets to correct either general or specific health problems that work well for many, such as blood type diets (D'Adamo 1998), Zone diets (Sears & Lawren 1995) and the GI factor diets (Brand-Miller *et al.* 1998). The Pritikin Diet helped reduce a whole generation's risk of heart disease by encouraging a higher legume and lower fat diet (Pritikin 1979).

There are some popular weight-loss diets like the Atkins Diet (Atkins 1992), which works well for short-term weight loss but can have long-term negative effects as it is too focused on high protein at the expense of carbohydrates. It is 'diets' like these that have changed the understanding of the original meaning of the word, so today the word 'diet' tends to be associated primarily with the weight-loss industry. It also has connotations of a short period of time and the elimination of many enjoyable foods or severe food restriction. Such 'diets' work well to lose weight for short periods of time with a specific purpose in mind, but are not suitable for the long term and do not offer the opportunity to alter lifestyle and improve health in significant ways. When choosing a diet and lifestyle package an individual's specific needs and family and cultural history should be considered. Climate is also a consideration as, for example, heavy, cooked, warming foods are not as suitable in hot weather.

Some diets or lifestyles are based on ancient specific philosophies. Macrobiotic and Ayurvedic diets have a long history of promoting health but are difficult to follow in western life as many of the foods are unfamiliar and eating habits are culturally significantly dissimilar. However, with a bit of dedication in learning and practising their principles on a daily basis, these diets can generate a major improvement in health, as they have done for thousands of years. For more information on Ayurveda see Chapter 1; Kushi (1985) and Pitchford (1993) have written excellent books on these topics.

Following the problem avoidance principle, diets for specific diseases are used by both orthodox and complementary medicine practitioners. These range from the low-sugar and low-fat diets to regulate diabetes and cardiovascular disease to the high-protein diets that can reduce seizures in epileptics. From a more functional perspective there are also diets to improve conditions such as arthritis (reducing animal products and the nightshade family while increasing the anti-inflammatory essential fatty acids), and diets to relieve auto-immune diseases such as psoriasis or rheumatoid arthritis, which often mean removing wheat and sugars. Sports performance can also be improved with dietary changes.

Overall, there are basic dietary guidelines for improving health, such as increasing the variety of foods, choosing organically grown foods and eating foods as close to the natural farm produce as possible, thereby reducing consumption of processed foods. By changing the foods eaten (and the way they are eaten) the body's functions can be manipulated to produce a desired result.

Quality issues

The main problems with modern diets and food supply are overeating and under-nutrition. The food supply has been changed by the use of technology, which provides the advantages of an abundant, consistent, low-cost food supply and great variety of foods, with massive transportation, communication and distribution networks. There also exists a huge range of convenience foods and high-speed cooking equipment, and technology has yielded a greatly increased knowledge of the body and its functions.

Weighed against this, technology has brought the disadvantages of increasing problems with smog, water, air and soil pollution and changed nutrient density of foods. Chemical additives are mixed with foods to preserve them, colour them, flavour them or change them in some way, and this is combined with lack of nutrients in the food itself as a result of agricultural and storage techniques. Seasonal foods (with optimal nutrient density) are not a priority as, with improved storage, food is available all year round. Agriculturally, monocultures have been built wherein foods are restricted to the most economically viable, which in turn leads to increasing demineralisation of soils and increasing use of pesticides/chemicals, with the creation of ecological imbalances. Genetic modification of foods is now being added to this mix.

These are some of the major problems with foods today that human ancestors never knew. Technology has far exceeded the human ability to adapt genetically to these changes and there is an imperative to rethink modern eating habits to regain and maintain health.

Recommended daily intakes/allowances

Australia, America and England (and 40 other countries) have developed a system of determining the minimum requirements of nutrients for health. In Australia this is called the 'recommended daily intake' (RDI), in other countries the 'recommended daily allowance' (RDA). The first Australian table was issued by the National Health and Medical Research Council in 1954. These RDIs have since been expanded several times, the last extensive review being published in 1990 (Truswell 1990). The RDIs are based on the historical concept of preventing major deficiency symptoms. However, these are only the acute and final consequences of a contrived period of insufficient nutrient supply. So even though the RDIs can be used as a guide, these are considered minimum requirements for a reasonably healthy person (or requirements for survival but not for optimal health), and greater amounts are often required by individuals or when the body is under some sort of environmental challenge.

There are many conflicting research papers on nutrition (and on medicine) and this creates significant debate. The overriding theme when dealing with humans and their health is that of bio-individuality. Not everyone who eats excess salt will have high blood pressure and dietary cholesterol will not raise everyone's blood cholesterol. There are many individual factors that need to be taken into account. What needs to be stressed is that each person must learn their family background as a guide to potential susceptibilities to illness. Individuals need to become aware of any small changes in their bodies so that any potential functional change can be dealt with early, in keeping with the ideal of preventive medicine.

The body's nutritional status varies for each individual, but optimal nutritional status occurs when the body has enough nutrients for both metabolic functions and for surplus stores that can be utilised during times of increased need. Individual nutritional needs vary according to genetic makeup, level of activity, general state of health, environment and drug consumption. Each individual's needs also vary with changing circumstances and diets should change to cope with this. The foods needed by an athlete, a grandmother, a growing girl or boy, a sedentary office worker or a pregnant mother, for example, are going to be vastly different and this needs to be accounted for in dietary choices. With the highly processed convenient foods available today, many nutritional lifestyles are out of balance with physiology. The goal is for optimal health, and with knowledge and conscious choice this goal is within reach.

Nutritional supplements

Vitamins and minerals are natural compounds that are indispensable for every living organism. However, as they have been freely available in the food of humans for millennia the ability to synthesise some of these micronutrients has been lost. For example, all animals apart from humans, fruit bats and hamsters can produce vitamin C from glucose. As human evolutionary diets were high in vitamin C the enzymes needed to manufacture it were lost. Several of the B vitamins can be manufactured in the digestive system in the presence of the correct bowel bacteria. Unfortunately, with the use of antibiotics, hormones (the oral contraceptive pill and hormone replacement therapy) and corticosteroids, which alter the bacterial balance in the gut, few people today have enough of the correct bacteria in the digestive system to be able to do this.

There is constant research being done on vitamins and minerals although this is hampered somewhat by difficulty obtaining research money, with no patentable product as the end result. No new vitamins have been discovered since the 1930s and no minerals since the 1970s. Newly discovered nutritional substances, however, are proving valuable, such as lipoic acid, s-adenosylmethionine and phosphatidyl serine. Despite the difficulties research has demonstrated the crucial importance of all these nutrients in disease prevention.

Vitamins and minerals are essential for life and for optimal human physical and mental health and wellbeing. Deficiencies of these nutrients develop through various stages. With increasing deficiency, the symptoms become more noticeable and specific and therefore easier to define and classify. In marginal deficiencies, tissue stores initially decline then biochemical changes start to take place; enzyme activity is reduced and indeterminate symptoms such as headaches, mood changes, anxiety, depression, irritability, fatigue and sleeplessness are experienced. In the early stages of deficiency, due to many confusing factors, including the interactive nature of the nutrients and the subjective nature of the complaints, the causal role of nutrient deficiencies is difficult to demonstrate. These are then called marginal deficiencies, and the resulting interactions complicate both the interpretation of the symptoms and the consequences for the individual. As the deficiency continues to worsen, clinical symptoms begin to appear and eventually these become pathological changes. Unfortunately many practitioners are more likely to prescribe drugs to counteract the

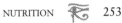

symptoms (now classified as a disease) rather than to look at the underlying deficiency that may be easily corrected.

Nutrient deficiencies occur for three major reasons:

1. **Biological risk factors: these are age related and reflect the varying nutritional demands of the different development stages of life.**
2. **Sociological risk factors: these derive from our contemporary lifestyles and habits. They include nutritional preferences (choices made about foods and fluids), as well as the quality of the daily nutrition available.**
3. **Requirements: these can be increased for both genetic and behavioural reasons. A person may have either a genetically greater need for specific nutrients (a genetic metabolic deficiency) or a dietary deficiency or both.**

In addition to these, chronic exposure to environmental pollutants needs to be included as an example of involuntary risk. In these situations a marginal deficiency of a single nutrient (e.g. vitamin A or zinc) may increase the damage.

Lifestyle and dietary choices influence requirements significantly. Those who drink alcohol, tea or coffee, smoke or take various drugs (prescription or otherwise) or who participate in high levels of exercise will have greater requirements of specific nutrients. For example, drinking alcohol requires larger amounts of B vitamins, zinc and magnesium for metabolism; because these are water-soluble nutrients they are also excreted more quickly with alcohol's diuretic effect.

Just as deficiencies do not affect the status of only a single nutrient at a time, so the underlying risk factors do not develop in isolation. The continual interaction of all different types of risk factors increases the cumulative damage. Today there are increasing numbers of people who are at risk of nutrient deficiency, in the affluent countries as well as the underdeveloped countries. The underlying factors here are both biological and sociocultural. Vitamin and mineral supplements are often necessary and are a cost-effective way to prevent health damage due to marginal (and severe) deficiencies. However, supplements are only ever meant as supplements to an already good diet. They are not intended to be taken instead of a good diet.

The micronutrients

Vitamins

Vitamins are complex organic food substances which are required in very small amounts by the body (Bridgman 2000). They are essential for growth, health, normal metabolism, physical wellbeing and life. Vitamins function as:

- **antioxidants—free-radical scavengers, both water soluble and fat soluble;**
- **cofactors of enzymes—without enzymes life would not proceed in a form that we recognise;**
- **regulators of metabolism—vitamins are essential in the regulation of biochemical reactions that convert absorbed foods into materials that can be used in the body, and for energy production (although they cannot themselves be metabolised for energy).**

Vitamins are classified on the basis of whether they are water soluble or fat soluble. This is useful because it gives an indication of the types of foods in which specific vitamins are found, the way the body can use them and the way they can be handled during food preparation to preserve maximum activity.

Water-soluble vitamins (vitamin C and B vitamins) have no precursors and can be leached out of foods easily by incorrect cooking, for example boiling or soaking. However, once absorbed they can travel freely in the water-soluble mediums of blood and lymph but minimal storage occurs except in lean tissues (e.g. muscles) for short periods. These tissues are actively exchanging materials with the body fluids at all times so the vitamins are easily dissolved and are excreted rapidly by the kidneys. Any substance that is diuretic can increase excretion and can generate deficiencies, but toxicity of water-soluble vitamins is unlikely unless they are pre-scribed at extremely high doses. A daily dietary source of the water-soluble vitamins is recommended because of their limited storage and rapid excretion.

The fat-soluble vitamins, A, D, E and K (and coenzyme Q10), are found in animal fats, fish oils, fish liver oils and plant oils. They often have precursors (provitamins); for example, beta carotene is the precursor to vitamin A. Losses of fat-soluble vitamins occur prior to absorption. If fat absorption is poor, or if a person is using mineral oils, laxatives or some cholesterol-lowering medication, fat-soluble vitamins will be lost in the stool. Once they have been absorbed through the digestive tract they are not excreted easily (they need replacing through usage). Being insoluble in water, fat-soluble vitamins require protein carriers to transport them from one part of the body to another, via the bloodstream or lymph (e.g. the zinc-dependent retinal-binding protein transports vitamin A), and they are stored in the fatty (adipose) tissues and in the liver in varying amounts. Because of this storage there is the potential for toxicity.

Minerals

Minerals are the essential inorganic elements that remain when tissue (plant or animal) is burnt, that is, the ash (Bridgman 2000). Minerals are locked into the earth's crust so our main link with these is through our diet of plants (and other animals that eat plants), which are able to extract minerals from the soil. Humans can manufacture some vitamins but if the minerals are not in the soil (or the foods we ingest) there is no replacement as they cannot be manufactured. Minerals are therefore essential in the diet. Humans require large amounts of some minerals (macro minerals) and smaller amount of others (trace minerals). As with all nutrients the amount required bears no relationship to their importance in the body and a deficiency of any mineral can be equally devastating.

The macro minerals make up no less than 0.01 per cent of body weight (i.e. more than 5 g) and include calcium, phosphorus, potassium, sulphur, sodium, chlorine and magnesium. The trace minerals include zinc, iron, selenium, manganese, copper, iodine, molybdenum, cobalt, chromium, fluorine, silicon, vanadium, nickel, tin, boron and so on. There are other minerals that are not believed useful at this stage, or we don't know what their uses are, including aluminium, lead, cadmium, arsenic and mercury. Many of these minerals (mainly heavy metals) have the potential to be toxic to humans, particularly in the doses we receive from our environment and foods. There is a huge amount of biochemical individuality associated with optimal mineral levels and these levels vary enormously from person to person. Speculation persists as to what the 'normal' levels should be. Clinical deficiency signs are still the best guide to requirements.

Minerals have both structural and functional roles. They are components of body tissues and fluids (iron), and work in combination with enzymes, hormones, vitamins and transport substances (zinc). Minerals are also involved in immunity (zinc and selenium), nerve transmission (magnesium and calcium), muscle contraction, cell permeability (phosphorus), tissue rigidity and structure (bone—calcium and phosphorus), blood formation, acid–base balance, fluid regulation and osmolarity (sodium and potassium) and protein (zinc) and sugar (chromium) metabolism. Minerals do not supply energy (calories) but are catalysts in the process of energy production.

Mineral balance is vital as minerals work in combination (synergistically) with each other, or as antagonists to each other. Some minerals compete with each other for absorption (zinc and copper), while others enhance the absorption of each other (zinc and manganese).

The body's concentration of minerals is maintained within very narrow limits through intake, absorption from the gastrointestinal tract, excretion (by the kidneys, bile and other intestinal secretions), storage, utilisation and mineral-to-mineral synergism or competition. Daily intakes vary enormously from one individual to another, the average adult male excreting 20–30 g of inorganic substances (minerals) each day. Chronic, low-grade as well as acute deficiencies can occur if the diet is inadequate or if a person has a genetically greater need for a particular mineral, and lifestyle choices and disease states can use up specific minerals very quickly.

Every essential element (mineral) has an optimal range. Too little can generate symptoms of deficiency, and all have potential toxicity at high doses. Overdoses

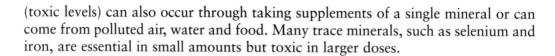

(toxic levels) can also occur through taking supplements of a single mineral or can come from polluted air, water and food. Many trace minerals, such as selenium and iron, are essential in small amounts but toxic in larger doses.

Reasons for requiring nutritional supplementation

Many believe that eating a fresh, well-balanced diet provides all the vitamins and minerals necessary for good health. In ideal circumstances this is the case. However, there are many reasons vitamin and mineral supplements are necessary to cope with living in the twenty-first-century environment. In addition to the food-growing and processing issues mentioned above, the following is a selection of reasons as to why supplementation may be necessary.

- **Poor digestion is a major issue as even if food intake is adequate, poor digestion can limit the body's absorption of vitamins and minerals. Eating too quickly can result in larger than normal food particles (macromolecules) which are too large to allow for the complete action of digestive enzymes. Many people with dentures also are unable to chew efficiently. Consuming foods or drinks (or drugs such as aspirin) that can cause inflammation of the digestive lining can result in a lowering of digestive enzymes and decreased extraction of vitamins and minerals from food.**
- **Alcohol in excess is known to damage the liver and pancreas, which are vital to digestion and metabolism. Alcohol can also damage the lining of the intestinal tract, adversely affecting the absorption of nutrients and leading to subclinical malnutrition. Regular heavy use of alcohol increases the body's needs for the B group vitamins, particularly B1 (thiamine), B3 (niacin), B6 (pyridoxine), folic acid and vitamin B12, and vitamin C. Alcohol also increases the need for the minerals zinc, magnesium and calcium and affects the availability, absorption, metabolism and excretion of all these nutrients.**
- **Smoking tobacco is an irritant to the mucous membranes of both the digestive tract and lungs, and increases metabolic requirements of vitamin C. Each cigarette uses up 25 mg of vitamin C and smokers need 30 per cent more than non-smokers. Smokers also have greater requirements for vitamin A, zinc and lecithin to repair lung membranes.**
- **Laxatives (or chronic diarrhoea) can result in poor absorption of vitamins and minerals from food, by hastening the intestinal transit time. Paraffin and other mineral oils increase losses of the fat-soluble vitamins A, D, E and K and essential fatty acids. Other laxatives used in excess can cause losses of minerals/electrolytes such as potassium, sodium and magnesium.**

- Fad 'diets' that leave out whole groups of foods can be seriously lacking in vitamins and minerals. Even the popular low-fat diets, if used too often or for too long a time, can generate a significant deficiency of the fat-soluble vitamins A, D, E and K and essential fatty acids. Vegan (and many vegetarian) diets must be very well planned to avoid iron, vitamin B12 and zinc deficiencies.

- Antibiotics, although valuable in fighting severe infections, also kill off the friendly bacteria in the gut, adversely affecting digestion. It is always important to take a lengthy course of B group vitamins and acidophilus or bifidobacteria for up to six weeks after antibiotics. Hormone replacement and the pill also decrease absorption of folic acid and increase the need for the vitamin B group, vitamin C, magnesium and zinc.

- Many people are on prescription drugs for a variety of conditions. While these may sometimes be lifesaving they can also increase the need for a variety of nutrients. For example, taking antacids will lower levels of calcium, iron, potassium, vitamin A and vitamin B1. Anti-inflammatory drugs increase the need for vitamins B6, C and E and iodine. Anti-hypertensive medication increases the need for vitamins B6 and B12, potassium and magnesium. Steroid medication increases the need for calcium, iron, zinc and vitamins B6, C and D. Even the humble aspirin increases the need for vitamin C.

- Burns lead to a loss of protein and essential trace nutrients. Surgery increases the need for zinc, vitamin E and other nutrients involved in the cellular repair mechanism. Vitamin C is vital to detoxify anaesthetics and prevent surgical shock (adrenal exhaustion). The repair of broken bones will be slowed by a deficiency of calcium, boron and vitamin C. The challenge of infection places a high demand on resources of zinc, magnesium and vitamins B3, B6, A, C and E.

- Chemical, physical and emotional stresses can increase the body's requirements for vitamins B2, B3, B5, B6 and C. Air pollution increases the requirements for vitamins A and E and the mineral zinc.

- The elderly have been shown to have a consistently low intake of nutrients, particularly protein, calcium, zinc and magnesium. Folic acid deficiency and vitamin B12 deficiency are common. Fibre intake is often low. Riboflavin (B2) and pyridoxine (B6) deficiencies have also been observed. Possible causes are low sense of taste and smell (a sign of zinc deficiency), reduction of digestive enzyme secretion, chronic disease and regular prescription drug use.

- Invalids, shift workers and those whose exposure to sunlight may be minimal can suffer from insufficient amounts of vitamin D, which is required for calcium metabolism, increasing the risk of osteoporosis.

Ultraviolet light is the stimulus for vitamin D production in the skin. Melatonin levels may also be lowered inducing insomnia and depression. This can be exacerbated by long hours on the computer or in a room with electromagnetic radiation (EMR).

- **Many agricultural soils are deficient in trace elements. Decades of intensive monocultures can overwork and deplete soils unless all the soil nutrients are replaced. Unfortunately only the ones known to produce larger crops are usually added. From the Earth Summit Report in Rio in 1992, figures showed that in the United States levels of essential minerals in crops were found to have declined over a 100-year period by up to 85 per cent, and Australian soils had (on average) a 55 per cent mineral depletion in that same timeframe.**

Research into nutrition

Since the 1920s there has been a huge interest in research into nutrition (from indigenous dietary patterns to specific nutrients and their effect on the human body) all around the world.

Overall, the research shows evidence 'that a poor diet is a risk factor for the major chronic diseases that are the leading causes of death, heart disease, stroke, hypertension, diabetes mellitus and some types of cancer' (Wardlaw & Insel 1990: 4). Today there are excellent international peer-reviewed journals specifically for research on nutrition such as the *American Journal of Clinical Nutrition*, the *European Journal of Clinical Nutrition*, the *Townsend Letter* and the *Cochrane Review*. These are just a few of the publications that feature extensive studies on nutritional medicine and further studies appear regularly in the mainstream medical and scientific journals.

Nutrition in practice

Patient compliance

The prevailing medical culture tends to promote the attitude 'for every ill, there's a pill', an easy way out whereby the person can negate any responsibility for their health or illness. It is also a culture whereby a person hands over the control of their health/illness to an external source, be it the doctor or the medical system. Changing food and lifestyle habits takes quite a lot of work. It also involves a change of philosophy and a change in the way individuals perceive themselves, since people often define themselves in terms of a specific lifestyle which involves the consumption of foods that fit that image.

Changing habits is a difficult thing to do. Humans are creatures of habit so changing something as fundamental as the foods we eat takes a huge shift of consciousness. Foods are often consumed (or not consumed) according to cultural or religious circumstances as well and this needs to be taken into account. For example, many Asian people who have never had dairy products as a part of their diet may not (in one lifetime) be able to adapt genetically to a diet high in milk and cheeses, and are likely to end up with dry, scaly skin conditions, acne or asthma if they adopt a diet high in these foods. Ritual fasting also needs to fit in with any nutritional program.

Applying nutrition in practice

Nutrition should form the basis of any complementary or orthodox medical practice as it is the basis of human health. Hence it is a vital component of any preventive healthcare system. While the benefits of nutrition are limited when illness is acute, the road to healing, the convalescent stage, can be dramatically speeded up if appropriate nutrition is put into operation. In chronic illness nutritional therapies and lifestyle changes can be very effective.

The study of nutrition is vitally important but it needs to be remembered that an ideal diet and nutrient supplementation may not be of use if the digestive system of the person is not functioning at its optimal level. If this is the case foods and nutrients will not be digested or absorbed correctly and are usually excreted.

Contraindications/precautions

If a diet is chosen appropriately there are few contraindications for nutritional therapies, although considerations regarding balance of nutrients is important if supplementing with single nutrients (especially minerals). However, when nutrients are used in orthomolecular doses (as drugs) more care needs to be taken, but even then the risk of side effects are minimal and transient when compared to pharmaceuticals.

There are food–drug interactions that can be important. It needs to be recognised that some foods can be powerful enough to alter the effectiveness of medical drugs (ADRAC 2002):

- **Grapefruit juice can increase the effectiveness of the statin drugs like Lipitor.**
- **Foods containing vitamin K (green leafy vegetables) can decrease the effectiveness of warfarin, a common blood-thinning drug, because vitamin K is involved with the production of blood-clotting factors.**

- **Fosamax, a drug for osteoporosis, can have its absorption reduced by 60 per cent if taken with fruit juice or stopped totally if taken with a meal.**

There is a wide range of nutrient and drug interactions (Buist 1984), so responsible administration of any supplement and/or drug requires thorough knowledge of both the supplement and pharmaceutical involved.

The place of nutrition

Medicine as it has been practised during the last century in the West pays little attention to the profound effects that can be obtained through correct nutrition. Orthodox medicine is based on regulating disease and uses as its tools/therapies pharmaceuticals, surgery and radiotherapy. The orthodox model has paid little attention to the concept of health and to the powerful role which food, the correct diet and nutritional supplementation (if appropriate) can play in improving health and therefore in disease resistance.

Nutrition and health

The best possible nutrition alone cannot ensure the best possible health, nor do the worst possible foods always cause the worst health; there are many other factors involved. However, the major cause of illness worldwide is poor nutrition. To summarise a consideration of the practice of nutrition, then, it is worth considering the elements of a diet that supports both the health of the person and the health of the planet. That diet should consist of:

- **Eating a wide variety of fresh foods, predominantly plant-based foods such as whole grains, fruit and vegetables.**
- **Choosing organically or biodynamically grown food, thereby reducing exposure to pesticides and herbicides and increasing nutrient density.**
- **Decreasing total fat intake especially saturated fats. Try frying foods in water (not fat/oil).**
- **Eating high levels of essential fatty acids (e.g. flaxseed oil and fish).**
- **Decreasing the consumption of sugar and refined carbohydrates, including hidden sugars.**
- **Limiting alcohol consumption. The occasional glass of red wine may confer some health benefits.**
- **Encouraging pure water intake. Water detoxifies the systems of the body and assists in waste removal; 2–3 litres per day is recommended.**

- **Reducing sodium (salt) intake.**
- **Ensuring adequate protein by increasing consumption of fish and using vegetable sources of protein such as soy, legumes and nuts, and by eating fewer animal products.**
- **Increasing fibre in the diet—both soluble and insoluble fibres. The best way to do this is by eating more unprocessed whole grains, nuts, seeds and legumes.**
- **Eliminate foods that cause allergy or intolerance.**
- **Minimising tea, coffee and chocolate intake. Try herbal teas and dandelion coffee instead. Green tea has benefits (antioxidants), improving liver and cardiovascular function.**
- **Eliminating processed foods where possible, reducing the intake of chemical food additives, flavourings and colourings (and, by default, increasing your nutrient density).**
- **Chewing food properly (until liquefied).**

'We are what we eat' (Bridgman 2000) is a truism. A diet high in sugars and simple carbohydrates will decrease energy, heighten disposition to headaches and increase the risk of developing type 2 diabetes. A diet high in fats or high in fried foods with little fish or vegetables may increase the risk of heart disease or cancer. Most degenerative diseases can be traced to a combination of genetic inheritance, diet and lifestyle. Informed manipulation of the nutritional components of a person's life can result in significant improvement of disease states and lead that person onto the road of optimal health.

Conclusion

The relationship between humans and food is rooted in evolution and over the millennia there have been periods of major change in that relationship. The first monumental shift was that from hunter-gatherer communities to that of agricultural communities. This was a process that had a profound effect on human health. Today a change of similar proportions is taking place, that of the development of technology. This is impacting agricultural practices, methods of storage and transportation of foods and contributing to the developing food technology industry. Foods can be altered or manufactured technologically either through processing that depletes the nutrients or the development of nutraceuticals where specific nutrients are added or increased in foods, and in the genetic manipulation of food.

Humans are facing enormous challenges today with the magnitude of this change in our relationship with food, for which there is no historical precedent. This change is being reflected in patterns of illness, particularly the development of degenerative diseases, 'the diseases of western civilisation'. Humans are no longer eating what is available, but now have to consider the health implications of what they choose to eat or drink and they are starting to realise that they can make good and bad choices that will be reflected in their health or illness. Along with this comes increasing research where knowledge of the human body and its requirements is at an all-time high. Translating this knowledge into everyday life and medical practice is a significant challenge. As food is the basis of not only survival on this planet, but also determines human health or disease, nutritional medicine including foods and nutrient supplementation is becoming a vital aspect of medicine. Medicine will increasingly rely on nutrition as a major tool in both preventive medicine and in therapeutics.

Recommended reading

Bridgman, K. 2000, *We Are What We Eat*, vols 1–3, 3rd edn, Starflower Pty Ltd, Sydney.

Bland, J. (ed.) 1999, *Clinical Nutrition: A Functional Approach*, Institute of Functional Medicine, Washington.

Eaton, S. *et al.* 1989, *The Stone Age Health Programme*, Angus & Robertson, Sydney.

Pitchford, P. 1993, *Healing with Whole Foods—Oriental Traditions and Modern Nutrition*, North Atlantic Books, California.

Wardlaw, G. and Insel, P. 1990, *Perspectives in Nutrition*, Times/Mirror/Mosby Publishing, St Louis.

14

Osteopathy
Nicholas Lucas, Robert Moran

Osteopathy, or osteopathic medicine, has been defined as 'a system of medical care with a philosophy that combines the needs of the patient with current practice of medicine, surgery and obstetrics, with an emphasis on the interrelationships between structure and function, and an appreciation of the body's ability to heal itself' (AACOM 1997).

Despite this definition, the practice of osteopathy is somewhat difficult to characterise, with many authorities holding differing views on what constitutes osteopathy (Cameron 1998). In order to understand the diverse nature of osteopathy it is necessary to understand the history of its development in, and outside of, the United States.

Development of osteopathy

United States

In the United States osteopaths have full medical licensure and are able to practise family medicine or pursue one of the various medical specialties. The official view of the American Osteopathic Association is that osteopathy is not a complementary medicine; rather, it is equal to, but separate from, orthodox medicine.

The term 'osteopathy' was first used in 1889 by Dr Andrew Taylor Still (1828–1917) to describe a system of medical practice that he had been developing since about 1874. Still learned medicine as an apprentice and later gained his medical doctorate (MD) degree in Kansas City. Still relates a number of events that led him to consider alternative methods to those that were in common use at the time like bloodletting, purgatives, emetics and addictive drugs. It is not hard to understand why he questioned such methods when the events of Still's life are considered. Three of his children died as a result of spinal meningitis despite the use of these common approaches. Further, Still's brother had become addicted to morphine, which had been prescribed as a medicinal substance (Peterson 1997).

Important in the development of Still's new system of medicine was an underlying belief that the body was created with all the necessary elements required to maintain health. He viewed many of the common medical treatments as useless and dangerous, and as causing more harm than help. He experimented with a variety of non-orthodox treatments of the day, including magnetic healing and bone-setting. Through his endeavours he came to believe that optimum mechanical alignment of the body's skeletal structure was necessary for optimum function of the body's systems. Still's term 'osteopathy' reflects the concept that the alignment and movement of bones (osteo-) was linked to disease (pathos). However, his model was not limited to the concept of bony alignment and his choice of the term 'osteopathy' has been criticised due to the implied limitation of dealing only with bones.

Still frequently referred to the importance of other body structures and systems and there was a strong emphasis on mechanistic reasoning from anatomical structure to physiological function. One of his most well-known quotes is that 'the rule of the artery is supreme', referring to the necessity of adequate blood supply for optimum health. On the basis of this single quote, many non-osteopathic authors have oversimplified osteopathy as a system focused on blood supply only. There were, however, other dimensions to Still's approach.

Still taught that osteopaths should know the exact pathway of every nerve from the spinal cord to its innervated tissues and look for any sites of compression that might obstruct the electrical and/or nutritive (axoplasmic) function of nerves. Statements such as 'every nerve should be free to act and do [its] part', 'the fascia is the place to look for the cause of disease', and 'all parts of the body have a direct or indirect connection with the diaphragm' (Kuchera & Kuchera 1994) further demonstrate that his theory of disease was not based solely on bony alignment or blood supply. Osteopathic practice was therefore characterised by the identification and manipulative treatment of bony misalignment, tight muscles, obstructed nerve supply, blood flow, fluid flow and the visceral organs. Surgery was performed when indicated and patients were advised about hygiene, healthy living and diet.

Still soon became overwhelmed with patients and realised that he would need to train new osteopaths in order to meet the demand. In 1892 Still and a colleague, Dr William Smith, opened the American School of Osteopathy in Kirksville, Missouri. Still decided that he would not offer the MD degree but would instead offer the Doctor of Osteopathy (DO) degree. This decision increased the difference between Still's system of osteopathy and orthodox medicine. There were hundreds of keen students and before long numerous other teaching institutions were established throughout the USA (Gevitz 1991).

During the first half of the twentieth century osteopaths sought to practise the full scope of medicine. The orthodox medical profession opposed this but osteopaths eventually gained full medical licensure in all American states. Advances in healthcare technology dominated medicine during the latter half of the twentieth century and this changed the practice of osteopathy in the United States (Gevitz 1991). The curriculum for both orthodox medical and osteopathic schools is almost identical and many argue today that there are few characteristics that distinguish physicians who hold an MD or a DO degree. Further, osteopathic students may complete their internships in regular teaching hospitals alongside their MD colleagues (Cameron 1998). The use of manipulative therapy by American osteopaths during the mid-twentieth century declined until it was practised by a minority who specialised in osteopathic manipulative medicine (see below). However, there has been renewed interest in these techniques within the American profession, with many orthodox medical doctors also wishing to learn musculoskeletal medicine (Palmer 2000).

Outside the United States, osteopathy is practised in 48 countries (Cameron 2002) and is recognisable as a system of healthcare that is based predominantly on osteopathic manipulative medicine.

Britain

The first osteopaths practising in Britain emigrated from America over 100 years ago, with the first recorded practice established in London in 1902. In 1917 John Martin Littlejohn, a graduate of the American College of Osteopathy, established the British School of Osteopathy, which has been in existence ever since.

Osteopathy was practised under British common law until 1993, when the *Osteopaths Act* was implemented to provide for the regulation of the profession. The Act also provided for the establishment of the General Osteopathic Council with which all practitioners using the title 'osteopath' must register. Registration is restricted to those graduates of approved institutions who meet registration requirements.

There are several British-based tertiary institutions providing four-year undergraduate degrees and postgraduate training programs in osteopathy. There are almost 3500 registrants of the General Osteopathic Council, with approximately 200 graduates joining the profession every year.

Since the *Osteopaths Act* of 1993 osteopathy has enjoyed wider recognition amongst the British healthcare community. The nature of funding for primary care has meant that general practitioners (GPs) have been able to purchase the services they consider best meet the needs of their patients and a number of GPs have contracted osteopaths to provide patient care. Similarly, some National Health Service (NHS) hospital trusts and community trusts have employed osteopaths on their staff. Approximately 0.7 million patients receive osteopathic treatment every year in Britain, placing osteopaths as the second largest provider of physical therapy after NHS physiotherapists, who treat one million per year. Osteopaths provide over half of all physical therapy treatments in the private sector in Britain and almost one-third in total (Rosen 1994; McIlwraith 2003).

Australia

The first American-trained osteopaths began practising in Australia around 1913 (Hawkins & O'Neill 1990). Their qualifications were not recognised in the medical act and they were prohibited from claiming to practise medicine or call themselves doctors. Subsequently, very few American osteopaths emigrated to Australia and those who did began to teach local Australians how to practise osteopathy. This style of practice was focused on manipulative therapy and not on surgery or pharmacology. This focus on osteopathic manipulative treatment formed the basis of osteopathic practice in Australia, as it did in Britain and New Zealand.

In Australia osteopathy is regulated at a state government level. In order to practise, osteopaths must register with and meet the requirements of the relevant state registration board. In terms of education, new registrants must have completed an accredited course of study at an approved Australian university. All such courses in Australia require five years of full-time study consisting of a three-year Bachelors degree followed by a two-year Masters degree. There are close to 1000 registered osteopaths practising in Australia and approximately 100 students graduate per year from accredited university courses.

Australian osteopaths practise almost exclusively in private clinics. New graduates are routinely employed as associates in existing practices, although a growing number of graduates are establishing their own practices (Hagi 1999). Osteopathic treatment is covered by many private health funds and government-sponsored schemes such as WorkCover and the Traffic Accident Commission (TAC).

New Zealand

The practice of osteopathy in New Zealand has not been regulated by any specific legislation. Until 1999 there had been no government-funded university courses in osteopathy, with only a few private colleges offering various modes of training. The first publicly funded tertiary program commenced in 1999. The program is similar in design to the British and Australian courses and follows the five-year double-degree model of training (Bachelors and Masters). The inclusion of education programs in public tertiary institutions will result in a rapid increase in the size of the profession.

The majority of osteopaths currently practising in New Zealand have trained at one of the British institutions. A group of osteopaths formed a voluntary registration body in 1973, called the New Zealand Register of Osteopaths (NZRO). This group has sought and gained recognition from various agencies such as the Accident Compensation Corporation and other third-party payers. There are approximately 250 members of the NZRO, with members adhering to codes of professional conduct and participating in continuing professional development programs. The unregulated nature of osteopathy in New Zealand makes it difficult to determine accurate numbers but it has been estimated that there are at least 300 practitioners who identify themselves as osteopaths.

Osteopathic principles and concepts

There are four general principles that have been put forward as those underpinning the practice of osteopathy (Seffinger 1997).

1. The body is a unit; the person is a unit of body, mind and spirit.
A contemporary example of this principle is the field of psychoneuroimmunology, which recognises that there is an integrated physiological relationship between a person's thoughts and their nervous and immune systems (Martin 1997; Willard *et al.* 1997). On a broader level, Engel (1977) coined the term 'biopsychosocial' to group together the influences that contribute to an individual's health status. He broadened the concept of biomedical disease causation and management to include social and behavioural influences.

2. The body is capable of self-regulation, self-healing and health maintenance.
This principle encompasses the physiological concept of homœostasis and emphasises the dynamic maintenance of the internal and external environments of the body under normal and challenging conditions. The processes of inflammation, healing and repair are relevant examples of this principle.

3. Structure and function are interrelated
Many of the basic sciences recognise the importance of structure–function relationships. For example, in biochemistry the structure of a molecule determines its function in terms of its affinity for the three-dimensional shape of receptor proteins in cell walls.

4. Rational treatment is based on an understanding of the basic principles of body unity, self-regulation and the interrelationship of structure and function.

Osteopathic manipulative medicine

Osteopathic manipulative medicine (OMM) is defined as 'a primary care specialty emphasising in-depth application of osteopathic philosophy and special proficiency in osteopathic diagnosis and treatment' (AACOM 1997). OMM encompasses:

1. **Assessing the patient from a holistic point of view, taking into account their lifestyle, working environment, home life and other psychosocial factors.**

2. **Forming diagnoses from the patient's history and clinical examination, supplemented where necessary with special investigations such as diagnostic imaging and laboratory testing.**
3. **Providing treatment that will alter the natural history of the disease or dysfunction, such as osteopathic manipulation, education and reassurance, medication or surgical intervention.**
4. **Providing a prognosis for the patient.**
5. **Advising the patient about prevention.**

Osteopathic diagnosis

Osteopaths utilise standard medical diagnostic procedures and specialised osteopathic procedures in order to understand the patient from an osteopathic perspective. Emphasis is placed on the assessment of the neuromusculoskeletal system with the aim of identifying gross pathological changes and/or somatic dysfunction. The search for abnormalities within the neuromusculoskeletal system is conducted with a view to implement treatment strategies that aim to improve the functioning of dysfunctional and/or pathological parts of the system.

Somatic dysfunction is a term used to describe a collection of observed and palpated changes within the neuromusculoskeletal system. It is defined as:

impaired or altered function of related components of the somatic (body framework) system: the skeletal, arthrodial, and myofascial structures, and related vascular, lymphatic and neural elements (World Health Organization 1992).

It is important to distinguish between pathology (such as arthritis or infection) and somatic dysfunction, in which no pathology is implied. Osteopaths therefore incorporate both pathological diagnoses and dysfunctional diagnoses into their total view of the patient. This allows osteopaths to design a management plan that addresses both the pathological and dysfunctional aspects of the patient's problem.

An illustrative example of an osteopathic diagnosis may be osteoarthritis (pathology) of the left hip joint and somatic dysfunction of the left foot. Management may include:

1. **The prescription and application of osteopathic manipulative techniques that aim to improve the functioning of the patient's left foot and hip.**
2. **The prescription of an analgesic if the pain is severe.**
3. **Education regarding the patient's condition and the pain they are feeling and advice regarding appropriate exercise and diet.**

4. **The osteopath listening to the patient in order to develop an understanding of the impact this condition has had on the patient's life.**

Osteopathic manipulative treatment

One of the defining features of osteopathic medicine is the use of osteopathic manipulative treatment (OMT). OMT is defined as 'the therapeutic application of manually guided forces by an osteopathic physician to improve physiologic function and/or support homœostasis' (AACOM 1997).

It is important to make the point that osteopathy is not limited to, or synonymous with, the use of manipulation. Osteopathic treatment in general can be defined as any treatment that takes into account the osteopathic principles discussed above, and by definition may include dietary advice, pharmaceuticals, surgery, counselling, exercise prescription and manipulative treatment.

Another term worth mentioning is manual therapy, which is a term used across disciplines to describe the various manipulative procedures used by osteopaths, physiotherapists, chiropractors and musculoskeletal physicians. Some osteopaths claim that the application of manual therapy is not 'osteopathic' unless it is applied according to the osteopathic principles. Osteopaths tend to avoid applying a 'protocol' of treatment for a 'condition' and rely instead on an assessment of the individual in order to implement a management plan that is designed to address the unique characteristics of the patient. To illustrate this view, standard osteopathic texts (Greenman 1995; Kuchera & Kuchera 1996; DiGiovanna & Schiowitz 1997; Ward 2003) do not provide chapters on specific pathological conditions with standardised treatment approaches. Rather, the texts are organised according to the identification and treatment of somatic dysfunction for each region. It is conceptualised that two patients with hip osteoarthritis may have entirely different patterns of somatic dysfunction. One patient may have somatic dysfunction of the foot (as in the above example), while the other may have somatic dysfunction of the pelvis and knee. A standardised best practice approach to the management of hip osteoarthritis may be taken, combined with an individualised approach to somatic dysfunction.

The following discussion about manipulative techniques used by osteopaths is taken broadly from the Glossary of Osteopathic Terminology (AACOM 1997).

Soft tissue manipulation

Soft tissue manipulation (STM) is any manual technique that is directed to non-skeletal structures. It encompasses massage, stretching, direct pressure, myofascial release and positional release techniques. The aims of STM are to specifically address abnormal changes within the soft tissues when these changes are considered to be a primary component of the patient's condition. These techniques are also commonly applied as preparatory techniques for the application of techniques directed to the joints, such as high-velocity, low-amplitude manipulation.

Articulation

Articulation is a technique in which a joint and its associated structures are rhythmically moved through a range of movement with the aim of improving joint motion, stretching joint tissues, enhancing the flow of fluid within and around the joint and activating the body's inherent analgesic systems. Mobilisation is a term used by other professions to describe a similar group of techniques.

High-velocity low-amplitude manipulation

During the application of a high-velocity, low-amplitude (HVLA) technique a very small (low-amplitude) but rapid (high-velocity) movement is directed toward a joint or joints. This technique is often associated with what is known as joint cavitation, which is the event thought to produce the audible 'popping' or 'cracking' sound that accompanies HVLA techniques. It is thought that cavitation occurs due to a rapid decrease in intra-articular pressure associated with the manipulation. The decrease in pressure leads to an implosion within the synovial fluid, producing a precipitation of small gas bubbles. The gas bubbles coalesce to form a larger bubble within the joint cavity that is visible on plain film radiographs. After approximately twenty minutes the gas dissolves back into the synovial fluid, and during this twenty-minute timeframe re-cavitation is not usually possible (Brodeur 1995).

There are a number of different situations in which a practitioner might choose to apply HVLA techniques:

1. **to improve a joint's range of motion (Surkitt et al. 2000);**
2. **to reduce the displacement of intra-articular meniscoids (Bogduk 1997);**
3. **to induce analgesia (Wright 2000);**
4. **to alter muscle tone (Evans 2002);**
5. **to disrupt the formation of adhesions (scar tissue) within joint capsules and ligaments (Stoddard 1969).**

Muscle energy techniques

Muscle energy techniques were first developed by North American osteopaths in the late 1940s and have been in common use since that time. The term muscle energy technique (MET) encompasses a range of treatment manoeuvres that are applied to joints and muscles. Application of the technique involves the specific positioning of the patient to assist localisation of the technique toward the target tissues. From this position the patient actively contracts against a counterforce provided by the osteopath. When used in this way the technique involves a patient-generated isometric muscle contraction. At the completion of the contraction it is proposed that post-isometric relaxation may be invoked in the contractile tissues. The techniques can be applied to almost any joint or muscle in the body, with the aim of improving a joint's range of motion and muscle function. Other effects of MET may include improving muscle recruitment and motor control, activating endogenous analgesia and improving fluid exchange in soft tissues and joints (Fryer 2000).

Positional release techniques

Positional release techniques are passive techniques in which the patient is positioned in such a way as to facilitate a relaxation of muscle, decrease in pain and improvement of fluid flow within the relevant tissues. There are a variety of positional release techniques and one of the more commonly used is 'strain-counterstrain' (SCS), which was developed by Lawrence Jones in 1955. In SCS the emphasis is on locating and relieving relevant tender points within myofascial structures associated with somatic dysfunction.

Osteopathy in the cranial field

In the early 1900s osteopath William Sutherland reported his discovery of movement at the cranial sutures and a palpable rhythm throughout the cranium, spinal column and extremities. He proposed several mechanisms to explain the basis of these observed phenomena and also developed a range of diagnostic and therapeutic techniques that were devised for use in the clinical setting. Unfortunately, many of Sutherland's early empirical observations and his proposed mechanisms have failed to be validated in contemporary experimental studies (Moran & Gibbons 2001; Hartman & Norton 2002). The underlying physiological mechanisms to explain the observed rhythmic phenomena have not been elucidated to date.

Practitioners usually apply their hands to the head and sacrum with the aim of detecting changes in the frequency and symmetry of the perceived rhythm. Any departure from what is considered normal is viewed within the context of the patient's condition and treatment is then directed toward the normalisation of the rhythm. The techniques typically involve the application of gentle contact pressures over the various cranial bones, sutures and sacrum.

Visceral techniques

Many visceral structures have myofascial, neural, vascular and lymphatic components and are theoretically considered to be subject to dysfunction. Viscera are relatively mobile within the abdominal cavity and mobility is a necessary requirement for normal function. The formation of adhesions following abdominal surgery and the resultant pain and loss of function is demonstrative of the important role that adequate visceral mobility may play in normal function. Visceral techniques are primarily aimed at maintaining or restoring mobility and involve the application of carefully directed contact pressures over the neck, chest and abdominopelvic region. Dysfunction of the gastrointestinal tract (e.g. gastric reflux, constipation, abdominal cramping) and improving the mobility of scar tissue following abdominal surgery are two of the more common presenting problems where visceral techniques may be indicated.

Osteopathy and evidence-based healthcare

Given more than 100 years of development it might be expected that the practice of osteopathy would be well supported by an established evidence base. However, this is not the case, with only a few outcome studies that specifically investigate the efficacy of osteopathic treatment being published in the peer-reviewed literature. This situation is largely due to the small size of a profession that is located primarily in the private sector, coupled with limited access to research funding and expertise. However, now that osteopaths are becoming increasingly more involved in third-party funded reimbursement, there is also an increasing awareness of the need for producing good quality outcome studies. This changing awareness is also reflected in the contemporary education of osteopaths, with training programs now including courses that aim to increase research literacy and promote models of patient management that are informed by clinical and applied research.

A recent example of clinical research specifically investigating an osteopathic approach to the treatment of low back pain has been reported in the literature. In 1999 Andersson *et al.* published a study that compared osteopathic spinal manipulation with standard medical care for patients with low back pain. The authors reported that at twelve weeks' follow-up both groups demonstrated similar levels of clinical improvement; however, those patients receiving osteopathic care required less medication than the group receiving standard medical care.

While there may be few studies directly investigating osteopathic treatment, there is an emerging literature that provides support for various aspects of the osteopathic concept. These include the performance of a skilled physical examination, the use of pain modification techniques, educating the patient about their condition, providing realistic goals and prognoses, helping the patient to overcome certain pain behaviours or beliefs that may be preventing their full recovery and encouraging patients to engage in moderate physical activity (Frank 1973; Gerteis *et al.* 1993; Achterberg 1996; Kendall *et al.* 1997; Linton 1998; NHMRC 1998; Waddell 1998). Other examples of research that is not uniquely osteopathic but that supports the osteo-pathic concept are available. For example, a recent randomised controlled trial led the investigators to conclude that manual therapy is a favourable treatment option for patients with neck pain compared with physical therapy or continued care by a general practitioner (Hoving *et al.* 2002).

Spinal manipulation has become a popular and widely accepted therapy in the treatment of low back pain, with several meta-analyses providing support for its use in both acute and chronic low back pain (Koes *et al.* 1991, 1996). Each of these reports a statistically significant effect for manipulation in terms of decreased pain and increased function. Further, spinal manipulation and manual therapy is recom-mended as a treatment for acute low back pain in evidence-based clinical guidelines issued by the American (AHCPR 1994), New Zealand (ACC 1997) and British (GSAC 1994; RCGP 1996) health authorities.

Similarly, in Australia spinal manipulation also forms part of a comprehensive treatment approach recommended for whiplash and associated disorders (grades 1 and 2) in the guidelines issued by the Motor and Accident Authority in New South Wales (MAA 2001).

Osteopathy in practice

Patients consult osteopaths for a range of problems, the most common being muscu-loskeletal pain. In several studies conducted in Britain low back pain was the most common presenting complaint, followed by cervical (neck) pain (Burton 1981; Pringle & Tyreman 1993; McIlwraith 2003).

Typically an initial consultation will last for between 30 minutes to one hour. During this time the osteopath will undertake a standard medical interview and ask specific questions which relate directly to the presenting complaint. The osteopath will then conduct a physical examination and, based on the history and physical examination findings, will formulate a diagnosis for which they will devise an appropriate management plan. Management typically involves osteopathic manip-ulative techniques, which may be coupled with physiological therapeutics, exercise prescription and dietary advice. Since many patients present with problems that are linked to posture or faulty movement patterns, osteopaths often attempt to encourage the patient to recognise the need for changes in posture and movement in order to rehabilitate the existing problem and prevent future recurrence. If the osteopath determines that treatment such as medication or further investigations such as diagnostic imaging are required, these will be arranged.

While there is no recognised specialisation system within osteopathy (outside the United States), practitioners invariably develop special interests in management of a particular problem or population. Such interests range across the full spectrum including the treatment of newborn infants and children, care of women during pregnancy, sporting injuries or workplace injury prevention and ergon omics.

Contraindications and risks

A thorough discussion of the specific risks and contraindications associated with osteopathic manipulative treatment (OMT) is beyond the scope of this text. In terms of risk associated with OMT, the necessary research has not been conducted. Therefore data on absolute risk, relative risk and the number of individual treatments needed before harm occurs for each of the treatment approaches are not available. There are limited data regarding the very small risk of vertebrobasilar accidents associated with HVLA techniques applied to the cervical spine. However, these data are based on retrospective cohort studies, case-control studies and reports in the literature of single case studies and do not constitute a sufficient level of evidence from which to draw valuable conclusions regarding risk.

In terms of contraindications, some general comments can be made. First, each case is considered on an individual basis and according to the clinical experience of the osteopath. In cases of fracture, active inflammation, bone-weakening diseases, neurological compromise, vascular compromise and bleeding disorders, the more forceful techniques such as HVLA are contraindicated. However, other osteopathic techniques may be permitted in such cases. Other general contraindications include lack of diagnosis, lack of patient consent and situations where the technique cannot be carried out because of patient pain or resistance. Relative contraindications include recent trauma, previous adverse reaction to OMT, inflammatory disease, pregnancy, anticoagulant use or long-term corticosteroid use, ligamentous laxity and psychological dependence on OMT (Gibbons & Tehan 2000).

Conclusion

Osteopathic medicine is a primary healthcare profession with an emphasis on the health of the neuromusculoskeletal system. In the United States, osteopaths have unlimited licensure; however, only a minority specialise in osteopathic manipulative medicine (Cameron 1998). In Australia, New Zealand and Britain (and Europe), osteopaths practise almost exclusively in osteopathic manipulative medicine without prescription rights or surgery, and use osteopathic manipulative techniques as their most common therapeutic tool.

Recommended reading

Gevitz, N. 1991, *The D.O.'s: Osteopathic Medicine in America*, Johns Hopkins University Press, Baltimore.

Greenman, P.E. 1995, *Principles of Manual Medicine*, Lippincott Williams & Wilkins, Baltimore.

Ward, R.C. (ed.) 2003, *Foundations for Osteopathic Medicine*, 2nd edn, Lippincott Williams & Wilkins, Baltimore.

Lederman, E. 1997, *Fundamentals of Manual Therapy*, Churchill Livingstone, Edinburgh.

Hartman, L.S. 1996, *Handbook of Osteopathic Technique*, 3rd edn, Chapman and Hall, London.

15

Yoga and meditation
Simon Borg-Olivier, Bianca Machliss

The word 'yoga' means 'union', 'joining' or 'to link together as one whole'. Yoga is the art and science of resolving the inherent opposition in all things to create a union of body, mind and soul. Meditation is an integral component, and the essence, of yoga.

Yoga is literally a holistic system. Iyengar (2001) describes yoga as 'the path, which integrates the body, senses, mind, and the intelligence, with the self'. Feuerstein (1996) describes the yoga approach as simplifying one's consciousness and energy to the point where one no longer experiences any inner conflict and is able to live in harmony with the world. In India yoga is traditionally thought of as a means to understanding the relationship between one's individual soul (*jivatma*) and the universal soul (*Paramatman*). In the dualist *Samkhya* philosophy, on which classical yoga was originally based, yoga is the result of joining *jivatma* with *Paramatman*. In the non-dualist *Vedanta* and *Tantric* philosophies, which modern yoga has absorbed, yoga is the process of realising that the *jivatma* and the *Paramatman* are in fact the same entity.

The paths to achieve yoga, or to realise yoga, are many. Hence, there are many types of yoga and each type has many styles. Essentially all the activities of yoga can be divided into two parts that can be referred to as 'physical yoga' and 'non-physical yoga'. Physical yoga consists of 'physical exercises' and 'breath control' and is often thought of as a static or slow-moving type of stretching and relaxation. However, it can also include strenuous exercises that tone muscles, tension nerves and stimulate the cardiovascular system (Raju *et al.* 1994). Physical yoga can be very fast and may include repetitive exercises that resemble western-style callisthenics and gymnastics. Physical yoga can also manipulate internal organs (Kuvalayananda 1925) and modify blood chemistry (Miyamura *et al.* 2002). Non-physical yoga consists of 'ethical disciplines' and 'meditative practices' and can help to expand the mind, explore the emotions and develop the relationships between oneself and the rest of the world.

History of yoga and meditation

The history of yoga and meditation is the subject of much controversy. Conventional belief is that yoga originated in India at least 5000 years ago (Ghosh 1999), but traditional Indian belief is that yoga itself is far older and was practised all over the world. Artwork depicting images of people or gods in advanced yoga postures are dated at 2700 BCE (Desikachar 1998). Buddhist yoga arose out of Indian yoga in about the fifth century BCE and slowly spread into the rest of Asia. Indian yoga came to China in about 500 CE and developed into Taoist yoga. Modern yoga has evolved and blended from two distinct and possibly unrelated sources, Vedic yoga and Tantric yoga.

Vedic yoga is one of six interrelated systems of classical Indian philosophical thought that are all interpretations of reality based on the *Vedas*, which most authors believe are India's most ancient texts. Vedic yoga, formalised in the *Patanjali-yoga-sutra*, is based on the dualist Samkhya School which says all things arise from two ultimate realities, spirit (*purusa*) and matter (*prakruti*). Vedic yoga includes jnana yoga ('yoga of self-knowledge'), which is based on the non-dualist Vedanta School which says there is only one ultimate reality (Brahman) making its appearance to our senses as an illusion (*maya*), and that all things are one, only appearing to be separate.

Tantric yoga is based on an important non-classical school of Indian philosophy called Tantra. Tantric texts (*Tantras*) are based on ancient texts called *Agamas*, which may pre-date the *Vedas* (Shah 2001). Tantra is non-dualist like Vedanta but is polarity based: everything consists of opposing and attractive forces such as male and female. Tantra is the base for most yoga and meditation practised today. Tantric yoga embraces all aspects of life and is often misunderstood as dealing only with sexual activity and black magic. However, hatha yoga, Buddhist yoga and Taoist yoga all have significant Tantric influences.

The first significant written mention of yoga is in the *Bhagavad-Gita*, which was written about the fifth century BCE and which extols the virtues of yoga (Desikachar 1998). The second major extant text on yoga is the *Patanjali-yoga-sutra*, which was written in the second century BCE. The *Patanjali-yoga-sutra* explains that the means to achieve yoga are by following an eight-limbed (*asta-anga*) path to the ultimate state of meditative absorption (*samadhi*). Most yoga can be classified in terms of astanga yoga. The eight (*asta*) limbs (*angas*) of astanga yoga (Iyengar 1988, 1993) are:

- *Yama* (our attitudes to our environment)
- *Niyama* (our attitudes towards ourselves)
- *Asana* (physical exercises)
- *Pranayama* (breath control)
- *Pratayahara* (meditative sense control)
- *Dharana* (meditative concentration)
- *Dhyana* (meditative contemplation)
- *Samadhi* (meditative absorption)

Table 15.1   Practical divisions of yoga based on the astanga yoga system

Functional divisions of the activities of yoga	Eight limbs of astanga yoga (All eight limbs can be applied to most types of yoga including hatha yoga and raja yoga)	Functional divisions of the activities of yoga
Non-physical yoga	1. *Yama* (our attitudes to our environment) 2. *Niyama* (our attitudes towards ourselves)	Ethical disciplines (which include the essence of jnana yoga, bhakti yoga and karma yoga)
Physical yoga	3. *Asana*	Physical exercises (including *asanas*, *vinyasas*, *bandhas*, *kriyas* and *mudras*)
	4. *Pranayama*	Breath control
Non-physical yoga	5. *Pratayahara* (meditative sense-control) 6. *Dharana* (meditative concentration) 7. *Dhyana* (meditative contemplation) 8. *Samadhi* (meditative absorption)	Meditative practices (including techniques of mantra yoga, yantra yoga and laya yoga)

Note: Each of the eight limbs of astanga yoga can be present while doing physical yoga.

Classifying the systems of yoga is problematic as there is considerable overlap between the various types of yoga. Table 15.1 shows the relationship between the traditional eight limbs of astanga yoga and the functional divisions of yoga. Various types of yoga are briefly described in Table 15.2.

Table 15.2   Types of yoga

Karma yoga	Yoga of action or 'work'
Jnana yoga	Yoga of self-knowledge
Bhakti yoga	Yoga of devotion
Mantra yoga	Yoga involving physical or mental recitation of sounds or chants
Yantra yoga	Yoga involving physical or mental visualisation of objects and symbols
Laya yoga	An advanced combination of mantra yoga and yantra yoga techniques
Kundalini yoga	The culmination of laya yoga
Hatha yoga	Yoga of physical forces, mainly using physical exercises to achieve yoga
Raja yoga	Yoga of the mind, mainly using meditative practices to achieve yoga

Yoga as it is practised in the western world can broadly be divided into two parts, hatha yoga and raja yoga. Hatha yoga is what most people in the West think of as physical yoga because it mainly uses physical exercises and breath control to achieve the meditative state. Hatha yoga was first described in the 2000-year-old text *Yoga-yajnavalkya-samhita* (Desikachar 2000) and is in essence a type of Tantric yoga. Although hatha yoga is typified by a series of exercises that are used to generate and manipulate physical and subtle forces in the body, its main aim is the same as every other form of genuine yoga, namely self-realisation. The *Gheranda-samhita* states that the sole reason to learn hatha yoga is as a path to raja yoga (Pranavananda 1992).

Raja yoga is what most people think of as meditation and is described in the yogic texts as the most difficult type of astanga yoga (Pranavananda 1992). Raja yoga is considered the non-physical approach to achieve yoga and mainly uses the meditative practices to achieve a meditative state. Raja yoga is essentially about controlling the mind and unifying one's intelligence with one's consciousness (Ghosh 1999). Raja yoga has little emphasis on physical work beyond sitting in a stable posture (*asana*) with an erect spine. However, the physical exercises of hatha yoga can help prepare one for the challenge of sitting comfortably for a long time in the raja yoga meditative state.

In the twenty-first century yoga is used to develop and maintain physical and mental health. The concept of using yoga as a healing tool for the body and the mind is not new. Yoga as a therapy had its first probable mention in the *Yoga-yaj-navalkya-samhita*, which dates to the second century BCE. More recent hatha yoga texts such as the *Hatha-yoga-pradipika* also mention the various therapeutic benefits of yoga (Vishnu-Devananda 1987).

Many of the world's complementary and physical therapies are yoga-based. Techniques resembling yoga and often derived from yoga are frequently used for therapy. Pilates is a yoga-based form of physical training that is especially popular as a therapy in the dance community. Pilates instructors and exercise-based physiotherapists even teach some concepts that are directly from the heart of traditional yoga. One example is the concept of 'core stabilisation', which is described in yoga texts as *bandha*, but which is often neglected or not known by many modern yoga teachers.

Physical yoga

In most conventional exercise, training for strength, flexibility and cardiovascular fitness are practised separately. In physical yoga, physical exercises and breath control can be used together to develop simultaneously strength, flexibility and relaxation, in conjunction with joint stabilisation, improved circulation and increased levels of energy. By working holistically, physical yoga can improve performance of functional tasks, while decreasing the effort involved.

Yogic physical exercises can increase the range of joint motion (ROM), increase muscle length and tension (stretch) *nadis* (nerves and other channels) while maintaining joint stability. Nerve reflexes can be utilised to develop muscular strength throughout the ROM and train muscles to be voluntarily active or relaxed at any length. Synergistic muscle activations can be used to maximise the distance between proximal and distal attachments of a muscle to increase flexibility. Muscle co-activations (*bandhas*) around the major joints can help stabilise these joints, assist in generation of energy and promote circulation. Yogic physical exercises can be 'weight bearing' on any part of the body including any part of the legs, arms, trunk, head or any combination of these parts. Weight-bearing exercises may minimise the risk of osteoporosis by maintaining bone mineral density in the area that is weight bearing (O'Brien 2001).

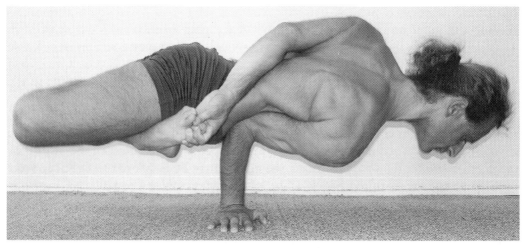

Eka Hasta Baddha Padma Mayurasana—'One-handed lotus balance' (Courtesy of Yoga Synergy)

Static postures (*asanas*)

Yogic texts suggest that there are more than 8 400 000 *asanas* (Vishnu-Devananda 1987). Although it is possible to perform any posture as an *asana*, a few classical postures offer the most benefits with the minimum of effort. Some *asanas* can be performed with completely relaxed muscles while others impose obligatory isometric muscle activations. In all *asanas* one can voluntarily activate any muscle in the body isometrically. Each *asana* may be held for anything from a few seconds to several hours depending on the level of difficulty.

Dynamic exercises (*vinyasas*)

Vinyasa is the term for a 'linked series of postures' and the 'linking movements between postures'. *Vinyasas* can vary in speed from being so slow that the movement is almost imperceptible to the eye to those that are too fast for the eye to follow. Concentric and eccentric muscle control is developed in *vinyasa* and, because one part of the body can resist against another, isokinetic muscle control can be developed.

Breath control (*pranayama*)

Breath control (*pranayama*) is considered the link between the body and the mind as it can be practised during both the physical exercises and the meditative practices. *Pranayama*, which literally means 'expansion and regulation' (*ayama*) of the 'life force in the breath' (*prana*) (Iyengar 1993), develops internal energy and very efficient breathing which can reduce the amount of oxygen required to do a specific amount of work (Bernardi *et al.* 2001a). The experienced 'yogin' can use 'breath control' to increase strength (Raghuraj *et al.* 1997), flexibility and cardiovascular fitness, to reduce blood pressure (Telles *et al.* 1996) and to regulate blood chemistry, hormone levels and the nervous system.

Yogic breathing is usually through both nostrils but can be done at times through the mouth or through individual nostrils. *Pranayama* can affect breathing by modifying the lengths of inhalation, inhalation retention (holding the breath in), exhalation and exhalation retention (holding the breath out). The sound of the breath, the position of one's tongue and regulation of one's diet all affect *pranayama*. Control of the muscles used for breathing and control of 'minute ventilation' (the amount of air breathed per minute) are the most important factors determining the outcome of breath control.

Adverse effects of incorrect yogic breathing, especially excessive breathing, can be extreme and dangerous (Teramoto *et al.* 1997). Yogic texts stress that physical exercises should be mastered before advanced breath control is attempted (Iyengar 1993). New practitioners of yoga who practise physical exercises while breathing naturally prepare their bodies and mind for the eventual practice of *pranayama*.

Yogic purification and energy control (*bandhas, mudras and kriyas*)

Breath control is also used in most of the unique exercises known as *sat-kriyas* (purificatory processes) and *mudras* (energy-control practices). *Sat-kriyas* are cleansing processes that literally purify the body inside and out. *Mudras* are special gestures, postures and muscle-control exercises that regulate the flow of energy in the body. Most *sat-kriyas* and *mudras* require the use of *bandhas* (muscle locks). *Bandhas, kriyas* and *mudras* are very powerful therapeutic agents but few teachers are qualified to teach them. On a physical level, a *bandha* is essentially the co-activation, or simultaneous tensing, of opposing (antagonistic) muscles across a 'joint complex'. *Bandhas* help to stabilise 'joint complexes' by balancing joint flexibility with muscular strength, and help generate and move energy through the body. Using the *bandhas* as a base, hatha yoga uses *kriyas* to 'cleanse and purify' the inside of the body and *mudras* to develop energy in the body and then channel it wherever it is needed. Probably the most powerful *kriyas* and *mudras* are those that apply all the main *bandhas* at the same time.

Effects of physical yoga

Many positive and some negative effects of yoga are reported in the literature. Reported long-term positive effects of yoga include increases in strength (Raghuraj & Telles 1997; Garfinkle *et al.* 1998; Dash & Telles 2001), flexibility (Moorthy 1982; Ray *et al.* 2001), cardiovascular fitness (Raju *et al.* 1986, 1994), anaerobic threshold, mental function (Ray *et al.* 2001) and wellbeing (Schell *et al.* 1994); and decreases in reaction times (Madanmohan *et al.* 1992) and blood pressure (Patel & North 1975; Selvamurthy *et al.* 1998).

Many of the well-documented benefits of the seated meditative practices, listed later in this chapter, can be obtained by practising purely physical yoga. This is because as one becomes more adept meditative states can be generated in any posture and even during movement (*vinyasa*). Physiological phenomena typical of those observed in seated meditative states, such as coherent synchronous EEG patterns (Aftanas & Golocheikine 2001) and hypoventilation (Travis & Pearson 2000), have been demonstrated in people practising physical yoga (Junker & Dworkis 1986; Kamei *et al.* 2000; Arambula *et al.* 2001; Vempati & Telles 2002).

Physical yoga can have a simultaneous effect on the brain and the immune system. Kamei *et al.* (2000) have demonstrated that during yoga exercises alpha waves increased while serum cortisol decreased. Yogic physical exercises can be thought of as a type of moderate exercise the long-term effects of which have been repeatedly shown to enhance the function of the immune system (Pedersen & Toft 2000; Fairey *et al.* 2002). Similarly, stress reduction and relaxation techniques probably derived from yoga have been shown to enhance immune function (Rood *et al.* 1993; Lowe *et al.* 2001).

An integral aspect of yoga is living in the present moment. Therefore it is important to note the immediate effects of intelligent and correctly performed practice of yogic physical exercises and breath control. These effects include increased circulation (Gardner *et al.* 2001), facilitation of neuromuscular control (Kocher 1976; Telles *et al.* 1993, 1994a), regulation of blood chemistry (Raju *et al.* 1986, 1994; Miyamura *et al.* 2002) and control over the nervous system (Vempati & Telles 2002) and the brain (Kamei *et al.* 2000).

Increased circulation through yoga

A main goal of yoga is to help integrate the body and mind as a whole. Therefore, one of the main physiological purposes of yoga is to improve the circulation of information, energy and matter throughout the body. Stimulation of body circulation is one of the main ways yoga works. The body's four circulatory systems (the cardio-vascular, lymphatic and nervous systems and the acupuncture meridian system) transport energy, matter and information through the body. In yoga terminology *nadis* are the channels of these four circulatory systems. Circulation is enhanced during a yoga practice by generating forces (*hatha*), in the form of high pressures (*ha*) and low pressures (*tha*), which act as circulatory 'pumps'. Yoga utilises five circulatory pumps to assist in the regulatory function of the heart. These pumps exist as a result of movement (*vinyasa*), breath control (*pranayama*), orientation to gravity (*viparita-karani*), posture (*asana*) and co-activation of opposing muscles across joints (*bandha*).

Yoga utilises the 'musculoskeletal pump' of circulation (Orsted *et al.* 2001) during movement. As muscles tense they increase local pressure in the veins and 'push' blood and intracellular fluid in the direction of the heart. One-way back-flow valves in the veins prevent movement of blood away from the heart in the veins. When a muscle relaxes it decreases local venous pressure and 'pulls' blood from regions more distal to the heart to that region. The 'respiratory pump' of circulation is also employed in yoga (Hillman & Finucane 1987) with breath control. Breath control can affect the pre-load of the blood into the heart, which can alter heart rate depending on whether the inhalation is directed to the thorax, which increases heart rate, or to the abdominal region, which decreases heart rate. A 'gravitational pump' also exists by virtue of *viparita-karani,* the inverted or semi-inverted postures. Simple postures such as resting the legs vertically up a wall and more advanced poses like *sirsasana* (headstand) reverse the natural flow of gravity and can offer the same benefits as the technique referred to as 'postural drainage' used in physiotherapy (Fink 2002). The 'postural pump' uses *asanas*, which are static postures. Relative to normal postures (such as anatomical position) *asanas* can physically compress (increase the pressure) at one region of the body while expanding or 'stretching' (decreasing the pressure) in another region of the body. Finally, the 'muscle co-activation pump' employs *bandhas* to create regions of high pressure (*ha-bandhas*) or regions of low pressure (*tha-bandhas*). Energy in the form of blood and heat (among other things) tries to move from the regions of high pressure to the regions of low pressure. Intelligent control of the formation of these *bandhas* during a yoga practice can regulate the circulation in any part of the body.

The five circulatory pumps also assist in the movement of food through the intestines, the absorption of nutrients and the elimination of wastes and can effectively massage internal organs and endocrine glands, assisting in their function.

Yogic facilitation of neuromuscular control

Another important way that yoga can effectively achieve union between body and mind is through integrated control and regulation of skeletal muscles and nervous system. This requires basic understanding and application of the principles of motor nerve reflexes and nerve tensioning.

A reflex is an automatic nerve response to some type of stimulus. There are three important reflexes which should be taken into account and which can be taken advantage of in any physical posture. The 'stretch (myotatic) reflex' is the reflex activation of a muscle whenever a muscle is sufficiently tensioned or stretched (Alter 1996). If the stretch reflex is activated during a stretching exercise then it will reduce the ability to stretch very far. If forced, the muscle may be damaged. The yogin tries to inhibit the stretch reflex by:

- **moving slowly into a stretch;**
- **exhaling while moving into a stretch;**
- **concentrating on the muscle being stretched; and**
- **activating antagonistic (opposing) muscles ('reciprocal innervation').**

In order to activate a muscle which is difficult to isolate the yogin can activate any of the muscles in the region of that muscle. They will exert a gentle 'pull' or stretch on neighbouring muscles that are joined by fascial connections and may then become activated via the stretch reflex.

The 'reciprocal relaxation reflex' is the reflex inhibition of a muscle due to the activation of its antagonist or opposing muscle (Alter 1996). The yogin can go deeper into a stretch by consciously activating the muscles opposing the muscles being stretched. An understanding of the reciprocal relaxation reflex gives the yogin the means to deeply relax a muscle, stretch it further and help to strengthen the opposing muscle. For example, in the 'hamstring stretch' the yogin activates and helps strengthen the knee extensors (e.g. quadriceps) in order to reciprocally relax and further stretch the knee flexors (e.g. hamstrings). The 'inverse myotatic reflex' is the reflex relaxation of a muscle after it has been subjected to a prolonged intense stretch (Alter 1996). This phenomenon, known as a 'lengthening reaction', is believed to take at least 12–15 seconds to take place if the stretched muscle is initially in a relaxed state. The lengthening reaction is most noticeable if a muscle is activated while being stretched. The yogin takes advantage of the inverse myotatic reflex by activating and helping to strengthen the muscles being stretched in order to inversely relax that muscle and subsequently help it relax and stretch further. After the active tension is released the muscle is usually seen to have stretched further.

Antagonistic muscle co-activation (*bandha*) has a variable effect on the nervous system depending on the individual. In some cases it may result in the activation of all three nerve reflexes mentioned above, leading to an overall stimulation of the nervous system. However, since co-activation is sometimes under voluntary control all the nerve reflexes may be inhibited, leading to an overall calming effect on the nervous system. Research has shown that during co-activation there is a significant interaction with the nervous system (Aagaard *et al.* 2000; Barbeau *et al.* 2000; Proske *et al.* 2000). However, further research is needed to establish exactly what is taking place in the nervous system both in the co-activations that are generated by the activities of everyday life and in the aware voluntary co-activations generated as *bandhas* by the experienced yogin.

Yogic use of nerve tensioning (stretching)

When yogic physical exercises create differential regions of pressure within the body *prana* ('life force' or 'vital energy') is made to move along the *nadis*. *Nadis* are subtle channels found within the body along which move *prana* and *citta* (consciousness) (Goswami 1980). When the body is stretched in a yoga practice it is not just muscles but also *nadis* that are stretched. Blood vessels and nerves are examples of gross manifestations of the *nadis* but are not actually the *nadis* themselves. More subtle *nadis* include acupuncture meridians of eastern medicine (Motoyama 1993).

When the *nadis* are stretched a significant proportion of the physical sensation that may be experienced results from nerves and acupuncture meridians being tensioned. An increased sense of wellbeing can result if nerves are carefully tensioned. Tensioning nerves mobilises and allows them to function more effectively as instigators of muscle activation. However, excessive tensioning or 'over-stretching' may result in nerve damage, pain or loss of muscle strength or control.

Certain postures or stretches require care in order not to over-tension the spinal cord or various nerves. All poses that include flexion of the neck, spine and hip with extension at the knees and ankles strongly tension the spinal cord and the sciatic nerves and can therefore be potentially damaging. In this category are all the straight-legged forward-bending hamstring stretches that may over-stretch the sciatic nerve and possibly the spinal cord if the head and neck are in a flexed position (i.e. chin brought to the chest). Similarly, risks exist in all lunging poses, including the front splits and other similar stretches of the front groin (hip flexor region). Also all postures in which the arms are outstretched and the neck is being moved may cause an over-stretch and perhaps damage to the brachial plexus and/or the median, radial and ulnar nerves.

Yogic control over blood chemistry

The yogin can significantly alter blood chemistry with breath control. Hyperventilation (increased breathing) leads to a decrease of carbon dioxide in the blood (hypocapnia) and an increase in pH or alkalinity, while hypoventilation (reduced breathing) leads to an increase of carbon dioxide in the blood (hypercapnia) and decrease in pH (increased acidity). Studies of yoga exercises have demonstrated changes in levels of noradrenaline (Bharucha *et al.* 1996), cortisol (Kamei *et al.* 2000) and lactate (Solberg *et al.* 2000) and changes in blood-clotting ability (Chohan *et al.* 1984). Yoga training has been shown to be comparable to submaximal endurance training in increasing levels of lactate dehydrogenase, a glycolytic enzyme utilised during exercise to provide energy to contracting muscles (Pansare *et al.* 1989).

Yogic regulation of the nervous system

Experienced yogins can regulate the autonomic nervous system (ANS) using physical exercises or breath control. Expansion of the chest while emphasising thoracic inhalations, or while practising *tha-uddiyana-bandha* with the breath held out, stimulates the sympathetic nervous system (SNS) and increases heart rate. This is due to the effects of the respiratory pump, which draws blood to the heart as the intra-thoracic pressure reduces with chest expansion. Lengthening exhalations stimulates the parasympathetic nervous system (PNS) and reduces heart rate (Zeier 1984). Another effect on the nervous system through breath control is via *mudra*. For example, in *maha-mudra* trunk muscles are activated while the breath is held in. This leads to an increase in blood pressure that is detected by the baroreceptors of the circulatory system. These baroreceptors then signal the PNS to slow the heart rate in order to reduce blood pressure.

Yogins can effectively regulate the ANS by selectively breathing through one nostril at a time through manipulation of the nasal passages with the fingers or tongue. Studies have shown that breathing through the right nostril stimulates the SNS (Mohan 1996) and increases body heat, oxygen consumption, blood pressure (Telles *et al.* 1996) and heart rate (Shannahoff-Khalsa & Kennedy 1993). It also stimulates the left cerebral hemisphere (Schiff & Rump 1995) and may stimulate verbal task performance (Jella & Shannahoff-Khalsa 1993). Breathing through the left nostril stimulates the PNS (Backon *et al.* 1990), decreasing body heat, heart rate and blood pressure (Telles *et al.* 1994b), stimulates the right cerebral hemisphere (Werntz *et al.* 1987) and increases spatial task performance (Jella & Shannahoff-Khalsa 1993). Alternate nostril breathing (*nadi-sodhana-Pranayama*) balances the ANS and the right and left cerebral hemispheres (Backon *et al.* 1990), increases alpha and beta brain waves (Stancak & Kuna 1994) and increases handgrip strength (Raghuraj *et al.* 1997). Yogic science has apparently had this type of knowledge for millennia (Ghosh 1999). However, most of the yogic information about this subject either has been lost or is not being taught by those who know about it because the ancient texts say that this information should be kept secret (Desikachar 1998).

Meditation—non-physical yoga

'Meditation' is a western term for a highly evolved process that can involve using various techniques of relaxation, sense control, concentration, contemplation and visualisation to control the mind, its thoughts and its emotions, until a state of clear, blissful, mental silence can be attained at will. Advanced yogins can even control the physiological functions of the body while in meditative states.

Physiological effects of meditation

There have been many studies on meditation but relatively few consistent effects are demonstrated between studies. The reason may be that there are many types of meditative states possible according to ancient texts, yet modern scientific literature considers meditation as one state. There are at least three distinct meditative states defined in the *Patanjali-yoga-sutra* (Iyengar 1993), seventeen meditative states according to the *Yoga-yajnavalkya-samhita* (Desikachar 2000) and even more if one includes the many stages of *samadhi* (meditative absorption). In addition, there are many ways to achieve these meditative states. The yogin can meditate using any posture. The meditation can be static or dynamic, done with or without breath control, and anything can be used as an object for meditation.

Jevning *et al.* (1996) have subjectively described meditation as a very relaxed but at the same time a very alert state. Lazar *et al.* (2000) describe meditation as a conscious mental process that induces a set of integrated physiological changes termed the relaxation response. Jevning *et al.* (1992) called meditation a 'wakeful hypo-metabolic integrated response'. However, studies of certain Tantric (Corby *et al.* 1978), Buddhist (Benson *et al.* 1990) and Taoist meditations (Peng *et al.* 1999) demonstrate stimulation of autonomic nervous activity.

The most consistent findings in the many studies of meditation are the presence of some sort of hypoventilation (Wolkove *et al.* 1984; Sudsuang *et al.* 1991; Peng *et al.* 1999) and coherent, synchronous brain wave patterns (Badawi *et al.* 1984; Travis & Pearson 2000; Arambula *et al.* 2001; Travis 2001) distinct from those of ordinary waking, hypnosis or sleep (Hewitt 1983). Additionally, various studies of meditation have reported the presence of levels of coherent EEG patterns in the delta (Stigsby *et al.* 1981), theta (Kubota *et al.* 2001), alpha (Dillbeck & Bronson 1981; Aftanas & Golocheikine 2001) and beta (Benson *et al.* 1990; Sim & Tsol 1992) ranges. For various reasons, foremost being the subjective nature of meditation, it is not always possible to determine which of the meditative practices are being examined in each scientific paper.

Other reported physiological effects of meditation include: muscle relaxation (Patel & North 1975; Narayan *et al.* 1990), lowered blood pressure (Wenneberg *et al.* 1997; Barnes *et al.* 1999, 2001), reduced heart rate, increased cardiac output

(Dillbeck & Orme-Johnson 1987), increased cerebral blood flow, reduction of carbon dioxide generation by muscle (Kesterson & Clinch 1989), decreased sensitivity to carbon dioxide (Wolkove *et al.* 1984), reduced oxygen consumption (Wilson *et al.* 1987), increased galvanic skin resistance, decreased spontaneous electrodermal response, increased sensory perception and attentiveness (Brown *et al.* 1984) and decreased reaction times (Sudsuang *et al.* 1991). Meditation training may also reduce the lactate response to exercise more effectively than simple relaxation does (Solberg *et al.* 2000).

Reported metabolic effects of meditation include:

- **increased blood pH during meditation but decreased arterial pH afterwards, resulting in a mild metabolic acidosis;**
- **decreased plasma lactate and changes in glucose metabolism (Herzog *et al.* 1990);**
- **decreased adrenocortical activity after 30 minutes of meditation and long-term decreased cortisol secretion (Sudsuang *et al.* 1991);**
- **changes in the secretion and release of several pituitary hormones (MacLean *et al.* 1997);**
- **increased concentrations of molecules thought to play an important role in learning and memory (Travis & Orme-Johnson 1989); and**
- **increased levels of melatonin (Tooley *et al.* 2000), which probably promotes analgesia and reduces stress and insomnia (Elias & Wilson 1995; Harte *et al.* 1995).**

Types of meditative practices

There are many types of meditation. Buddhist monks are reported to have thousands of meditative techniques (Yeshe 1999). Each meditative technique can be done with or without breath control (*pranayama*) and can be a starting point to move into all the meditative states. All of these meditations can progress to the ultimate state of meditative absorption (*samadhi*) where the breath is not controlled but is in the state of prolonged hypoventilation with breathing so minimal that it appears as apnoea (no breathing).

The meditative state can be achieved in any static posture and during movement. Most of the studies on meditation have mainly focused on meditative states obtained in seated or supine positions. Only a few studies have described meditative states in other yoga postures (Junker & Dworkis 1986; Kamei *et al.* 2000). Styles of Taoist yoga including Tai Chi and Qi Gong have been described as dynamic meditations (Liu *et al.* 1990; Jin 1992). The yogic texts recommend new yogins to work initially with physical exercises and breath control, then work with the physical yoga approaches to the meditative practices and finally progress to the seated meditative practices.

The ancient yoga texts are clear in stating that *citta* (mind or consciousness) and *prana* (essential life force in the breath) move as one and are always together in the body (Iyengar 1993). Raja yoga texts such as the *Patanjali-yoga-sutra* describe yoga as 'stillness of the mind' (Iyengar 1993), while the *Hatha-yoga-pradipika* describes yoga as 'stillness in the breath' (Vishnu-Devananda 1987). Therefore, when there is stillness in the mind there should be stillness in the breath and vice versa. From this philosophical point arise the two approaches to achieve yoga and reach a meditative state, the raja yoga approach and the hatha yoga approach. These two approaches lead to a meditative state that is physiologically similar in terms of brain wave patterns and physiological responses.

In the raja yoga approach, which mainly uses the meditative practices of non-physical yoga, the yogin stills the mind, generating synchronous brain waves (Corby *et al.* 1978; Aftanas & Golocheikine 2001). The body then responds with a state of hypoventilation in which the breath is almost imperceptible or spontaneously absent (Farrow & Herbert 1982; Badawi *et al.* 1984; Gallois 1984; Travis & Wallace 1997). Hatha yoga mainly uses physical yoga to bring stillness to the breath that is seen as some form of hypoventilation (Stanescu *et al.* 1981; Miyamura *et al.* 2002). The mind then responds with a calmness that is associated with the presence of coherent and synchronous brain waves (Stancak *et al.* 1993; Arambula *et al.* 2001).

Mantra yoga

Mantra yoga is a popular method of meditation that uses chanting of sounds and phrases to induce a meditative state. Chanting can be done audibly as a type of breath control or mentally with or without breath control. Types of mantra yoga are used in Vedic, Tantric and Buddhist meditative practices and are used in the devotional practices of Christians, Muslims, Jews and tribal cultures around the world. Yogins can chant mantras aloud or recite them mentally during exhalation. Mental or visual recitation of mantras occurs during inhalation or breath retention. Chanting is a practice that develops the left side of the brain.

In a study by Bernardi *et al.* (2001b) it was found that both rosary prayer (recitation of the Ave Maria in Latin) and mantra caused synchronous increases in existing cardiovascular rhythms when recited aloud six times a minute. Baroreflex sensitivity also increased significantly. The imposed breath-control pattern of six breaths per minute induced favourable psychological and possibly physiological effects (Bernardi *et al.* 2001b).

Following a clinical trial of seven experienced meditators it was deduced that mantra meditation (mental chanting of 'om') caused an increase in mental alertness and relaxation (as shown by the reduced heart rate) (Telles *et al.* 1995). Mantra meditation was found to be more effective at reducing anxiety than either relaxation techniques (Dillbeck 1977) or meditative concentration (Eppley *et al.* 1989). Similar brain wave patterns as seen during meditation are also apparent during certain important stages of sleep (Sei & Morita 1996; Benca *et al.* 1999; Cantero *et al.* 1999; Parrino *et al.* 2001). This may support Krishnamacharya's often-quoted statement that yoga and meditation can replace sleep (Desikachar 1998).

Beneficial effects of meditation

The reported psychological effects of meditation used as a therapy are not based on properly randomised and controlled trials and placebo comparisons for meditation are problematic. Atwood & Maltin (1991) described how meditation helps one to develop patience, to be aware of a problem before attempting to solve it, to promote a non-judgemental attitude and to be comfortable with ambiguity, ignorance and uncertainty. Meditators learn to recognise and trust their inner nature and wisdom. Meditation also fosters the recognition of personal responsibility.

Reports claim that meditation helps improve memory (Atwood & Maltin 1991), increases vigour (Kutz *et al.* 1985a, b) and enhances compassion, acceptance and tolerance of self and others (Dua & Swinden 1992). Shapiro (1992) found that 88 per cent of subjects reported greater happiness and joy, positive thinking, increased self-confidence, effectiveness and better problem-solving skills (Dillbeck & Vesely 1986). Other reported beneficial effects include better ability to control feelings, more relaxation, greater resilience (Scheler 1992) and increased life expectancy (Wallace *et al.* 1982; Alexander *et al.* 1989).

Adverse effects and dangers of meditation

Many people are not initially able to practise or do not have the predisposition for static sitting meditation. Adverse effects of seated meditation described in the literature include anxiety, panic, tension, boredom, pain, confusion, disorientation, decreased motivation, impaired sense of reality, fear, anger, apprehension and despair (Kutz *et al.* 1985a, b; Craven 1989; Shapiro 1992).

Ancient texts such as the *Patanjali-yoga-sutra* are clear that the eight steps of astanga yoga should be followed in some sequence. It is safer for most people to practise the techniques of physical yoga, including simple relaxation, first, then once established in these progress to the meditative practices (Iyengar 1993; Mohan 2000). In a controlled clinical trial by Wood (1993) comparing effects of relaxation, visualisation (*dhyana*) and physical yoga, normal volunteers found that physical yoga produced a significantly greater increase in perceptions of mental and physical energy and feelings of alertness and enthusiasm than the other two procedures. Relaxation and visualisation made subjects more sleepy and sluggish than physical yoga, and visualisation made them less content than physical yoga and more upset than relaxation. Wood (1993) thus found that a simple 30-minute program of physical yoga which is easy to learn and which could be practised even by the elderly had a markedly invigorating effect on perceptions of both mental and physical energy and increased positive mood in the participants.

The evidence on effectiveness of yoga and meditation

A Medline literature search on yoga reveals that there are 604 'scientific' articles regarding yoga, written from 1965 to December 2002. These articles claim that benefits of yoga range from improvements in strength (Madanmohan et al. 1992), flexibility (Ray et al. 2001) and aerobic ability (Balasubramanian & Pansare 1991) to improvements in muscle tone, rheumatoid arthritis, lung function, concentration, poor eyesight, obesity, indigestion, back pain, hypertension, various respiratory diseases, sinusitis, arthritis, diabetes (types 1 and 2), as well as anxiety, nervousness, attention deficit and memory loss. Many of these articles make interesting reading and may be correct in their claims regarding yoga, but very few articles represent 'valid' scientific proof of the benefits of yoga. Only 23 articles were randomised controlled trials on yoga, and some of these report that either yoga has 'no effect' (e.g. Kroner-Herwig et al. 1995) or that the effect is 'not significant' (Shaffer et al. 1997). Similarly, a Medline search on meditation reveals that there are 852 scientific articles regarding meditation, written from 1965 to December 2002. Of these, only 26 were randomised controlled trials.

Randomised controlled trials of yoga have shown that it is effective in increasing joint flexibility (Ray et al. 2001), increasing regression of coronary atherosclerosis (Manchanda et al. 2000), coping with exam stress (Malathi & Damodaran 1999), management of hypertension (Patel & North 1975), management of stress in epilepsy (Panjwani et al. 1995), relief in hand osteoarthritis (Garfinkel et al. 1994), increasing ability to perform complex tasks (Manjunath & Telles 2001), long-term management of bronchial asthma (Nagarathna & Nagendra 1985) and reduction of medication in asthma (Singh et al. 1990). A randomised, controlled trial of specialised breath control (unilateral nostril breathing) was found to increase spatial memory (Naveen et al. 1997).

While there is a paucity of valid scientific research published on yoga, there are many well-researched papers on the scientific elements of yoga. Medline searches on topics such as the following can reveal many papers which provide tangible evidence regarding the benefits of yoga and meditation: isometric exercise (e.g. Monteiro Pedro et al. 1999), breathing exercise (e.g. Yan & Sun 1996), stretching (e.g. Herbert & Gabriel 2002), relaxation (e.g. Weber 1996), stretching, posture (e.g. Cholewicki et al. 1997), one-legged exercises (e.g. Kannus et al. 1992), antagonistic muscle co-activation (e.g. Glasscock et al. 1999), aerobic conditioning, unilateral forced nostril breathing (Naveen et al. 1997), 'Valsalva' (Bazak 1990) and 'Mueller' manoeuvres (Gioia et al. 1995), visualisation (Kominars 1997) and mental imagery (e.g. Hudetz et al. 2000).

The practice of yoga and meditation

Patient compliance, or to put it more in yoga-like terms, the student's ability to attend class or maintain a regular practice, depends on the nature of the yoga teacher (guru), the student (sisya) and the relationship between guru and sisya. To be of use as a teacher the guru must be able to offer more information to the sisya than they already know. It is ideal if the guru has a better understanding of yoga, anatomy, physiology and psychology than the sisya. The guru must be able to encourage the sisya to strive to work to their personal maximum and to advise the sisya when it is time to back off in order to avoid physical or psychological injury. If a student does not make an effort in their practice that is close to their personal maximum, which will vary from day to day, then they will not get the full short- and long-term benefits of their practice and they may become bored and discontinue the practice. If a student overworks with either physical exercises, breath control or their meditative practices then physical, physiological or psychological injury is possible. Excessive discomfort on any level either during or after practice because of overwork during practice may cause a student to abandon their pursuit of yoga.

Anyone can practise some type of yoga in every situation provided one makes appropriate adaptation and modifications. Only three conditions apply. First, the teacher must have sufficient understanding and experience in yoga, anatomy, physiology and psychology. Second, the student must be willing to learn. Third, it is important that a good relationship exists between yoga teacher and student.

Yoga is primarily about relationships and communication. Ultimately, yoga is the realisation of the fundamental relationship and identity between the individual soul (*jivatma*) and the universal soul (*Paramatman*). However, at the commencement of one's yoga the relationships that are most important to develop are those of the self (e.g. the connections between body and mind) and the relationship between guru and sisya. Unless there is a functional relationship between guru and sisya the yoga may be of limited value (Desikachar 1998).

Contraindications in yoga

A good yoga teacher can tailor an individual yoga practice to suit anybody. However, few people can safely practise all aspects of yoga as described in this chapter without years of training. To learn yoga a student has a choice of a mixed-level open class, a beginner or higher-level closed course or individual tuition. Traditionally, yoga instruction was a one-to-one interaction between teacher and student, but very few yoga teachers work this way now. A good yoga teacher can safely guide a student through an individually modified yoga practice in a group class provided they are aware of that student's injuries or medical conditions. Attendance at group yoga classes is not recommended unless the teacher is able to adapt and modify the yoga to accommodate each student's special needs. Students who should be particularly aware and who need to have special instructions and individual guidance include those with:

- **cancer and other diseases**
- **cardiovascular problems**
- **nervous system disorders**
- **endocrine system disorders**
- **pregnancy**
- **spinal abnormalities**
- **intervertebral disc bulging**
- **spondylolisthesis**
- **spinal nerve entrapment**
- **sciatica**
- **musculoskeletal problems**
- **joint instability**
- **respiratory problems**

Yoga can affect all the body systems and has the potential to help people with specific musculoskeletal problems and medical conditions. However, very few teachers have the necessary combination of a theoretical understanding of the body and the practical application of yoga to help everyone. Most yoga teachers are still advised to refer patients on to medical practitioners and physiotherapists unless their problems are very straightforward.

Yoga and the medical community

Over the years many people have been injured during yoga practice or in classes. Yoga-based injuries have especially increased over the last decade as more people have been drawn to the more dynamic and demanding styles of yoga such as astanga-vinyasa (Dembner 2003). Injuries are due in part to the limitations of the western body. Yoga was initially designed for Indian bodies, which have developed strength and flexibility from sitting cross-legged on the floor, squatting to go to the toilet and often carrying large weights on their heads. Lack of understanding of yoga and anatomy, physiology and psychology by yoga teachers and students are also causes of yoga-based injuries.

Depending largely on the teacher, yoga can have an efficient relationship with physiotherapists, doctors, chiropractors, osteopaths and naturopaths.

Ethical disciplines (*Yama* and *Niyama*)

The effects of yoga can vary according to the way one practises and the attitude one has when practising. These attitudes are trained by the yogic ethical disciplines, *Yama* and *Niyama*, which form the most fundamental differences between yoga and conventional exercise.

Yama and *Niyama*, the first two stages of astanga yoga, hold the key to yoga and the fulfilment of one's life. *Yama* includes the principles of non-violence, truthfulness, non-stealing, continence and non-covetousness. On the simplest level, one quickly learns these principles during a yoga practice. For example, to prevent physical or psychological injury during yoga one must practise without aggression, with an honest recognition of one's limitations and without a competitive nature. *Niyama* includes the principles of purity, contentment, fervour, self-study and devotion or love. On the simplest level, this means to rid oneself of things that are not needed and to be ultimately content with one's limitations but nevertheless to strive to keep improving one's body and mind through self-study and devotion.

To achieve complete success in yoga one must embrace at least part of the philosophy behind it. Yoga is such that its ongoing practice can teach the ethical disciplines behind it. Success in yoga may be seen when the ethical disciplines enter into one's daily life.

Conclusion

The practice of yoga is a means to enhance all aspects of one's life but, ideally, yoga can also be a way of life. Correct application of the physical aspects of yoga, namely physical exercises (*asana*) and breathing exercises (*pranayama*), has been shown to improve one's physical health and fitness. Mindfulness of the non-physical aspects of yoga, namely ethical disciplines (*Yama* and *Niyama*) and meditative practices (*pratayahara, dharana, dhyana* and *samadhi*), has been shown to augment one's mental and emotional wellbeing.

When one practises physical yoga, even basic stretching exercises, the best effects are achieved when ethical disciplines such as the principle of non-aggression (*ahimsa*) and meditative practices such as meditative concentration (*dharana*) are applied simultaneously. Conversely, when one practises non-physical yoga, in particular meditative contemplation (*dhyana*), the greatest benefits for the mind and emotions can be more easily achieved while engaging in a physical yoga practice involving breathing (*pranayama*), posture (*asana*) and even movement (*vinyasa*).

The ongoing practice of physical yoga, in particular correct posture, movement and breathing, can translate to one's everyday life. Some can eventually obtain the physical benefits of physical yoga through the activities of daily life alone. In a similar fashion ethical disciplines such as truthfulness, self-study and devotion, and meditative practices such as meditative sense-control and meditative concentration of non-physical yoga can also translate to everyday life. The mental and emotional benefits of non-physical yoga may also be eventually replaced by the activities of everyday life.

Therefore, even though the paths of yoga are many, there is really only one type of yoga. Yoga is the integration of one's actions and deeds, via the interplay between one's posture, movement and breathing, with one's thoughts, attitudes and feelings, and the effects one has on people and the environment.

Recommended reading

Alter, M.J. 1996, *Science of Flexibility*, Human Kinetics, South Australia.

Borg-Olivier, S.A. and Machliss, B.E. 2003, *Applied Anatomy and Physiology of Hatha Yoga*, 9th edn, Yoga Synergy Pty Ltd, Sydney.

Coulter, H.D. 2001, *Anatomy of Hatha Yoga: Body and Breath*, Honesdale, PA, USA.

Iyengar, B.K.S. 2001, *Yoga: The Path to Holistic Health*, Dorling Kindersley Limited, London.

CONCLUSION

Challenges facing integrated medicine
Stephen P. Myers

The purpose of this final chapter is to stimulate thought, encourage discussion and engender debate on the challenges facing an integrated system of medicine. Given the extent of community utilisation of complementary medicine it could be argued that we already have an integrated health system. Currently, the primary integrators are health consumers, individuals that choose from both sides of the available spectrum to treat their condition. Many of these individuals utilise conventional approaches to healthcare alongside complementary medicine approaches and in doing so practice integrated medicine at the grassroots level. Many health professions have also developed, or joined, integrated health practices incorporating general practitioners, naturopaths, chiropractors, counsellors and other therapists. These practices provide integrated medicine through cross-referral, co-management and collegial support and interaction. Even where practices are not integrated, professional dialogue is beginning to occur between the various health professionals spanning the spectrum from complementary to conventional. The integration of naturopaths into Australian pharmacy practice is an example of newly developing collaborations. Little integration has yet occurred, however, at the health policy level and there are only a few isolated instances of complementary medicine being integrated into conventional healthcare delivery through placement in public or private hospitals. Complementary medicine is currently not being incorporated into community healthcare planning or health budgets and the potential of integrated medicine will not be fully realised until public health decision makers see complementary medicine as a component of effective healthcare delivery.

Finding a common vision

Part of the challenge of integrated medicine is in finding a common vision. What one individual or sector of the healthcare community considers to be effective integration may to another individual or sector not only be ineffective but detrimental. An integrated healthcare system depends on professional perspective. However, a medical doctor may have a very different understanding of what this means from a naturopathic practitioner, massage therapist or homœopath. Given the conflicting voices it appears obvious that it is unlikely that any one perspective will totally dominate, nor possibly should it. The rise of complementary medicine is evidence enough that the biomedical approach to healthcare has not served all the health needs of the community. Yet complementary medicine, for all its value, would be a poor replacement for conventional medicine. It is difficult to imagine a world without trauma surgery or life-saving drugs. It is also difficult to imagine a world without massage or herbal medicine.

Quite simply, an integrated healthcare system requires integration. This means that every sector of the healthcare community needs to work together in a co-operative way. The development of an integrated system would be much more immediate if all the participants in the health sector were able to reach a consensus on how integration should be advanced. The fundamental challenge in the development of an integrated health system is to find a shared vision between the participants. Where does one start in finding such a vision from such a diverse group of participants? It is often easier, and more productive, to search for existing commonality rather than focus on differences. This is how the Collaboration for Healthcare Renewal Foundation (CHRF) approached this challenge. The CHRF is a US group dedicated to enhancing healthcare of individuals through promoting collaborative activity among healthcare leaders to generate solutions to the complex operational and clinical challenges facing organisations providing integrated healthcare, education and research. The CHRF is a collaboration of hospitals and health systems, professional associations (currently massage therapists, acupuncturists, naturopaths and chiropractors), employers and healthcare purchasers, integrative medical clinics, academic medical institutions, educators and researchers from licensed complementary medicine professions, health maintenance organisations, complementary-focused provider organisations and individual and corporate philanthropists.

A working group of the CHRF took the guiding principles from 47 organisations and blended them into one set of principles to be used as a blueprint for an approach to an integrated health system. The organisations chosen for this assessment included the Institute of Medicine of the National Academy of Sciences, complementary medicine professional organisations, hospitals, the American Holistic Medical Association and the American Holistic Nurses Association. Ten draft principles were developed (see below) that provide a framework on which to approach the development of an integrated health system. The CHRF has put these principles forward to act as a starting point for individuals and organisations in meeting the challenges of integration. It is the belief of the CHRF that these principles are a necessary and practical step in developing integrated healthcare.

Design principles of healthcare

Preamble

Core principles drive the way healthcare operates and is experienced. Times of change and disturbance call us to examine, clarify and commit to renew our individual and community practices. The following set of principles emphasises the integrative nature of optimal healthcare. Such care seeks to create health by engaging new and old approaches to health for the individual, system, community and environment. Integrative care is grounded in relationships, seeks sustainability, is energised by the unknown and crafted through continuous exploration of strategies for uniting the best of the world's evolving practices, outcomes and traditions.

These principles, based on the missions and visions of diverse stakeholders, are an initial expression of an effort to create a unifying view of a renewed system for healthcare delivery and payment. These principles are meant not as ideals but as working tools of design, application, evaluation and alignment. They are offered here for community review, revision and amendment by the *ad hoc* Task Force on the Principles of Healthcare which grew out of the Vision Group of the Integrative Medicine Industry Leadership Summit 2000.

The design principles for accelerating health and wellbeing in individuals, and in the health system, are:

1. Honour wholeness and interconnectedness in all actions.

Body, mind, spirit, community and environment are an integral whole that cannot be separated into isolated parts. All are involved in healing. Healthcare interventions, regardless of their focus, affect the whole.

2. Enhance the capacity for self-repair and healing.

The innate capacity for healing and the individual's personal empowerment in supporting these natural processes are fundamental considerations in all healthcare decisions.

3. Prioritise care in accordance with a hierarchy of treatment.

Care, and the leveraging of resources to affect care, are prioritised along diagnostic and therapeutic hierarchies which begin with education and empowerment in healthy choices, then move to the least invasive approaches and escalate, as necessary, to approaches linked to increased likelihood of adverse effects or higher costs. The starting point for intervention is established through clarifying, with the individual receiving care, the risks associated with forgoing, and with undertaking, more invasive approaches. Chronology and cause are fundamental aspects of this healing order.

4. Improve care through continuously expanding the evidence base.

Healthcare is a combined art and science in which personal practices and clinical choices and services are continuously evaluated and improved, by practitioners, users and organisations, based on diverse evidence. Included are the desires, perceptions and outcomes experienced by the individuals at the centre of care, the clinical experience and understandings of all members of a provider team and, particularly, systematically gathered evidence of experience and outcomes. More stringent evidentiary standards are associated with higher risk or more costly interventions.

5. Embrace the fullness of diverse healthcare systems.

Conventional, traditional, indigenous, complementary and alternative models of care, and their bodies of knowledge, have contributions to make to the healthcare which is culturally most appropriate and effective for individuals and communities. Best practices are discovered through exploring diverse structures for integration, including parallel, collaborative and assimilative models.

6. Partner with patients, their families and other practitioners.

Care givers profoundly enhance healing and strengthen shared accountability through supporting the informed decision making of the individuals/ families/loved ones they serve, and through inclusive, respectful partnerships with other practitioners with whom they collaborate in care provision.

7. Use illness and symptoms as opportunities for learning and growth.

Illness represents an opportunity in which healing and balance are always possible even when curing is not. Symptoms are guides to health.

8. Explore integration in one's own care.

Practitioners, administrators and individuals are most effective in understanding and delivering integrative healthcare, and in embracing these design principles, when they follow these principles in their own care choices.

9. Align resource investment with these healthcare principles.

The renewal of our healthcare payment and delivery systems is fostered by aligning resource investment, in the personal, public, philanthropic and private sectors, with these principles. Humble willingness to work to resolve the tensions between one's personal and professional interests, and those shared interests expressed in these principles, is required of all participants. The renewed healthcare system is a partnership between an expanded commitment to the public health and a thriving industry of health creation.

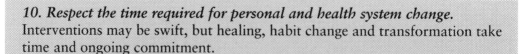

10. Respect the time required for personal and health system change. Interventions may be swift, but healing, habit change and transformation take time and ongoing commitment.

Source: Design Principles Healthcare Renewal Workgroup. Draft. Workgroup Co-Chairs—Pamela Snider ND and Alan Dumoff JD MSW. A National Working Group of the Collaboration for Healthcare Renewal Foundation, Seattle 2001.

Apart from the CHRF, the general healthcare community does not share a common vision and pragmatically it will take time and a massive effort on behalf of the policy advocates among the professions at large to reach such a vision. Until this fundamental challenge is met the process of integration is more likely to happen organically. In planning for integration it is important to realise that the field of complementary medicine itself represents a large and diverse community of different approaches to health and healing. An appropriate first step is to bring these groups together to establish their common goals. Incorporation of the conventional health disciplines is more likely to occur after this first step has been taken.

The future of integrated medicine

The future is defined as 'relating to or connected with time to come' (Delbridge & Bernard 1998). While it may be possible to predict some aspects of the future by projecting the past and the present, the future is formless. What will happen is truly uncertain. Chinese philosophy suggests that the only thing in the universe that is certain is change. We can be certain, then, that the future will bring change but how that change will come about remains unknown. Such uncertainty has given rise to fear in some complementary therapists that the future of integrated medicine is bleak and will give rise to the dominance of complementary medicine by orthodox medicine.

In this projected 'bleak future', complementary medicine has not vanished but has become distorted. It has been absorbed into the mainstream health disciplines as an adjunct to current practice without having affected the fundamental nature of that practice. The basic approach to healthcare is still aimed at taking care of the unwell and the sick and the main focus of practice is on the physical body. Complementary medicines, such as St John's wort and saw palmetto, and some complementary medicine practices, such as acupuncture, are well integrated into the healthcare system; however, the scope of their use has been significantly narrowed. Acupuncture is only used to control nausea and for musculoskeletal pain and discomfort. St John's wort is confined to mild depression and is never used for other conditions. The rich tradition that flourished in the late twentieth and early twenty-first centuries is gone. Complementary medicine practitioners have been forced underground due to restrictive practice legislation outlawing them from practising. Crystals, feathers and the traditional approach to herbal medicine are all coloured with the same brush and there is no attempt to distinguish between them. Complementary medicine is unidimensional and monochromatic and the health system is the antithesis of pluralistic.

The other extreme to this bleak perspective is to look at the future with rose-coloured glasses and paint a picture of a health system dominated by complementary medicine. In the 'rosy future', complementary medicine is completely integrated into contemporary healthcare. Rapid change occurred at the turn of the twenty-first century as the conventional health system fell deeply into crisis. The conventional approach to health was seen as too narrow and health decision makers looked for more effective approaches to healthcare delivery. Complementary medicine was embraced by conventional care givers and natural therapists invited to work within the conventional hospital system. Over time the hospital environment changed and reflected holistic principles of management. The majority of hospital patients are now enrolled in educational programs looking at lifestyle options that will enhance their overall health. Herbal and nutritional medicine form the primary basis on which most diseases are treated and pharmaceutical agents and surgery are used as therapies of last resort. The focus of the health system is on health enhancement and community wellbeing. Complementary medicine is multidimensional and polychromatic and the health system is truly pluralistic.

Neither the bleak future nor the rosy future is likely to occur in the immediate future and both are probably unlikely to occur in any future. Their value is that they can guide us on the road to integration. The fears that give rise to the bleak future are real and need to be addressed. There has been a long history of professional animosity within the health disciplines which give such fears a basis on which to flourish. The benefit of these fears is that they serve to encourage vigilance as to how the process of integration is moving and the direction in which it is heading. The benefit of the rosy future is that it can act as a utopian ideal to follow, the magnetic north to which compasses are set as society sails into the uncertain future.

The pressures of integration are going to raise challenges for both complementary and orthodox professions and the medicine they practise. How those challenges are met will determine how the future unfolds.

Evidence-based medicine

Evidence-based medicine (EBM) is a phenomenon that is sweeping through all fields of health. The concept was given impetus from the ground-breaking work of Chalmers, Enkin and Keirse in their review of the practices used in pregnancy and childbirth (Chalmers *et al.* 1989). This review led to a reassessment of clinical practice. Their argument was that knowledge, not tradition, should drive practice; the premise being that if something does not work it should be discontinued no matter how long it has been practised. As such, they recommended that many practices that had a long tradition in obstetrics be discontinued. This concept was an idea whose time had come and it has swept through the field of medicine like wildfire. The coining of the term 'evidence-based medicine' is ascribed to Professor Gordon Guyatt, who at the time was a graduate student of Dr David Sackett from McMaster University in Canada. Sackett describes EBM as 'the conscientious, explicit and judicious use of current best evidence in making decisions about the care of individual patients' (Sackett *et al.* 1996: 71). Sackett saw that EBM should be a balance between the best external evidence and clinical expertise. He wrote:

> without clinical expertise, practice risks becoming tyrannized by external evidence, for even excellent external evidence may be inapplicable to or inappropriate for an individual patient. Without best external evidence, practice risks becoming rapidly out of date, to the detriment of patients (Sackett *et al.* 1996: 72).

It appears certain that the concept of EBM has and will revolutionise the field of healthcare. The challenge for complementary medicine will be to come to terms with what is emerging as 'evidence-based complementary medicine' (Wilson & Mills 2002). Some of the practices within complementary medicine, such as nutritional supplementation, fall directly within the domain of science and are immediately subject to the concept of evidence-based utilisation. However, many of the practices of complementary medicine are based on traditional knowledge and have never been the subject of systematic investigation. This will place significant pressure on complementary medicine as the concept of tradition is not sacrosanct within the field of EBM. Tradition will not be accepted as a reason not to subject practices to appropriate assessment. The fundamental concept that underlies EBM is that medicine should be based on proof. The principal implication of this concept is that if proof does not exist then research should be undertaken. EBM considers it inappropriate to do the same thing over and over because that is what you have always done. This is, however, the basis on which much traditional medicine stands. How the various sectors of complementary medicine come to terms with the challenge of EBM will be a major determinant of their acceptability within conventional health disciplines and their likely integration and acceptance into the mainstream health system.

In addition to pressure from the conventional health disciplines, complementary medicine will be under pressure from consumers as they too become informed about the concept of EBM. The consumer has a right to ask questions about the products and services they purchase. These questions might include: 'Is this a high-quality product?', 'Is it safe?' and, most importantly, 'Does it work?'. As consumers become empowered by an understanding that they have a right to proven healthcare, it is inevitable that complementary health products and practices that can provide such evidence will be under high demand. Given a choice between one product or service with a tradition of use for a given condition and another with both tradition of use and scientific evidence of its effectiveness and safety, it is highly likely the consumer will purchase the product or service with both tradition and science. This choice will also be reflected in the products and services used by conventional health professionals.

Research

The need for research to be undertaken within complementary medicine is compounded by the challenge of EBM. There is little doubt that research needs to be undertaken, but 'what needs to be researched' and 'in what priority' are questions that have not been broadly addressed. In established sciences research occurs as an organic process with thousands of researchers working within a particular discipline pushing the knowledge barriers in a myriad of different directions simultaneously. Gradually, like termites building a hive grain by grain, knowledge is distilled and advanced. Occasionally, a major advance is made by an individual or research group that leads to a quantum leap in knowledge. After this advance, however, the gradual process of advancement commences again. It is highly probable that this is how complementary medicine will gradually be researched, with individual researchers each contributing their own grains to the mass of evidence. While this of itself will be valuable, there are some within the complementary medicine research community that are interested in setting a broader agenda and trying to define priorities and how they can best be addressed. This approach is likely to produce greater fruits at an earlier time, provided that such an agenda can attract the funding required to undertake these priority projects and the research community to engage in this priority research.

The challenge is to build the human resources required to undertake this research. Currently, the majority of people undertaking research in complementary medicine are within conventional medical science. Like all disciplines, complementary medicine needs to develop its own cadre of researchers, individuals that understand complementary medicine and have the skills required to undertake research. In order to do this it is essential that educational institutions provide research training at both an undergraduate and postgraduate level. This requires educational modules on research, Masters and doctoral programs, research facilities, qualified staff capable of supervising research students and the development of a research culture within the institutions. As formal research has not been part of the educational culture of complementary medicine a special effort is required to build this research culture. The critical factor for educational institutions is the employment of key staff members who have the capacity and the vision required to commence this work.

The significant challenge of having the majority of researchers outside the area of complementary medicine is that the research they undertake will not be in a complementary medicine context. By way of example, immunologists are interested in the effect of a given agent or practice on immune modulation. Their methods will generally not entail researching complementary medicine within its holistic practice where multiple interventions are undertaken simultaneously. Such researchers use a reductionist approach where extraneous variables are reduced to the minimum in order to be able to assess the effect of a single variable. The majority of research on traditional medicine has been pharmaceutical and nearly all of this has been to look at the effect of a specific agent on a given condition. While this research has definite benefit it is not research that supports the practice of complementary medicine within its traditional context where interventions are multiple and individualised. Little such research has been undertaken, due to a variety of factors among which are a lack of researchers interested in this topic and a lack of funding to undertake such research. It is essential that complementary medicine be researched within the context of its practice as this is the only way to assess if it is truly effective and safe.

Pharmaceuticalisation

The vast majority of the research undertaken in complementary medicine is on the pharmacological activity of complementary medicines, especially herbal medicines. This research is generally undertaken on the role of single herbs for specific conditions at a determined dose. Understanding the pharmacological effect of complementary medicines is not in and of itself wrong. This research has led to the development of herbal medicines with a high level of evidence for their effectiveness and safety. However, to undertake such research to the exclusion of understanding complementary medicine in its broader context is to reduce complex therapeutic traditional systems to a series of scientifically proven medicinal agents.

A number of issues arise from this process of pharmaceuticalisation. First, there is concern that this represents what one author has referred to as 'bio-medical cherry picking from the complementary field' (St George 2001). This reduces traditional systems of medicine with thousands of years of history to a few medications to be used within conventional medicine. Such an outcome does not fulfil the promise that complementary medicine aroused within the community for a more holistic approach to healthcare. Second, research of this type often fixates both the medical community and consumers on one association between a complementary medicine and a health outcome. A good example is St John's wort (*Hypericum perforatum*) and depression. Over 25 randomised controlled trials have been undertaken to assess this association

(Linde & Mulrow 2001). While this plant has been used for centuries as an anxiolytic, and research on its role in depression follows its traditional use, it has also been used as a respiratory medicine, a gastrointestinal medicine and a wound healer. While these other uses have not been the subject of rigorous systematic investigation it is essential that they are not overlooked. To do so would be to dismiss the complexity of plant medicines and to fail to understand their full therapeutic potential.

Holistic practice

Very little research has been undertaken into the practice of complementary medicine within its own domain. An individual going to a Traditional Chinese Medicine (TCM) practitioner would often be given individualised acupuncture, Chinese herbs and dietary and lifestyle advice based on Chinese medicine theory. Some TCM practitioners would supplement this with Chinese massage and recommend the individual to take up therapeutic exercises such as Tai Chi or Qi Gong. This treatment would be undertaken against a background of traditional diagnostic methods and TCM principles of management. The same individual could go to a naturopath and receive dietary and lifestyle advice, based on a synthesis of traditional naturopathic approaches and modern science, together with individualised herbal therapy and nutritional agents. Some naturopaths would supplement this with tactile therapies, intensive counselling and exercise therapy. This treatment would be undertaken against a background of western diagnosis and physiological assessment coupled with naturopathic management principles. These two approaches to treatment, while extremely different, are based on holistic models of practice with an emphasis on individualisation of treatment. Little is known about the outcomes of this holistic practice applied to a cohort of individuals homogenised according to western diagnostic labels. Such research is necessary to underpin the validity of any approach to treatment that does not follow the dominant biomedical paradigm. Neither is anything understood about the effects of a cohort of individuals homogenised according to traditional diagnostic labels to assess the internal consistency of the theory and its predictive treatments.

Professional issues

The future of any collaboration between health disciplines to some extent rests on past history. It is unfortunate that the history between complementary medicine and conventional medicine is littered with animosity and apprehension on both sides. Like many things in life, time is likely to be the greatest healer of the rifts that have occurred. The newer generation of complementary medicine practitioners and conventional health professionals are not tainted with the bias of past hostilities and it is on their shoulders that the future of integrated medicine will rest. This history of hostility underlies the fear evident in some complementary therapists who see a bleak future. The history of medicine has seen many instances where newer professions have been subsumed or ostracised. In only recent times a number of prominent medical organisations lost an anti-trust suit for a concerted campaign to undermine chiropractic medicine in the United States (Wilk 1996). Against this background it is essential that the utilisation of complementary medicine by the conventional health disciplines is approached with an understanding and respect for the complementary medicine disciplines that are the primary custodians of these therapies. The development of professional dialogue between complementary health professionals and conventional health professionals is a challenge facing integrated medicine. While this is happening spontaneously between individuals the development of dialogue between their respective professional associations and policy forming bodies is a larger challenge.

Education for conventional health professionals

A review into TCM in Australia (Bensoussan & Myers 1996) demonstrated that the development of short courses in acupuncture for other health professions had created two distinct tiers of education. This was reflected in a survey of the Australian TCM workforce undertaken in 1996 as part of the review process. In this survey the reported length of education for TCM practitioners ranged from 50 hours to eight years, with an average for primary TCM practitioners (individuals identifying TCM as their primary practice, mainly non-medical) of 43.6 months, and for non-primary TCM practitioners (mainly medical) of eight months. A controversial finding of the TCM report was that a significant difference was found between medical and non-medical practitioners in the adverse event rate per year of full-time TCM practice ($p < 0.001$). Medical practitioners reported more than double the adverse event rate of non-medical practitioners. While there may be a number of reasons for this difference, one interpretation is that education provided by short courses is inadequate for safe practice (Bensoussan *et al.* 2000). A recommendation from the Australian TCM review arising from these findings was:

> That professional associations representing practitioners of registered health occupations (including medicine, nursing, physiotherapy, chiropractic and osteopathy) who utilise TCM, review and upgrade the minimum qualifications required of their members for safe practice, particularly in acupuncture and Chinese herbal medicine (Bensoussan & Myers 1996: 175).

This recommendation reflects the spirit of a 1993 report on complementary medicine by the British Medical Association (BMA 1993) which recommended that:

Medically qualified practitioners wishing to practise any form of non-conventional therapy should undertake recognised training in that field approved by the appropriate regulatory body, and should only practise the therapy after registration (BMA 1993: 148).

Increasingly, members of the medical and other health professions are realising the value of complementary medicine and wish to incorporate it into their practice. To do this effectively and sensitively it is essential that issues of professional boundaries be resolved and that appropriate training programs be established to ensure safe and effective practice for these professions.

Education for complementary medicine health professionals

The field of complementary medicine education is not without problems. Dr Stephen Fulder points out that:

> There are basically two ways to learn the healing arts. At one extreme is the apprenticeship in which students learn their skills through a gradual process of osmosis from long periods of working with accomplished therapists. At the other extreme is the highly formal and standardised training, as in modern medicine today. At one time complementary therapies, such as traditional medicine, were all taught by apprenticeship . . . The knowledge was passed down as a semi-secret art from master to disciples, whose entrance requirements were aptitude, enthusiasm, and endurance. Under these circumstances, there was every opportunity to be very good or very bad . . . However for the main therapeutic systems, the last 30 years saw the establishment of small formal colleges which varied widely in quality of training, depending on the competence and ability of their founders. They often taught different interpretations of each therapy, fragmenting the knowledge and preserving the fragments with professional rivalries. Attempts in the past to set up common standards were fruitless, and possibly unnecessary as therapists could practise anyway under common law. There was no chance of formal recognition and the medical profession successfully marginalised complementary medicine. Therapists therefore arrived at the end of the 1980's as a mixture of the highly competent and less competent, highly trained and untrained, and with widely differing interpretations of each therapeutic modality (Fulder 1996: 53).

While Dr Fulder is describing the training of complementary medicine practitioners in Britain, this paralleled the rise of complementary medicine in other western countries. Wide discrepancy of standards is still in evidence today and the challenge for the future is to narrow this distance. In the process leading to the Victorian *Chinese Medicines Act 2000* in Australia, the TCM profession made a landmark decision that they would set the minimum standard of education for their profession as an undergraduate degree. This was courageous at a time when there were only four degree programs in the country which were far outweighed by numerous private colleges providing diploma-level education. Appropriate educational standards are required of all health professions working within mainstream healthcare delivery and a major challenge for complementary medicine is to set and meet these standards. These standards will be critical in the regulation of these professions, especially if they are to take their place as equal members in an integrated healthcare system.

Meeting the challenge

Complementary medicine has made major advances over the past three decades wherein it has moved from a fringe activity to a healthcare practice with an opportunity for integration into mainstream health delivery. The movement of complementary medicine education into the university sector, the establishment of the initial Office of Alternative Medicine in the US Institutes of Health (which has since become the National Center for Complementary and Alternative Medicine) and an Office of Complementary Medicines in the Australian Therapeutic Goods Administration are all examples of change that was previously unexpected. In truth they were a reaction to the health consumers pursuit of what appears to be a gentle, safe and effective therapeutic practice. The consumer led the process of transition by making a choice and voting with their bodies and health dollars. The response of universities and government was a reflection of these community trends.

The complementary medicine movement consisting of consumers, practitioners and industry has risen to the challenges that needed to be overcome to get to where it is today. However, while complementary medicine has made major advances, if it wants to enter mainstream healthcare as an equal and integrated partner, it now needs to confront the challenges that faces it today.

Recommended reading

Bensoussan, A. and Myers, S.P. 1996, *Towards a Safer Choice*, Faculty of Health, University of Western Sydney, Sydney.

Lewith, G., Jonas, W.B. and Walach, H. 2002, *Clinical Research in Complementary Therapies. Principles, Problems and Solutions*, Churchill Livingstone, Edinburgh.

Fulder, S. 1996, *The Handbook of Alternative and Complementary Medicine*, Oxford University Press, Oxford.

REFERENCES

Introduction The evolving medical paradigm

Bensoussan, A. 1999, 'Complementary medicine—where lies its appeal?' *Medical Journal of Australia* 170: 247–8.

Brown, T. 2000, *The Historical and Conceptual Foundations of the Rochester Biopsychosocial Model*, Department of History, University of Rochester <www.history.rochester.edu>, 12/11/2002.

Campbell, J. 1993, *The Hero With a Thousand Faces*, Fontana Press, London.

Conlan, R. 1999, *States of Mind*, John Wiley and Sons, New York.

Datamonitor 2002, 'US Nutraceuticals 2002', <www.datamonitor.com>, 16/10/2002.

Eisenberg, D.M., Kessler, R.C., Van Rompay, M.I., Kaptchuk, T.J., Wilkey, S.A., Appel, S. and Davis, R.B. 2001, 'Perceptions about complementary therapies relative to conventional therapies among adults who use both: results from a national survey' *Annals of Internal Medicine* 135(5): 344–51.

Fields, W.S. 1991, 'The history of leeching and hirudin' *Haemostasis* 21(suppl 1): 3–10.

Foss, L. 2002, *The End of Modern Medicine*, State University of New York Press, Albany.

Hyland, M.E. 2001, 'The intelligent body' *New Scientist* 170(2292): 32–3.

MacLennan, A.H., Wilson, D.H. and Taylor, A.W. 2002, 'The escalating cost and prevalence of alternative medicine' *Preventive Medicine* 35: 166–73.

Michaelsen, A., Moebus, S., Spahn, G., Esch, T., Laughorst, J. and Dobos, G.J. 2002, 'Leech therapy for symptomatic treatment of knee osteoarthritis' *Alternative Therapy in Health and Medicine* 8(5): 84–8.

Mills, S.Y. 2001, 'Regulation in complementary and alternative medicine' *British Medical Journal* 322: 158–60.

Nahin, R.L. and Straus, S.E. 2001, 'Research into complementary and alternative medicine: problems and potential' *British Medical Journal* 322: 161–4.

Nuland, S.B. 2000, *The Mysteries Within*, Touchstone, New York.

Prince Charles, HRH 2001, 'The best of both worlds' *British Medical Journal* 322: 181.

Rees, L. 2001, 'Integrated medicine' *British Medical Journal* 322: 119–20.

Reuters 2002, 'UK's Prince Charles urges free alternative therapy' *Reuters Health* 21 May.

Rivera, J.O., Ortiz, M., Lawson, M.E. and Verma, K.M. 2002, 'Evaluation of the use of complementary and alternative medicine in the largest United States–Mexico border city' *Pharmacotherapy* 22(2): 256–64.

Schafer, T., Riehle, A., Wichmann, H.E. and Ring, J. 2002, 'Alternative medicine in allergies—prevalence, patterns of use and costs' *Allergy* 57: 694–700.

Theobald, R. 1999, *Visions and Pathways for the 21st Century*, Southern Cross University Press, Lismore, Australia.

Timeline 1926, 'Physician of the future to keep patients well' *Science Newsletter* 1 May.

Tudge, C. 2001, 'The best medicine' *New Scientist* 172(2317): 40–3.

United Kingdom Parliament 2001, *Select Committee on Science and Technology: Sixth Report*, http://www.parliament.the-stationery-office.co.uk [date of access 6 April 2002].

Von Peter, S., Ting. W., Scrivani, S., Korkin, E., Okvat, H., Gross, M., Oz, C. and Balmaceda, C. 2002, 'Survey on the use of complementary and alternative medicine among patients with headache syndromes' *Cephalalgia* 22: 395–400.

Whitfield, J. 2002, 'Botanists probe medieval medicine' *Nature Science Update* 22 July.

World Health Organization 2002a, 'Traditional and alternative medicine', *Fact Sheet 271*.

World Health Organization 2002b, 'Traditional medicine—growing needs and potential' *WHO Policy Perspectives On Medicine* No. 2, May.

Chapter 1 Ayurveda

Dash, B. and Junius, M. 1983, *A Handbook of Ayurveda*, Concept Publishing Company, New Delhi.

Frawley, D. 1997, *Ayurveda and the Mind*, Lotus Press, Wisconsin.

Frawley, D. and Ranade, S. 2001, *Ayurveda: Nature's Medicine*, Lotus Press, Wisconsin.

Lad, V. 1985, *Ayurveda: The Science of Self-healing*, Lotus Press, Wisconsin.

Svoboda, R. 1992, *Ayurveda: Life Health and Longevity*, Arkana, London.

Chapter 2 Indigenous healing

Adelson, N. 2000, *'Being Alive Well': Health and the Politics of Cree Well-Being*, University of Toronto Press, Toronto.

Bell, D. 1983, *Daughters of the Dreaming*, Allen & Unwin, Sydney.

Berndt, C. 1982, 'Sickness and health in Western Arnhem Land: a traditional perspective', in J. Reid (ed.) *Body, Land and Spirit: Health and Healing in Aboriginal Society*, University of Queensland Press, St Lucia.

Cambie, R.C. and Ash, J. 1994, *Fijian Medicinal Plants*, CSIRO, Australia.

Connor, L., Asch, P. and T. 1996, *Jero Tapakan: Balinese Healer*, Ethnographics Press, Los Angeles.

Das, V. 1990, 'What do we mean by health?', in J. Caldwell (ed.) *What We Know About the Health Transition: The Cultural, Social and Behavioural Determinants of Health: Proceedings of an International Workshop*, The Health Transition Centre, Australian National University, Canberra, 1: 27–46.

Frankel, S. and Lewis, G. (eds) 1989, *A Continuing Trial of Treatment: Medical Pluralism in Papua New Guinea*, Kluwer Academic Publishers, Boston.

Franklin, M.-A. and White, I. 1991, 'The history and politics of Aboriginal health', in J. Reid and P. Trompf (eds) *The Health of Aboriginal Australia*, Harcourt Brace Jovanovich, Sydney.

Evans-Pritchard, E. 1937, *Witchcraft, Oracles and Magic among the Azande*, Clarendon Press, Oxford.

Keesing, R. 1981, *Cultural Anthropology: A Contemporary Perspective*, Holt Rinehart and Winston, New York.

Kleinman, A. 1980, *Patients and Healers in the Context of Culture*, University of California Press, Berkeley.

Lewis, G. 2000, *A Failure of Treatment*, Oxford University Press, Oxford.

Macintyre, M. 1987, 'Flying witches and leaping warriors: supernatural origins of power and matrilineal authority in Tubetube society', in M. Strathern (ed.) *Dealing with Inequality: Analysing gender relations in Melanesia and Beyond*, Cambridge University Press, Cambridge.

Macintyre, M. 1990, 'Christianity, cargo cultism and the concept of the spirit in Misiman cosmology', in J. Barker and C. Forman (eds) *Christianity in Oceania, Ethnographic Perspectives*, ASAO Monograph Series, University Press of America, Washington.

Malinowski, B. 1932, *The Sexual Life of Savages in North-Western Melanesia*, Routledge and Kegan Paul, London.

Mobbs, R. 1991, 'In sickness and in health: the sociocultural context of Aboriginal well-being, illness and healing', in J. Reid and P. Trompf (eds) *The Health of Aboriginal Australia*, Harcourt Brace Jovanovich, Sydney.

Reid, J. 1983, *Sorcerers and Healing Spirits: Continuity and Change in an Aboriginal Medical System*, Australian National University Press, Canberra.

Strathern, A. and Stewart, P.J. 2000, *Curing and Healing: Medical Anthropology in Global Perspective*, Carolina Academic Press, Durham, North Carolina.

Tonkinson, M. 1982, 'The *Mabarn* and the hospital: the selection of treatment in a remote Aboriginal community', in J. Reid (ed.) *Body, Land and Spirit: Health and Healing in Aboriginal Society*, University of Queensland Press, St Lucia.

Chapter 3 Naturopathic medicine

Boon, H. 1998, 'Canadian naturopathic practitioners: holistic and scientific world views' *Social Science and Medicine* 46(9): 1213–25.

Cody, G. 1999, 'History of naturopathic medicine', in J. Pizzorno and M. Murray (eds) *Textbook of Natural Medicine*, 2nd edn, Churchill Livingstone, New York.

Eisenberg, D.M., Kessler, R.C., Van Rompay, M.I., Kaptchuk, T.J., Wilkey, S.A., Appel, S. and Davis, R.B. 2001, 'Perceptions about complementary therapies relative to conventional therapies among adults who use both: results from a national survey' *Annals of Internal Medicine* 135(5): 344–51.

Evans, S. 2000, 'The story of naturopathic education in Australia' *Complementary Therapies in Medicine* 8: 234–40.

Fulder, S. 1996, *The Handbook of Alternative and Complementary Medicine*, 3rd edn, Oxford University Press, Oxford.

Hippocrates 1987, *Hippocratic Writings* (translated by F. Adams), Encyclopaedia Britannica Inc., Chicago.

Hunter, A. 2002, 'Natural therapies: how good is the training?' *Diversity* 2(7): 40–7.

Lewith, G.T. 1984, Foreword, in R. Newman Turner *Naturopathic Medicine. Treating the Whole Person*, Thorsons Publishers, Wellingborough.

Kirchfeld, F. and Boyle, W. 1994, *Nature Doctors*, Buckeye Naturopathic Press, Ohio.

Martyr, P. 2002, *Paradise of Quacks*, Macleay Press, Sydney.

MacLennan, A.H., Wilson, D.H. and Taylor, A.W. 2002, 'The escalating cost and prevalence of alternative medicine' *Preventive Medicine* 35: 166–73.

Newman Turner, R. 1984, *Naturopathic Medicine. Treating the Whole Person*, Thorsons Publishers, Wellingborough.

Pizzorno, J. and Snider, P. 1999, 'Naturopathic medicine', in M. Micozzi (ed.) *Fundamentals of Complementary and Alternative Medicine*, 2nd edn, Churchill Livingstone, New York.

Snider, P. and Zeff, J. 1988, *Report to the AANP House of Delegates: Select Committee on the Definition of Naturopathic Medicine*.

Smith, M.J. and Logan, A.C. 2002, 'Naturopathy' *Complementary and Alternative Medicine* 86(1): 173–84.

Whorton, J.C. 1999, 'The history of alternative and complementary medicine', in W.B. Jonas and J.S. Levin (eds) *The Essentials of Complementary and Alternative Medicine*, Lippincott, Williams & Wilkins, Philadelphia.

Zeff, J. 1997, 'The process of healing: A unifying theory of naturopathic medicine' *Journal of Naturopathic Medicine* 8: 62–5.

Chapter 4 Traditional Chinese Medicine

Bellavite, P., Semizzi, M., Lussignoli, S., Andrioli, G. and Bartocci, U. 1998, 'A computer model of the "five elements" theory of Traditional Chinese Medicine' *Complementary Therapies in Medicine* 6: 133–40.

Bensoussan, A. and Myers, S.P. 1996, *Towards a Safer Choice: The Practice of Traditional Chinese Medicine in Australia*, University of Western Sydney, Sydney.

Bensoussan, A., Talley, N.J., Hing, M., Menzies, R., Guo, A. and Ngu, M. 1998, 'Treatment of irritable bowel syndrome with Chinese herbal medicine' *Journal of the American Medical Association* 280(18): 1585–9.

Chan, K. 2002, 'The historical evolution of Chinese medicine and orthodox medicine in China', in K. Chan and H. Lee (eds) *The Way Forward for Chinese Medicine*, Taylor & Francis, London.

Chan, K. and Lee, H. 2002, 'The progress of Chinese medicine in the United Kingdom', in K. Chan and H. Lee (eds) *The Way Forward for Chinese Medicine*, Taylor & Francis, London.

Freeman, L.W. and Lawlis, G.F. 2001, *Mosby's Complementary and Alternative Medicine: A Research-Based Approach*, Harcourt Health Sciences Company, St Louis.

Helms, J.M. 1987, 'Acupuncture for the management of primary dysmenorrhea' *Obstetrics and Gynecology* 69(1): 51–6.

Hesketh, T. and Zhu, W.X. 1997, 'Health in China: traditional Chinese medicine: one country, two systems' *British Medical Journal* 315: 115–17.

Hui, K.K., Yu, J.L. and Zylowska, L. 2002, 'The progress of Chinese medicine in the United States of America', in K. Chan and H. Lee (eds) *The Way Forward for Chinese Medicine*, Taylor & Francis, London.

Kaptchuk, T. 1993, *Chinese Medicine: The Web That Has No Weaver*, Rider, London.

Liu, Y. 1995, *The Essential Book of Traditional Chinese Medicine*, Vol. 1, Theory, Columbia University Press, New York.

Liu, Z.W. 2002, 'Philosophical aspects of Chinese medicine from a Chinese medicine academician', in K. Chan and H. Lee (eds) *The Way Forward for Chinese Medicine*, Taylor & Francis, London.

Loh, L., Nathan, P.W., Schott, G.D. and Zilkha, K.J. 1984, 'Acupuncture versus medical treatment for migraine and muscle tension headaches' *Journal of Neurology, Neurosurgery and Psychiatry* 47(4): 333–7.

MacLennan, A.H., Wilson, D.H. and Taylor, A.W. 2002, 'The escalating cost and prevalence of alternative medicine' *Preventive Medicine* 35: 166–73.

Maciocia, G. 1995, *The Foundations of Chinese Medicine: A Comprehensive Text for Acupuncturists and Herbalists*, Churchill Livingstone, Edinburgh.

Maciocia, G. 1998, *Obstetrics and Gynecology in Chinese Medicine*, Churchill Livingstone, New York.

Ni, M. (trans.) 1995, *The Yellow Emperor's Classic of Medicine: A New Translation of the Neijing Suwen with Commentary*, Shambhala, Boston.

Sheehan, M.P. and Atherton, D.J. 1992, 'A controlled trial of traditional Chinese medicinal plants in widespread non-exudative atopic eczema' *British Journal of Dermatology* 126(2): 179–84.

Veith, I. (trans.) 1972, *The Yellow Emperor's Classic of Internal Medicine*, Pelanduk Publications, Selangor Darul Ehsan.

Weatherall, D. 1997, *Science and the Quiet Art: Medical Research and Patient Care*, Oxford University Press, Oxford.

Wiseman, N. and Ellis, A. 1996, *Fundamentals of Chinese Medicine*, Paradigm Publications, Brookline.

Zhang, Y.H. and Rose, K. 1999, *Who Can Ride the Dragon: An Exploration of the Cultural Roots of Traditional Chinese Medicine*, Paradigm Publications, Brookline.

Chapter 5 Acupuncture

Bensky, D. and Gamble, A. 1993, *Chinese Herbal Medicine Materia Medica*, Eastland Press, Seattle.

Cai, G., Chao, G., Chen, D. *et al.* (eds) 1995, *State Administration of Traditional Chinese Medicine, Advanced Textbook on Traditional Chinese Medicine and Pharmacology*, Vol. I, New World Press, Beijing.

Cai, J., Chao, G., Chen, D. *et al.* (eds) 1997, *State Administration of Traditional Chinese Medicine, Advanced Textbook on Traditional Chinese Medicine and Pharmacology*, Vol. IV, New World Press, Beijing.

Cardini, F. and Huang, W. 1998, 'Moxibustion for correction of breech presentation. A randomised controlled trial' *Journal of the American Medical Association* 280(8): 1580–4.

Cheng, X. (chief ed.) 1987, *Chinese Acupuncture and Moxibustion*, Foreign Languages Press, Beijing.

Deadman, P., Al-Khafaji, M. and Baker, K. 1998, *A Manual of Acupuncture*, Journal of Chinese Medicine Publications, East Sussex, England.

Easthope, G., Beilby, J. and Tranter, B. 1998, 'Acupuncture in Australian general practice: practitioner characteristics' *Medical Journal of Australia* 167: 197–200.

Eisenberg, D.M., Davis, R.B., Ettner, S.L., Appel, S., Wilkey, S., Van Rompay, M. and Kessler, R.C. 1998, 'Trends in alternative medicine use in the United States, 1990–1997. Results of a follow-up national survey' *Journal of the American Medical Association* 280(18): 1569–75.

Ellis, N. 1993, 'A pilot study to evaluate the effect of acupuncture on nocturia in the elderly' *Complementary Therapies in Medicine* 1: 164–7.

Ellis, N., Briggs, R. and Dawson, D. 1990, 'The effect of acupuncture on nocturnal urinary frequency and incontinence in the elderly' *Complementary Medical Research* 4: 16–17.

Filshie, J. and White, A. 1998, 'The clinical use of, and evidence for, acupuncture in medical systems', in J. Filshie and A. White (eds) *Medical Acupuncture. A Western Scientific Approach*, Churchill Livingstone, Edinburgh.

Gerber, R. 1988, *Vibrational Medicine*, Bear and Co., Sante Fe.

Ghaly, R.G., Fitzpatrick, K.T. and Dundee, J.W. 1987, 'Antiemetic studies with traditional Chinese acupuncture—comparison of manual needling with electrical stimulation and commonly used emetics' *Anaesthesia* 42(10): 1108–10.

Gunn, C.C. 1998, 'Acupuncture and the peripheral nervous system', in J. Filshie and A. White (eds) *Medical Acupuncture. A Western Scientific Approach*, Churchill Livingstone, Edinburgh.

Helms, J.M. 1987, 'Acupuncture in the management of primary dysmenorrhoea' *Obstetrics and Gynecology* 69(1): 51–6.

Hester, J. 1998, 'Acupuncture in the pain clinic', in J. Filshie and A. White (eds) *Medical Acupuncture. A Western Scientific Approach*, Churchill Livingstone, Edinburgh.

Kaptchuk, T. 1983, *Chinese Medicine: The Web That Has No Weaver*, Rider, London.

Lewith, G.T. and Vincent, C.A. 1998, 'The clinical evaluation of acupuncture', in J. Filshie and A. White (eds) *Medical Acupuncture. A Western Scientific Approach*, Churchill Livingstone, Edinburgh.

Li, W.X., Xue, C.L. and Li, J.H. 2000, *Easy Locating of Acupuncture Points*, 4th edn, Shanghai Book Company Ltd, Hong Kong.

Linde, K., Vickers, A., Hondras, M. *et al.* 2001, 'Systematic reviews of complementary therapies—an annotated bibliography. Part 1: Acupuncture', <www.pubmedcentral.nih.gov/artic*der.fcgi?tool=pubmed&pubmedid=11513758>, 28 July 2002.

NHMRC 1989, 'National Health and Medical Research Council, Acupuncture: a working party report', Australian Government Publishing Service, Canberra, in A. Bensoussan and S.P. Myers 1996, *Towards a Safer Choice: The Practice of Traditional Chinese Medicine in Australia*, University of Western Sydney, Sydney.

Qiu, M.L., Zang, S.C., Yu, Z.Q. *et al.* 1993, *Chinese Acupuncture and Moxibustion*, Churchill Livingstone, Edinburgh.

Strauss, A.J. and Xue, C.C.L. 2001, 'Acupuncture for chronic non-specific lower back pain: a case series study' *China Journal of Integrative Medicine* 7(3): 190–4.

Vincent, C. and Furnham, A. 1997, *Complementary Medicine. A Research Perspective*, Wiley, Chichester, England.

World Health Organization 1986, *Ottawa Charter for Health Promotion*, World Health Organization, Geneva.

Xue, C.C.L. 1993, 'Clinical research of acupuncture combination with Chinese herbal medicine for 108 cases of hemiplegia' *Guangdong Medical Journal* [in Chinese] 3: 149–50.

Xue, C.C.L. 1998, 'Prof. Yang Wen Hui's academic achievement in acupuncture—the emphasis of the combination of acupuncture and Chinese herbal medicine in clinical management', in X.S. Lai and J.W. Zhang (eds) *A Compendium of Clinical Experience of Acupuncture Experts in South China* [in Chinese], 1st edn, China Medical Technology Publishing House, Beijing.

Xue, C., English, R., Zhang J.J., Da Costa, C. and Li, C.G. 2002, 'Effects of acupuncture in the treatment of seasonal allergic rhinitis: a randomised controlled clinical trial' *The American Journal of Chinese Medicine* 30(1): 1–11.

Xue, C.C.L. and Yang, W.H. 1990, 'Meridian research', in X.J. Cheng and J.H. Wang (eds) *Research on Traditional Chinese Medicine Theory* [in Chinese], 1st edn, Press of South China University of Technology, Guangzhou.

Yan, Z.Y. (ed.) (1984), *High Education in Chinese Medicine*, Shanghai Science and Technology Press, Shanghai.

Chapter 6 Aromatherapy

Battalgia, S. 1997, *The Complete Guide to Aromatherapy*, The Perfect Potion, Queensland, Australia.

Bowles, E.J. 2000, *The Basic Chemistry of Aromatherapeutic Essential Oils*, 2nd edn, Bowles, Sydney.

Buchbauer, G., Jiroveta, L., Jager, W., Dietrich, H. and Plank, C. 1991, 'Aromatherapy: evidence for sedative effects of the essential oil of lavender after inhalation' *Zeitschrift fur Naturfurschung* 46(11–12): 1067–72.

Carson, C.F. and Riley, T.V. 1995, 'Anti-microbial activity of the major components of the essential oil of *Melaleuca alternatifolia*' *Journal of Applied Bacteriology* 78(3): 264–9.

Cooksley, V.G. 2002, *Aromatherapy: Soothing Remedies to Restore, Rejuvenate and Heal*, Prentice Hall Press, USA.

Cornwell, P.A. and Barry, B.W. 1994, 'Sesquiterpene components of volatile oils as skin penetration enhancers for the hydrophilic permeant 5-flourouracil' *Journal of Pharmacy and Pharmacology* 46(4): 261–9.

Diego, M.A., Jones, N.A., Field, T., Hernandez-Reif, M., Schanberg, S., Kuhn, C., McAdam, V., Galamaga, R. and Galamaga, M. 1998, 'Aromatherapy positively affects mood, EEG patterns of alertness and math computations' *International Journal of Neuroscience* 96(3–4): 217–24.

Etherington, K. 2000, *Anatomica*, Random House, Australia.

Fischer-Rizzi, S. 1990, *Complete Aromatherapy Handbook*, Sterling Publishing Company Inc., New York.

Franchomme, P. and Pénoël, D. 1990, *L'aromatherapie exactment*, Roger Jollois, Limoges, France.

Gearon, V. 2002, 'Commentary' *Aromatherapy Today* 24 (12.02): 31–2.

Guba, R. 2000, 'Toxicity myths—the actual risks of essential oil usage' *International Journal of Aromatherapy* 10(1/2): 37–49.

Hay, I.C., Jamieson, M. and Ormerod, A.D. 1998, 'Randomized trial of aromatherapy. Successful treatment for alopecia areata' *Archives of Dermatology* 134(11): 1349–52.

Holmes, C., Hopkins, H., Hensford, C., MacLaughlin, V., Wilkinson, D. and Rosenvinge, H. 2002, 'Lavender oil as a treatment for agitated behaviour in severe dementia: a placebo controlled study' *International Journal of Geriatric Psychiatry* 17: 305–8.

Holmes, P. 1992, 'Lavender oil' *International Journal of Aromatherapy* 4(4): 20–1.

Hongratanaworakit, T., Heuberger, E. and Buchbauer, G. 2000, *Effects of Sandalwood Oil and a–Santalol on Humans II: Percutaneous Administration*, Institute of Pharmaceutical Chemistry, Vienna.

Johnson, G. 2003, 'Growing essential oil crops in New Zealand' *Aromatherapy Today* 25(03.03): 24.

Jurgens, U.R., Stober, M., Schmidt-Schilling, L., Kleuver, T. and Vetter, H. 1998, 'Anti-inflammtory effects of eucalyptus (1,8 cineole) in bronchial asthma inhibition of arachidonic acid metabolism in human blood monocytes ex vivo' *European Journal of Medical Research* 3(9) 407–12.

Kerr, J. 2002, 'Research project—using essential oils in wound care for the elderly' *Aromatherapy Today* 23(10.02): 14–19.

Lawrence, B. 1987/1988, 'Lavender oil' *Perfume and Flavourist* 12(6): 56.

Leffingwell, J.C. 1999, 'Smell and the olfactory system', Leffingwell & Assoc., <www.leffingwell.com/olfaction.htm>, 17/12/02.

Lester, A., Touche, J., Linas, R. and Derbesy, M. 1986, 'Haute-provence French lavender essential oil' *Proceedings of the 9th International Congress Of Essential Oils*, Singapore, 127–3.

Lis-Balchin, M. and Hart, S. 1999, 'Studies on the mode of action of the essential oil lavender (*Lavandula angustifolia* P Miller)' *Phytotherapy Research* 13(6): 540–2.

McCabe, P., Ramsay, L. and Taylor, B. 1994, *Complementary Therapies in Relation to Nursing Practice in Australia*, Discussion Paper No. 2, Royal College of Nursing Australia.

Marieb, E.N. 2000, *Essentials of Human Anatomy and Physiology*, Addison Wesley Longman Inc., USA.

Myers, S., O'Connor, J., Brooks, L., Cheras, P., Paul-Brent, P., Orrock, P. and Church, P. 2002, 'The acute effects of sandalwood oil and massage on physiological and psychological parameters' *Proceedings of the Australian Centre for Complementary Medicine Education and Research (ACCMER) Complementary Medicine Research Symposium*, 35–6.

Noonan, T. 1997, 'Effects of massage techniques on the autonomic nervous system, endocrine system and other systems', <www.softspeak.com.au/maspap98.htm>, 6/9/02.

Primmer, J. 2002, 'Case study—healing skin tear with essential oils' *Aromatherapy Today* 23(10.02): 20–1.

Quirk, L. 2003, 'Practical nursing skills in residential aged care', in press.

Schnaubelt, K. 1999, *Medical Aromatherapy—Healing with Essential Oils*, Frog, Berkley.

Shepherd, G.M. 1983, *Neurobiology*, Oxford University Press, Oxford.

Sheppard-Hanger, S. 1995, *The Aromatherapy Practitioners Manual*, Vols 1 and 2, Aquarius, Willeton.

Tisserand, R. 1997, *The Art of Aromatherapy*, Destiny Books, USA.

Tisserand, R. and Balacs, T. 1995, *Essential Oil Safety—A Guide for Health Care Professionals*, Churchill Livingstone, Edinburgh.

Ulmer, W.T. and Schott, D. 1991, 'Chronic obstructive bronchitis. Effects of Gelomyrtol Forte in placebo-controlled double blind study' *Fortschritteder Medizin* 109(27): 547–50.

Williams, A.C. and Barry, B.W. 1991, 'Terpenes and the lipid-protein-partitioning theory of skin penetration enhancement' *Pharmaceutical Research* 8(1): 17–24.

Zhang, X. and Firestein, S. 2002, 'The olfactory receptor gene superfamily of the mouse', *Nature Neuroscience* 5(2): 124–33.

Zola, A. and Le Vanda, J.P. 1979, 'Le Lavandin Grosso' *Perfumerie, Cosmetique et Aromes* 25: 60–2.

Chapter 7 Chiropractic

Adams, M.A. and Hutton, W.C. 1980, 'The effect of posture on the role of the apophyseal joints in resisting intervertebral compressive force' *Journal of Bone and Joint Surgery* 62(B): 358–62.

Association of Chiropractic Colleges 1996, 'Position paper #1' *Journal of Manipulative and Physiological Therapeutics* 19: 634–7.

Bartsch, T. and Goadsby, P.J. 2002, 'Stimulation of the greater occipital nerve induces increased excitability of dural afferent input' *Brain* 125(7): 1496–509.

Bowers, L.J. and Mootz, R.D. 1995, 'The nature of primary care: the chiropractor's role' *Topics in Clinical Chiropractic* 2(1): 66–84.

Briggs, C.A. and Chandraraj, S. 1996, 'Variations in the lumbosacral ligament and associated changes in the lumbosacral region resulting in compression of the fifth dorsal root ganglion and spinal nerve' *Clinical Anatomy* 9(4): 278–9.

Brumagne, S., Cordo, P., Lysens, R., Verschueren, S. and Swinnen, S. 2000, 'The role of paraspinal muscle spindles in lumbosacral position sense in individuals with and without low back pain' *Spine* 25: 989–94.

Brumagne, S., Lysens, R., Swinnen, S. and Verschueren, S. 1999, 'Effect of paraspinal muscle vibration on position sense of the lumbosacral spine' *Spine* 24: 1328–31.

Budgell, B.S. 2000, 'Reflex effects of subluxation: the autonomic nervous system' *Journal of Manipulative and Physiological Therapeutics* 23: 104–6.

Budgell, B. and Hirano, F. 2001, 'Innocuous mechanical stimulation of the neck and alterations in heart-rate variability in healthy young adults' *Autonomic Neurosciences* 91(1–2): 96–9.

Budgell, B.S., Hotta, H. and Sato, A. 1998, 'Reflex responses of bladder motility after stimulation of interspinous tissues in the anesthetized rat' *Journal of Manipulative and Physiological Therapeutics* 21: 593–9.

Budgell, B. and Sato, A. 1996, 'Modulations of autonomic functions by somatic nociceptive inputs' *Progress in Brain Research* 113: 525–39.

Budgell, B. and Sato, A. 1997, 'The cervical subluxation and regional cerebral blood flow' *Journal of Manipulative and Physiological Therapeutics* 20: 103–7.

Budgell, B., Sato, A., Suzuki, A. and Uchida, S. 1997, 'Responses of adrenal function to stimulation of lumbar and thoracic interspinous tissues in the rat' *Neuroscience Research* 28(1): 33–40.

Budgell, B. and Suzuki, A. 2000, 'Inhibition of gastric motility by noxious chemical stimulation of interspinous tissues in the rat' *Journal of the Autonomic Nervous System* 80(3): 162–8.

Chance, M.A. 1996, 'Australians draft chiropractic clinical parameters' *Dynamic Chiropractic* 15 January, and at <www.chiroweb.com/archives/14/02/01.html>.

Chapman-Smith, D. 1998, 'Cost-effectiveness—the second Manga report', in D. Chapman-Smith (ed.) *The Chiropractic Report* 12(2): 1–8.

Chapman-Smith, D. 2001a, 'The chiropractic profession', in D. Chapman-Smith (ed.) *The Chiropractic Report* 15(6): 1–8.

Chapman-Smith, D. 2001b, 'Safety and effectiveness of cervical manipulation', in D. Chapman-Smith (ed.) *The Chiropractic Report* 15(3): 1–8.

Chapman-Smith, D. 2002, 'A new analysis of work-related chronic back pain', in D. Chapman-Smith (ed.) *The Chiropractic Report* 16(2): 1–8.

Coulter, I.D. 1999, *Chiropractic. A Philosophy for Alternative Health Care*, Butterworth Heinemann, Oxford.

Coulter, I.D., Danielson, C.D. and Hays, R.D. 1996, 'Measuring chiropractic practitioner satisfaction' *Topics in Clinical Chiropractic* 3(1): 65–70.

Coulter, I.D., Hurwitz, E.L., Adams, A.H., Genovese, B.J., Hays, R. and Shekelle, P.G. 2002, 'Patients using chiropractors in North America: who are they and why are they in chiropractic care?' *Spine* 27: 291–6. Discussion 297–8.

Dolan, P. and Adams, M.A. 2001, 'Recent advances in lumbar spinal mechanics and their significance for modelling' *Clinical Biomechanics* 16 (suppl. 1): S8–16.

Ebrall, P.S. 1992a, 'Mechanical low-back pain: a comparison of medical and chiropractic management in Victoria' *Chiropractic Journal of Australia* 22: 47–53.

Ebrall, P.S. 1992b, 'Utilisation of chiropractic services by the members of one private health fund in Victoria, 1990' *Chiropractic Journal of Australia* 22: 122–8.

Ebrall, P.S. 1993, 'A descriptive report of the case-mix within Australian chiropractic practice, 1992' *Chiropractic Journal of Australia* 23: 92–7.

Ebrall, P.S. 1995a, 'A review of the practice of medicine in 1895' *Chiropractic Journal of Australia* 25: 93–100.

Ebrall, P.S. 1995b, 'A review of the neurological concepts of 1895' *Chiropractic Journal of Australia* 25: 56–60.

Ebrall, P.S. 1996a, 'Clinical parameters: what do they mean to you?', in *Proceedings, Chiropractors' Association of Australia (Ltd) National Conference. Perth, WA, Sept 1996.* CAA (National) Ltd, Faulconbridge. E3.

Ebrall, P.S. 1996b, 'A user's guide to the clinical parameters of Australian chiropractic practice', in *Proceedings, Chiropractors' Association of Australia (Ltd) National Conference. Perth, WA, Sept 1996.* CAA (National) Ltd, Faulconbridge. E4.

Ebrall, P.S. 1996c, 'Clinical parameters: where to now?', in *Proceedings, Chiropractors' Association of Australia (Ltd) National Conference. Perth, WA, Sept 1996.* CAA (National) Ltd, Faulconbridge. E5.

Ebrall, P.S. 2001, 'A survey of sets of principles of chiropractic' *Chiropractic Journal of Australia* 31: 58–69.

Ebrall, P.S. (in press), *Assessment of the spine*, Churchill Livingstone, Edinburgh.

Faye, L.J. 1986, *Spinal motion palpation and clinical considerations of the lumbar spine and pelvis* [Lecture notes], Huntington Beach, Motion Palpation Institute.

Firth, J.N. 1948, *A Text-Book on Chiropractic Diagnosis*, 5th edn, James N. Firth, Indianapolis.

Forster, A.L. 1920, *Principles and Practice of Chiropractic*, 2nd edn, The National Publishing Company, Chicago.

Fujimoto, T., Budgell, B., Uchida, S., Suzuki, A. and Meguro, K. 1999, 'Arterial tonometry in the measurement of the effects of innocuous mechanical stimulation of the neck on heart rate and blood pressure' *Journal of the Autonomic Nervous System* 75(2–3): 109–15.

Gatterman, M.I. 1992, 'The vertebral subluxation syndrome: is a rose by any other name less thorny?' *Journal of the Canadian Chiropractic Association* 36(2): 102–4.

Gatterman, M.I. 1995a, 'Advances in subluxation terminology and usage', in D.J. Lawrence (ed.) *Advances in Chiropractic*, Vol. 2, Mosby, St Louis.

Gatterman, M.I. 1995b, 'A patient centered paradigm: a model for chiropractic education and research' *Journal of Alternative and Complementary Medicine* 1: 415–32.

Gatterman, M.I. 1995c, *Foundations of Chiropractic: Subluxation*, Mosby, St Louis.

Gatterman, M.I. 1997, 'Teaching chiropractic principles through patient centered outcomes' *Journal of the Canadian Chiropractic Association* 41(1): 27–35.

Gatterman, M.I. and Hansen, D.T. 1994, 'Development of chiropractic nomenclature through consensus' *Journal of Manipulative and Physiological Therapeutics* 17(5): 302–9.

Gaumer, G., Koren, A. and Gemmen, E. 2002, 'Barriers to expanding primary care roles for chiropractors: the role of chiropractic as primary care gatekeeper' *Journal of Manipulative and Physiological Therapeutics* 25: 427–49.

Gaumer, G.L., Walker, A. and Su, S. 2001, 'Chiropractic and a new taxonomy of primary care activities' *Journal of Manipulative and Physiological Therapeutics* 24: 239–59.

Gillet, H. 1972, 'Gillet talks about Illi' *Journal of the Australian Chiropractor's Association* 6(2): 16–18.

Gillet, J.J. and Gaucher-Peslherbe, P.L. 1996, 'New light on motion palpation [commentary]' *Journal of Manipulative and Physiological Therapeutics* 19(1): 52–9.

Haldeman, S., Chapman-Smith, D. and Petersen, D. 1992, *Guidelines for Chiropractic Quality Assurance and Practice Parameters*, Gaithersburg, Aspen.

Haldeman, S., Carey, P., Townsend, M. and Papadopoulos, C. 2001, 'Arterial dissections following cervical manipulation: the chiropractic experience' *Canadian Medical Association Journal* 165(7): 905–6.

Haldeman, S., Kohlbeck, F.J. and McGregor, M. 1999, 'Risk factors and precipitating neck movements causing vertebrobasilar artery dissection after cervical trauma and spinal manipulation' *Spine* 24: 785–94.

Haldeman, S., Kohlbeck, F.J. and McGregor, M. 2002a, 'Unpredictability of cerebrovascular ischaemia associated with cervical spine manipulation therapy: a review of sixty-four cases after cervical spine manipulation' *Spine* 27: 49–55.

Haldeman, S., Kohlbeck, F.J. and McGregor, M. 2002b, 'Stroke, cerebral artery dissection, and cervical spine manipulation therapy' *Journal of Neurology* 249(8): 1098–104.

Harrison, E. 1820, 'Remarks upon the different appearances of the back, breast and ribs, in persons affected with spinal diseases: and on the effects of spinal distortion on the sanguineous circulation' *London Medical Physicians Journal* 14: 365–78.

Hartvigsen, J., Sorensen, L.P., Graesborg, K. and Grunnet-Nilsson, N. 2002, 'Chiropractic patients in Denmark: a short description of basic characteristics' *Journal of Manipulative and Physiological Therapeutics* 25: 162–7.

Hawk, C., Lawrence, D. and Nyiendo, J. 1996, 'The role of chiropractors in the delivery of interdisciplinary health care in rural areas' *Journal of Manipulative and Physiological Therapeutics* 19: 82–91.

Hayes, B.M. and Gemmell, H.A. 2001, 'Patient satisfaction with chiropractic physicians in an independent physicians' association' *Journal of Manipulative and Physiological Therapeutics* 24: 556–9.

Henderson, D., Chapman-Smith, D., Mior, S. and Vernon, H. 1994, 'Clinical guidelines for chiropractic practice in Canada' *Journal of the Canadian Chiropractic Association* Suppl., 38(1).

Hertzman-Miller, R.P., Morgenstern, H., Hurwitz, E.L., Yu, F., Adams, A.H., Harber, P. and Kominski, G.F. 2002, 'Comparing the satisfaction of low back pain patients randomised to receive medical or chiropractic care: results from the UCLA low back pain study' *American Journal of Public Health* 92: 1628–33.

Holm, S., Indahl, A. and Solomonow, M. 2002, 'Sensorimotor control of the spine' *Journal of Electromyography and Kinesiology* 12(3): 219–34.

Homewood, A.E. 1981, *The Neurodynamics of the Vertebral Subluxation*, 3rd edn, The Parker Chiropractic Research Foundation, Fort Worth.

Hurwitz, E.L., Aker, P.D., Adams, A.H., Meeker, W.C. and Shekelle, P.G. 1996, 'Manipulation and mobilization of the cervical spine. A systematic review of the literature' *Spine* 21: 1746–59. Discussion 1759–60; Comment 22: 1676–7.

Hurwitz, E.L., Coulter, I.D., Adams, A.H., Genovese, B.J. and Shekelle, P.G. 1998, 'Use of chiropractic services from 1985 through 1991 in the United States and Canada' *American Journal of Public Health* 88(5): 771–6.

Indahl, A., Kaigle, A.M., Reikeras, O., Sten, H. and Holm, S. 1997, 'Interaction between the porcine lumbar intervertebral disc, zygapophysial joints, and paraspinal muscles' *Spine* 22: 2834–40.

Jamison, J.R. 1996, 'Patient satisfaction: exploring a new dimension' *Chiropractic Journal of Australia* 21: 15–20.

Jamison, J.R. 2002, 'Health information and promotion in chiropractic clinics' *Journal of Manipulative and Physiological Therapeutics* 25: 240–5.

Janse, J. 1948, 'The vertebral subluxation' *The National Chiropractic Journal* 18(10): 9–11, 66, 67.

Janse, J., Houser, R.H. and Wells, B.F. 1947, *Chiropractic Principles and Technic*, National College of Chiropractic, Chicago.

Jarvis, K.B., Phillips, R.B. and Danielson, C. 1997, 'Managed care preapproval and its effect on the cost of Utah worker compensation claims' *Journal of Manipulative and Physiological Therapeutics* 20: 372–6.

Jarvis, K.B., Phillips, R.B. and Morris, E.K. 1991, 'Cost per case comparison of back injury claims of chiropractic versus medical management for conditions with identical diagnostic codes' *Journal of Occupational Medicine* 33(8): 847–52.

Jull, G., Trott, P., Potter, H., Zito, G., Niere, K., Shirley, D., Emberson, J., Marschner, I. and Richardson, C. 2002, 'A randomised controlled trial of exercise and manipulative therapy for cervicogenic headache' *Spine* 27: 1835–43.

Kassak, K. and Sawyer, C.E. 1993, 'Patient satisfaction with chiropractic care' *Journal of Manipulative and Physiological Therapeutics* 16: 25–32.

Keating, J.C. 1992, 'The evolution of Palmer's metaphors and hypotheses' *Philosophical Constructs for the Chiropractic Profession* 2(1): 9–19.

Keating, J.C., Caldwell, S., Nguyen, H., Saljooghi, S. and Smith, B. 1998, 'A descriptive analysis of the *Journal of Manipulative and Physiological Therapeutics* 1989–1996' *Journal of Manipulative and Physiological Therapeutics* 21: 539–52.

Koes, B.W., van Tulder, M.W., Ostelo, R., Burton, A.K. and Waddell, G. 2001, 'Clinical guidelines for the management of low back pain in primary care: an international comparison' *Spine* 26: 2504–12.

Koumantakis, G.A., Wistanley, J. and Oldham, J.A. 2002, 'Thoracolumbar proprioception in individuals with and without low back pain: intratester reliability, clinical applicability, and validity' *Journal of Orthopaedic and Sports Physical Therapy* 32(7): 327–35.

Lantz, C.A. 1989, 'The vertebral subluxation complex' *ICA International Review of Chiropractic* Sept/Oct: 37–61.

Lantz, C.A. 1995a, 'A review of the evolution of chiropractic concepts of subluxation' *Topics in Clinical Chiropractic* 2(2): 1–10.

Lantz, C.A. 1995b, 'The vertebral subluxation complex', in M.I. Gatterman *Foundations of Chiropractic: Subluxation*, Mosby, St Louis.

Lawrence, A. 2002, Letter to the Chiropractors Registration Board of Victoria dated 18 June 2002, Chiropractors Association of Australia (National) Limited, Penrith.

Long, C.R. and Hawk, C. 2001, 'Patient satisfaction with the chiropractic clinical encounter: report from a practice based research program' *Journal of the Neuromusculoskeletal System* 4: 109–17.

McCrory, D.C., Penzien, D.B., Hasselblad, V. and Gray, R.N. 2001, *Evidence Report: Behavioural and Physical Treatments for Tension-Type and Cervicogenic Headaches*, Foundation for Chiropractic Education and Research, Des Moines.

Manga, P. and Angus, D. 1993, *The Effectiveness and Cost-Effectiveness of Chiropractic Management of Low Back Pain*, Pran Manga and Associates, University of Ottawa, Ontario.

Manga, P. and Angus, D. 1998, *Enhanced Chiropractic Coverage Under OHIP as a Means of Reducing Health Care Costs. Attaining Better Health Outcomes and Proving the Public's Access to Cost-Effective Health Services*, University of Ottawa, Ontario.

Meade, T.W., Dyer, S., Browne, W., Townsend, J. and Frank, A.O. 1990, 'Low back pain of mechanical origin: randomised comparison of chiropractic and hospital treatment' *British Medical Journal* 300: 31–7.

Meeker, W.C. and Haldeman, S. 2002, 'Chiropractic: a profession at the crossroads of mainstream and alternative medicine' *Annals of Internal Medicine* 136: 216–27.

Newcomer, K., Laskowski, E.R., Yu, B., Johnson, J.C. and An, K.N. 2000, 'Differences in repositioning error among patients with low back pain compared with control subjects' *Spine* 25: 2488–93.

Palmer, B.J. 1966, *Our Masterpiece*, Vol. XXXIX, Palmer College of Chiropractic, Davenport.

Palmer, D.D. 1910, *The Science, Art and Philosophy of Chiropractic*, Portland Publishing House, Portland.

Peters, R.E. and Chance, M.A. 1996, 'Chiropractic in Australia: the first forty years (1905–1945)' *Chiropractic History* 16(1): 28–38.

Piovesan, E.J., Kowacs, P.A., Tatsui, C.E., Lange, M.C., Ribas, L.C. and Werneck, L.C. 2001, 'Referred pain after painful stimulation of the greater occipital nerve in humans: evidence of convergence of cervical afferences on trigeminal nuclei' *Cephalgia* 21(2): 107–9.

Roberts, L., Little, P., Chapman, J., Cantrell, T., Pickering, R. and Langridge, J. 2002, 'The Back Home trial' *Spine* 27: 1821–8.

Rome, P.L. 1996, 'Usage of chiropractic terminology in the literature: 296 ways to say "subluxation": complex issues of the vertebral subluxation' *Journal of Chiropractic Technique* 2(8): 49–60.

Rosner, A.L. 2002, 'FCER responds to PBS broadcast' *Advances* Summer: 4, 30.

Sato, A. 1992, 'The reflex effects of spinal somatic nerve stimulation on visceral function' *Journal of Manipulative and Physiological Therapeutics* 15: 57–61.

Seaman, D.R. and Winterstein, J.F. 1998, 'Dysafferentation: a novel term to describe the neuropathophysiological effects of joint complex dysfunction. A look at likely mechanisms of symptom generation' *Journal of Manipulative and Physiological Therapeutics* 21: 267–80.

Sigrell, H. 2002, 'Expectations of chiropractic treatment: what are the expectations of new patients consulting a chiropractor, and do chiropractors and patients have similar expectations?' *Journal of Manipulative and Physiological Therapeutics* 25: 300–5.

Sjolander, P., Johansson, H. and Djupsjobacka, M. 2002, 'Spinal and supraspinal effects of activity in ligament afferents' *Journal of Electromyography and Kinesiology* 12(3): 167–76.

Smart, L.J. and Smith, D. 2001, 'Postural dynamics: clinical and empirical implications' *Journal of Manipulative and Physiological Therapeutics* 24: 340–9.

Smith, O.G., Langworthy, S.M. and Paxson, M.C. 1906, *Modernized Chiropractic*, Lawrence Press, Cedar Rapids.

Smith, M. and Stano, M. 1997, 'Costs and recurrences of chiropractic and medical episodes of low back care' *Journal of Manipulative and Physiological Therapeutics* 20: 5–12.

Solomonow, M., Zhou, B.H., Harris, M., Lu, Y. and Baratta, R.V. 1998, 'The ligamento-muscular stabilizing system of the spine' *Spine* 23: 2552–62.

Sportelli, L. 2000, *A Natural Method of Healthcare: An Introduction to Chiropractic*, 10th edn, Practice Makers, Palmerton, PA.

Stano, M. 1993, 'A comparison of health care costs for chiropractic and medical patients' *Journal of Manipulative and Physiological Therapeutics* 16: 291–9. Comment 16: 615.

Stano, M. 1994, 'Further analysis of health care costs for chiropractic and medical patients' *Journal of Manipulative and Physiological Therapeutics* 17: 442–6.

Stano, M. and Smith, M. 1996, 'Chiropractic and medical costs of low back care' *Medical Care* 34(3): 191–204.

Stephenson, R.W. 1948, *Chiropractic Textbook*, Palmer School of Chiropractic, Davenport.

Symons, B.P., Leonard, T. and Herzog, W. 2002, 'Internal forces sustained by the vertebral artery during spinal manipulative therapy' *Journal of Manipulative and Physiological Therapeutics* 25: 504–10.

Taimela, S., Kankaanpää, M. and Luoto, S. 1999, 'The effect of lumbar fatigue on the ability to sense a change in lumbar position' *Spine* 24: 1322–7.

Terrett, A.G.J.T. 1987, 'The search for the subluxation: an investigation of medical literature to 1985' *Chiropractic History* 7(1): 29–33.

Terrett, A.G.J.T. 1995, 'The cerebral dysfunction theory', in M.I. Gatterman *Foundations of Chiropractic: Subluxation*, Mosby, St Louis.

Terrett, A.G.J.T. 2002, 'Did the SMT practitioner cause the arterial injury?' *Chiropractic Journal of Australia* 32: 99–110.

Vear, H.J. 1981, *An Introduction to Chiropractic Science*, Monograph, Western States College of Chiropractic, Portland.

Waddell, G. 1998, *The Back Pain Revolution*, Churchill Livingstone, Edinburgh.

Wardwell, W.I. 1992, *Chiropractic—History and Evolution of a New Profession*, Mosby, St Louis.

Wilk et al. v. AMA et al. US District Court Northern District of Illinois Eastern Division, No. 76 C 3777, Getzendanner J. Judgment dated 27 August 1987.

World Federation of Chiropractic 1999, *Proceedings*, World Education of Chiropractic Conference, Auckland 1999, World Federation of Chiropractic, Toronto, Ontario.

Chapter 8 Counselling

Akeret, R.U. 1997, *The Man Who Loved a Polar Bear*, Penguin, Harmondsworth.

Andrew, S.D. 2000, 'A challenge to the accuracy and efficacy of the concept of "addiction" when applied to problem gambling behaviour' *The Australian Journal of Counselling Psychology* 2(1): 22–9.

Astin, J.A. 1998, 'Why patients use alternative medicine: results of a national survey' *Journal of the American Medical Association* 279: 1548–53.

Bach, E. and Wheeler, F.J. 1979, *The Bach Flower Remedies*, Keats, Connecticut.

Barnhart, R.K. 1995, *The Barnhart Concise Dictionary of Etymology*, HarperCollins, New York.

Barrett-Leonard, G. 1993, 'The phases and focus of empathy' *British Journal of Medical Psychology* 66: 3–14.

Beck, A.T. and Weishaar, M.E. 1989, 'Cognitive therapy', in R.J. Corsini and D. Wedding (eds) *Current Psychotherapies*, 4th edn, F.E. Peacock, Itasca, Illinois.

Bohart, A.C. and Tallman, K. 1999, *How Clients Make Therapy Work: The Process of Active Self-Healing*, American Psychological Association, Washington.

Brown, J.A.C. 1979, *Freud and The Post-Freudians*, Penguin, Harmondsworth.

Brown, N.O. 1970, *Life Against Death*, Sphere, London.

Cain, D.J. 2002, 'Defining characteristics, history, and evolution of humanistic psychotherapies', in D.J. Cain and J. Seeman (eds) *Humanistic Psychotherapies: Handbook of Research and Practice*, American Psychological Association, Washington.

Caplin, E. 2001, *Mind Games: American Culture and the Birth of Psychotherapy*, University of California Press, Berkeley.

Corsini, R.J. 1981, *Handbook of Innovative Psychotherapies*, John Wiley & Sons, New York.

Corsini, R.J. 1989, 'Introduction', in R.J. Corsini and D. Wedding (eds) *Current Psychotherapies*, 4th edn, F.E. Peacock, Itasca, Illinois.

Corsini, R.J. and Wedding, D. (eds) 1989, *Current Psychotherapies*, 4th edn, F.E. Peacock, Itasca, Illinois.

de Botton, A. 2000, *The Consolations of Philosophy*, Hamish Hamilton, London.

Egan, G. 1998, *The Skilled Helper: A Problem-Management Approach to Helping*, Brooks/Cole, Pacific Grove.

Ellis, A. 1995, *How to Stubbornly Refuse to Make Yourself Miserable About Anything, Yes Anything!*, Sun/Pan MacMillan, Sydney.

Feltham, C. 1999, 'Controversies in psychotherapy and counselling', in C. Feltham (ed.), *Controversies in Psychotherapy and Counselling*, Sage, London.

Frank, J.D. 1977, *Persuasion and Healing: A Comparative Study of Psychotherapy*, Schocken Books, New York.

Frankl, V.E. 1970, *The Will to Meaning: Foundations and Applications of Logotherapy*, New American Library, New York.

Freud, A. 1986, 'Human sexuality: Introduction', in S. Freud *The Essentials of Psychoanalysis*, Penguin, Harmondsworth.

Freud, S. 1916–1917, 'Introductory lectures in psycho-analysis', in *The Standard Edition of the Complete Psychological Works of Sigmund Freud*, 1963 Vols XV and XVI, Hogarth Press, London.

Freud, S. 1920, 'Beyond the pleasure principle', in S. Freud, 1986, *The Essentials of Psychoanalysis*, Penguin, Harmondsworth.

Freud, S. 1926, 'The question of lay analysis', in *The Standard Edition of the Complete Psychological Works of Sigmund Freud*, 1986, Vol. XX, Hogarth Press, London.

Freud, S. 1937, *The New Introductory Lectures on Psycho-analysis*, 2nd edn, Hogarth Press/Institute of Psychoanalysis, London.

Gay, P. 1998, *Freud: A Life For Our Time*, W.W. Norton, New York.

Geldard, D. and Geldard, K. 2001, *Basic Personal Counselling*, 4th edn, Prentice-Hall, Sydney.

Gotlib, I.H. and Colby, C.A. 1987, *Treatment of Depression: An Interpersonal Systems Approach*, Pergamon Press, New York.

Grof, S. 1985, *Beyond The Brain*, State University of New York, Albany.

Grof, S. 1988, *The Adventure of Self-Discovery*, State University of New York Press, Albany.

Hearnshaw, L.S. 1989, *The Shaping of Modern Psychology*, Routledge, London.

Heil, J. 1995, 'Philosophical relevance of psychology', in T. Honderich (ed.) *The Oxford Companion to Philosophy*, Oxford University Press, Oxford.

Hellinger, B. 1989, *Love's Hidden Symmetry*, Zeig, Tucker & Co., Phoenix.

Heyn, B. 1987, *Ayurvedic Medicine*, Thorsons Publishers, Wellingborough.

Hillman, J. 1991, *A Blue Fire*, Harper & Row, New York.

Hillman, J. 1992a, *Re-Visioning Psychology*, HarperCollins, New York.

Hillman, J. 1992b, 'Dialogue', in J. Hillman and M. Ventura *We've Had a Hundred Years of Psychotherapy and the World's Getting Worse*, HarperCollins, New York.

Howe, D. 1993, *On Being a Client*, Sage, London.

Hubble, M.A., Duncan, B.L. and Miller, S.D. (eds) 2000, *The Heart and Soul of Change*, American Psychological Association, Washington.

Ivey, A.E. 1988, *Intentional Interviewing and Counseling*, 2nd edn, Brooks/Cole, Pacific Grove.

Juhan, D. 1987, *Job's Body*, Station Hill Press, New York.

Jung, C.G. 1916, *The Collected Works of C.G. Jung*, Vol. 7: *Two Essays on Analytical Psychology*, 2nd edn, 1966, Bollingen Foundation, New York.

Jung, C.G. 1921, 'Psychological types', in *The Collected Works of C.G. Jung*, Vol. 6, 1971, Bollingen Foundation, New York.

Jung, C.G. 1934/1954, 'The archetypes and the collective unconscious', in *The Collected Works of C.G. Jung*, 2nd edn, Vol. 9, part I, 1968, Bollingen Foundation, New York.

Jung, C.G. 1949, Foreword, in R. Wilhelm (trans.), 1989, *I Ching or Book of Changes*, Arkana/Penguin, Harmondsworth.

Jung, C.G. 1960, *The Collected Works of C.G. Jung*, Vol. 3: *The Psychogenesis of Mental Disease*, Bollingen Foundation, New York.

Jung, C.G. 1966, *The Collected Works of C.G. Jung*, Vol. 16: *The Practice of Psychotherapy*, 2nd edn, Bollingen Foundation, New York.

Jung, C.G. 1983, *Memories, Dreams, Reflections*, HarperCollins, London.

Kent, J.T. 2000, *Repertory of the Homœopathic Materia Medica*, reprint edn, B. Jain Publishers, New Delhi.

Kirschenbaum, H. and Henderson, V.L. 1989, 'A more human world', in C.R. Rogers *The Carl Rogers Reader*, Houghton Mifflin, New York.

Kopp, S.B. 1976, *If You Meet Buddha On The Road, Kill Him!*, Bantam, New York.

Kovel, J. 1978, *A Complete Guide to Therapy: From Psychoanalysis to Behaviour Modification*, Penguin, Harmondsworth.

Kurtz, R. 1990, *Body-Centred Psychotherapy*, Life Rhythm, California.

Lambert, M.J., Shapiro, D.A. and Bergin, A.E. 1986, 'The effectiveness of psychotherapy', in S.L. Garfield and A.E. Bergin *Handbook of Psychotherapy and Behavior Change*, 3rd edn, John Wiley and Sons, New York.

Latner, J. 1976, *The Gestalt Therapy Book*, Bantam, New York.

Lee, R.R. and Martin, J.C. 1991, *Psychotherapy After Kohut: A Textbook of Self Psychology*, The Analytic Press, Hillsdale, New Jersey.

Litwack, L., Litwack, J.M. and Ballou, M.B. 1980, *Health Counseling*, Appleton-Century-Crofts, New York.

Luborsky, L., Singer, B. and Luborsky, L. 1975, 'Comparative studies of psychotherapies: is it true that "everyone has won and all must have prizes"' *Archives of General Psychiatry* 32: 995–1008.

McLeod, J. 1998, *An Introduction to Counselling*, 2nd edn, Open University Press, Buckingham.

Maguire, M. 1995, *Men, Women, Passion and Power*, Routledge, London.

Marcuse, H. 1974, *Eros and Civilization*, Beacon Press, Boston.

Marinoff, L. 2000, *Plato, Not Prozac!*, Quill, New York.

Maslow, A.H. 1968, *Toward a Psychology of Being*, Van Nostrand Reinhold, New York.

Maslow, A.H. 1978, *The Farther Reaches of Human Nature*, Penguin, Harmondsworth.

Maslow, A.H. 1987, *Motivation and Personality*, 3rd edn, Harper & Row, New York.

Masson, J.M. 1988, *Against Therapy*, Atheneum, New York.

May, R. 1989, *The Art of Counselling*, Souvenir Press, London.

Milkman, H.B. and Sunderwirth, S.G. 1993, *Pathways to Pleasure: The Consciousness and Chemistry of Optimal Living*, Lexington Books, New York.

Miller, S.D., Duncan, B.L. and Hubble, M.A. 1997, *Escape From Babel: Towards a Unifying Language for Psychotherapy Practice*, W.W. Norton, New York.

Moore, T. 1994, *Care of The Soul*, HarperCollins, New York.

Moore, T. 2002, *The Soul's Religion*, HarperCollins, New York.

Moustakis, C.E. 1967, *Creativity and Conformity*, Van Nostrand Reinhold, New York.

Murphy, M. 1992, *The Future of The Body*, Jeremy P. Tarcher, Inc., Los Angeles.

Nathan, P.E. and Gorman, J.M. (eds) 1998, *A Guide to Treatments That Work*, Oxford University Press, New York.

Neville, B. 1989, *Educating Psyche*, Collins Dove, Blackburn, Victoria.

Nolen-Hoeksema, S. 2004, *Abnormal Psychology*, 3rd edn, McGraw-Hill, New York.

Norcross, J.C. (ed.) 1986, *Handbook of Eclectic Psychotherapy*, Brunner/Mazel, New York.

Nye, R.D. 1992, *The Legacy of B.F. Skinner*, Brooks/Cole, California.

Ouspensky, P.D. 1978, *The Psychology of Man's Possible Evolution*, Routledge & Kegan Paul, London.

Peck, M.S. 1996, *The Road Less Travelled*, Arrow, London.

Raskin, N.J. and Rogers, C.R. 1989, 'Person-centred therapy', in R.J. Corsini and D. Wedding (eds) *Current Psychotherapies*, 4th edn, F.E. Peacock, Itasca, Illinois.

Rogers, C.R. 1942, 'The use of electronically recorded interviews in improving psychotherapeutic techniques', in H. Kirschenbaum and V.L. Henderson (eds) 1989, *The Carl Rogers Reader*, Houghton Mifflin, Boston.

Rogers, C.R. 1957, 'The necessary and sufficient conditions of therapeutic personality change', in H. Kirschenbaum and V.L. Henderson (eds) 1989, *The Carl Rogers Reader*, Houghton Mifflin, Boston.

Rogers, C.R. 1958, 'The characteristics of a helping relationship', in H. Kirschenbaum and V.L. Henderson (eds) 1989, *The Carl Rogers Reader*, Houghton Mifflin, Boston.

Rogers, C.R. 1960, 'Dialogue between Martin Buber and Carl Rogers', in H. Kirschenbaum and V.L. Henderson (eds) 1989, *Carl Rogers: Dialogues*, Constable, London.

Rogers, C.R. 1962, 'The interpersonal relationship: the core of guidance', in C.R. Rogers and B. Stevens 1967, *Person to Person: The Problem of Being Human*, Real People Press, Utah.

Rogers, C.R. 1973, 'Some new challenges' *American Psychologist* 28(5): 379–87.

Rogers, C.R. 1980, *A Way of Being*, Houghton Mifflin, Boston.

Rogers, C.R. 1982, *On Becoming a Person: A Therapist's View of Psychotherapy*, Constable, London.

Rogers, C.R. 1986, 'Client-centred therapy', in I.L. Kutash and A. Wolf (eds) *Psychotherapist's Casebook*, Jossey-Bass, San Francisco.

Rogers, C.R. 1989, 'Person-centred therapy', in D. Wedding and R.J. Corsini (eds) *Current Psychotherapies*, F.E. Peacock, Itasca, Illinois.

Rogers, C.R. and Sanford 1989, 'Client-centred psychotherapy', in H.I. Kaplan and B.J. Sadock (eds) *Comprehensive Textbook of Psychiatry*, 5th edn, William & Wilkins, Baltimore.

Rowan, J. 1992, 'The myth of therapist expertise—rebuttal', in W. Dryden and C. Feltham *Psychotherapy and its Discontents*, Open University Press, Buckingham.

Skinner, B.F. 1976, *Beyond Freedom and Dignity*, Penguin, Harmondsworth.

Smith, M.J. 1988, *When I Say No, I Feel Guilty*, Bantam, Toronto.

Snyder, C.R., Michael, S.T. and Cheavens, J.S. 2000, 'Hope as a psychotherapeutic foundation of common factors, placebos, and expectancies', in M.A. Hubble, B.L. Duncan and S.D. Miller, *The Heart and Soul of Change*, American Psychological Association, Washington.

Spinelli, E. 1997, *Tales of Un-Knowing*, New York University Press, New York.

Spinelli, E. 1999, 'If there are so many different psychotherapies how come we keep making the same mistakes?' *Psychotherapy in Australia* (6)1: 16–22.

Szasz, T.S. 1974, *The Ethics of Psychoanalysis*, Routledge & Kegan Paul, London.

Szasz, T.S. 1977, *The Myth of Mental Illness*, Paladin, Frogmore, St Albans.

Therapeutic Guidelines Limited 2000, *Therapeutic guidelines: Psychotropic*, 4th edn, Therapeutic Guidelines Limited, Melbourne.

Travis, J.W. and Ryan, R.S. 1988, *Wellness Workbook*, 2nd edn, Ten Speed Press, California.

Wedding, D. and Corsini, R.J. (eds) 1989, *Case Studies in Psychotherapy*, 4th edn, F.E. Peacock, Itasca, Illinois.

West, W. 2000, *Psychotherapy and Spirituality*, Sage, London.

Wilber, K. 1993, 'Psychologia perennis: the spectrum of consciousness', in R. Walsh and F. Vaughan (eds) *Paths Beyond Ego*, Tarcher/Putnam, New York.

Wilber, K. 1997, *The Eye of Spirit*, Shambhala, Boston.

Wilber, K. 2000, *Integral Psychology: Consciousness, Spirit, Psychology, Therapy*, Shambhala, Boston.

Worell, J. and Remer, P. 2003, *Feminist Perspectives in Therapy*, 2nd edn, John Wiley and Sons, Hoboken, New Jersey.

Worwood, V.A. 1996, *The Fragrant Mind*, Doubleday, London.

Yalom, I.D. 1974, *Every Day Gets a Little Closer*, Basic Books, New York.

Chapter 9 Flower essences: Bach Flowers/Australian Bush Flower Essences

Bach Flowers

Bach, E. 1931, *Heal Thyself*, C.W. Daniel, Saffron Waldon, Essex.

Bach, E. 1933, *The Twelve Healers*, C.W. Daniel, Saffron Waldon, Essex.

Barnard, J. 1997, *Collected Writings of Edward Bach*, Ashgrove Press, London.

Howard, J. 1990, *The Bach Flower Remedies Step by Step: A Complete Guide to Prescribing*, C.W. Daniel, Saffron Waldon, Essex.

Howard, J. and Ramsell, J. 1990, *The Original Writings of Edward Bach*, C.W. Daniel, Saffron Waldon, Essex.

Hyne Jones, T.W. 1976, *Dictionary of the Bach Flower Remedies—Positive and Negative Aspects*, C.W. Daniel, Saffron Waldon, Essex.

Vlamis, G. 1990, *Flower Remedies to the Rescue: The Healing Vision of Dr Edward Bach*, Thorsons, London.

Weeks, N. 1973, *The Medical Discoveries of Edward Bach, Physician*, Keats Publishing, Connecticut.

Weeks, N. and Bullen, V. 1990, *The Bach Flower Remedies: Illustrations and Preparations*, C.W. Daniel, Saffron Waldon, Essex.

Wheeler, F.J. 1952, *The Bach Remedies Repertory*, C.W. Daniel, Saffron Waldon, Essex.

Australian Bush Flowers

Arroyo, S. 1975, *Astrology, Psychology and the Four Elements*, CRCS Publications, Sebastopol, California.

Baker, M., Corringham, R. and Dark, J. 1986, *Native Plants of the Sydney Region*, Three Sisters Productions, Sydney.

Brennan, K. 1986, *Wildflowers of Kakadu*, G. Brennan, Jabiru.

Brock, J. 1988, *Top End Native Plants*, John Brock, Darwin.

Caddy, E. 1971, *God Spoke to Me*, Findhorn Press, Findhorn.

Caddy, E. 1976, *Footprints on the Path*, Findhorn Press, Findhorn.

Cunningham, D. 1992, *Flower Remedies Handbook*, Sterling Publishing Company Inc., New York.

Dyer, W.W. 1993, *Everyday Wisdom*, Hay House, Inc., Carson.

Eggenberger, R. and M.H. 1988, *The Handbook on Plumeria Culture*, The Plumeria People, Houston, Texas.

Gardener, C.A. 1959, *Wildflowers of Western Australia*, St George Books, Perth.

Gerber, R. 1988, *Vibrational Medicine for the 21st Century*, Bear & Co., Sante Fe.

Gibran, K. 1923, *The Prophet*, Random House Inc., New York.

Goodman, L. 1972, *Linda Goodman's Sun Signs*, Pan Books, London.

Goodman, L. 1987, *Star Signs: The Secret Codes of the Universe*, St Martins Press, New York.

Greenaway, K. 1978, *The Illuminated Language of Flowers*, MacDonald and James, London.

Gurudas 1983, *Flower Essences*, Brotherhood of Life, Albuquerque, New Mexico.

Guttman, A. and Johnson, K. 1993, *Mythic Astrology: Archetypal Powers in the Horoscope*, Llewellyn Publications, St Paul, Minnesota.

Hand Clow, B. 1994, *Chiron: Rainbow Bridge between the Inner and Outer Planets*, Llewellyn Publications, St Paul, Minnesota.

Harvey, C. and Cochrane, A. 1995, *The Encyclopaedia of Flower Remedies*, Thorsons, London.

Hawkins, G.S. 1965, *Stonehenge Decoded*, Dorset Press, New York.

Hay, L. 1976, *Heal Your Body*, Specialist Publications, Sydney.

Hay, L. 1984, *You Can Heal Your Life*, Hay House, Santa Monica.

Hayward, S. (ed.) 1985, *A Guide for the Advanced Soul*, In-Tune Books, Sydney.

Hayward, S. and Cohan, M. (eds) 1988, *A Bag of Jewels*, In-Tune Books, Sydney.

Johnson, R. 1991, *Owning Your Own Shadow*, Harper, San Francisco.

Krystal, P. 1989, *Cutting the Ties that Bind*, Element Book Ltd, Shaftesbury.

Kushi, M. 1978, *Oriental Diagnosis*, Sunwheel Publications, London.

Lofthus, M. 1983, *A Spiritual Approach to Astrology*, CRCS Publications, Sebastopol, California.

McIntre, A. 1996, *The Complete Floral Healer*, Gaia Books Limited, London.

Maltz, M. 1960, *Psycho-Cybernetics*, Prentice-Hall, New Jersey.

Mann, A.T. 1989, *Astrology and the Art of Healing*, Unwin Hyman Ltd, London.

Nixon, P. 1987, *The Waratah*, Kangaroo Press, Sydney.

Noontil, A. 1994, *The Body is the Barometer of the Soul*, Noontil, Nunawading.

Odent, M. 1984, *Birth Reborn*, Pantheon Books, New York.

Pert, C. 1997, *Molecules of Emotions*, Simon & Schuster, London.

Ray, S. 1985, *Ideal Birth*, Celestial Arts, Berkeley.

Roberts, J. 1974, *The Nature of Personal Reality*, Prentice-Hall, New Jersey.

Ruhela, S.P. (ed.) 1996, *Immortal Quotations of Bhagavan Sri Sthya Sai Baba*, BR Publishing Corporation, Delhi.

Sagan, S. 1996, *Planetary Forces, Alchemy and Healing*, Clairvision School Foundation, Sydney.

Sams, J. and Carson, D. 1998, *Medicine Cards*, Bear & Co., Santa Fe.

Setzer, C. 1994, *The Quotable Soul*, The Stonesong Press Inc., USA.

Sharamon, S. and Baginski, B.J. 1989, *Cosmobiological Birth Control*, Lotus Light Publications, Wilmont.

Stevenson, I. 1980, *Twenty Cases of Reincarnation*, 2nd edn, University Press, Virginia.

Stevenson, I. 1987, *Children Who Remember Past Lives: A Question of Reincarnation*, University Press, Virginia.

Stevenson, I. 1997, *Where Reincarnation and Biology Intersect*, Praeger, Westport, Connecticut.

The Essence 1999, June, Newsletter of the Australian Bush Flower Essences.

Trenorden, J. 1991, *The Essences and Chironic Healing*, Chironic Enterprises Pty Ltd, Warrnambool, Victoria.

Tresidder, A. 2000, *Lazy Persons Guide to Emotional Healing*, New Leaf, Dublin.

Urban, A. 1990, *Wildflowers and Plants of Central Australia*, Southbank Editions, Melbourne.

Valles, C.G. 1987, *Unencumbered by Baggage*, X. Diaz del Rio, Gujarat, India.

Verny, T. 1981, *The Secret Life of the Unborn Child*, Sphere Books, London.

Weinburg, S.L. (ed.) 1986, *Ramtha*, Sovereigny Inc., Washington.

White, I. 1991, *Australian Bush Flower Essences*, Bantam Books, Sydney.

White, I. 1996, *Australian Bush Flower Remedies*, revised edn, Australian Bush Flower Essences (ABFE), Sydney.

White, I. 1999, *Australian Bush Flower Healing*, Bantam Books, Sydney.

Zolar, 1972, *The History of Astrology*, W. Foulsham & Co. Ltd, London.

Chapter 10 Herbal medicine

Barnes, J., Mills, S.Y., Abbot, N.C., Willoughby, M. and Ernst, E. 1998, 'Different standards for reporting ADRs to herbal remedies and conventional OTC medicines: face-to-face interview with 515 users of herbal remedies' *British Journal of Clinical Pharmacology* 45: 496–500.

Barrett, B., Kiefer, D. and Rabago, D. 1999, 'Assessing the risks and benefits of herbal medicine: an overview of scientific evidence' *Alternative Therapies in Health & Medicine* 5: 40–9.

Bryant, B., Knights, K. and Salerno, E. 2003, *Pharmacology for Health Professionals*, Mosby, Sydney.

Carraro, J.-C., Raynaud, J.-P., Koch, G., Chisholm, G.D., Di Silverio, F. and Teillac, P. 1996, 'Comparison of phytotherapy (Permixon®) with finasteride in the treatment of benign prostate hyperplasia: a randomized international study of 1,098 patients' *The Prostate* 29: 231–40.

Delbridge, A. (ed.) 1990, *The Macquarie Encyclopedic Dictionary*, Macquarie Library, Sydney.

Drew, A.K. and Myers, S.P. 1997, 'Safety issues in herbal medicine: implications for the health professions' *Medical Journal of Australia* 166: 538–41.

Farnsworth, N.R., Akerele, O. and Bingel, A.S. 1985, 'Medicinal plants in therapy' *Bulletin of the World Health Organization* 63: 965–81.

Federspil, G. and Sicolo, N. 1994, 'The nature of life in the history of medical and philosophic thinking' *American Journal of Nephrology* 14: 337–43.

Griggs, B. 1997, *New Green Pharmacy—The Story of Western Herbal Medicine*, Vermillion, London.

Huffman, M.A., Ohigashi, H., Kawanaka, M., Page, J.E., Kirby, G.C., Gasquet, M., Murakami, A. and Koshimizu, K. 1998, 'African great ape self-medication: a new paradigm for treating parasite disease with natural medicines?', in H. Ageta, N. Aimi, Y. Ebizuka, T. Fujita and G. Honda (eds) *Towards Natural Medicine Research in the 21st Century*, Elsevier Science, Amsterdam.

Johne, A., Schmider, J., Brockmoller, J., Stadelmann, A.M., Stormer, E., Bauer, S., Scholler, G., Langheinrich, M. and Roots, I. 2002, 'Decreased plasma levels of amitriptyline and its metabolites on comedication with an extract from St. John's wort *(Hypericum perforatum)*' *Journal of Clinical Psychopharmacology* 22: 46–54.

Johns, T. 1990, '*With Bitter Herbs They Shall Eat It—Chemical Ecology and the Origins of Human Diet and Medicine*', University of Arizona Press, Tuscon, Arizona.

Mann, J. 1992, *Murder, Magic and Medicine*, Oxford University Press, Oxford.

Mills, S.Y. 1991, *Out of the Earth: The Essential Book of Herbal Medicine*, Viking, Harmondsworth.

Mills, S. and Bone, K. 2000, *Principles and Practice of Phytotherapy*, Churchill Livingstone, Edinburgh.

Priest, A.W. and Priest, L.R. 1982, *Herbal Medication: A Clinical and Dispensary Handbook*, L.N. Fowler & Co. Ltd, London.

Seaman, D.R. 1999, 'Antiquated concepts related to chiropractic technique. Part II: A case against the chiropractic variety of vitalism and innate intelligence' *Chiropractic Technique* 11: 101–7.

Solecki, R.S. 1975, 'Shanidar IV, a neanderthal flower burial in northern Iraq', *Science* 190: 880–1.

Woelk, H. 2000, 'Comparison of St John's wort and imipramine for treating depression: randomised controlled trial' *British Medical Journal* 321: 536–9.

Wohlmuth, H. 2002, 'Herbal medicines—an ethnobotanical survey', in *Proceedings of Complementary Medicine Symposium, Brisbane, 26 March 2002*, Australian Centre for Complementary Medicine, Lismore/Brisbane.

Wohlmuth, H., Oliver, C. and Nathan, P.J. 2002, 'A review of the status of western herbal medicine in Australia' *Journal of Herbal Pharmacotherapy* 2: 33–46.

Chapter 11 Homœopathy

Allen, H.C. 1910, *The Materia Medica of the Nosodes*, Boericke and Tafel, Philadelphia.

Allen, J.H. 1910, *Chronic Miasms*, Vol. I, *Psora and Pseudo-psora*, J.H. Allen, Chicago.

Baker, D. 2002, 'Avogadro's number: a homœopathic metaphor' *Journal of the Australian Traditional-Medicine Society* 8(3): 113–15.

Boger, C.M. (trans.) 1983, *Boenninghausen's Characteristics and Repertory*, B. Jain, New Delhi.

Coulter, H.L. 1994, *Divided Legacy: A history of the Schism in Medical Thought*, 2 vols, Centre for Empirical Medicine Washington.

Culpeper, N. 1995, *Culpeper's Complete Herbal*, Wordsworth Reference, Hertfordshire.

Eskinazi, D. 1999, 'Homœopathy revisited. Is homœopathy compatible with biomedical observations?' *Archives in Internal Medicine* 159: 1981–7.

Haehl, R. 1985, *Samuel Hahnemann, His Life and Work*, 2 vols, B. Jain, New Delhi.

Hahnemann, S. 1880, *Materia Medica*, Hahnemann Publishing House, London.

Hahnemann, S. 1896, *The Chronic Diseases—Their Peculiar Nature and Homœopathic cure*, Vol. 1, B. Jain, New Delhi.

Hahnemann, S. 1990, *Organon of the Medical Art*, edited and annotated by Wenda Brewster O'Reilly; based on a translation by Steven Decker, Birdcage Books, Redmond, Washington.

Hahnemann, S. 1996, *Organon of Medicine*, translated from the fifth edition, with an appendix by R.E. Dudgeon; with additions and alterations as per sixth edition translated by William Boericke; and introduction by James Krauss, B. Jain, New Delhi.

Hippocrates 1952, *Hippocratic Writings*, translated by Francis Adams; *On the Natural Faculties by Galen*, translated by Arthur John Brock, Encyclopaedia Britannica, Chicago.

Jacobs, J. 2002, 'Homœopathic research—a review of the evidence' *American Journal of Homœopathic Medicine* 95(1): 28–34.

Kaplan, B. 2001, *The Homœopathic Conversation. The Art of Taking the Case*, Natural Medicine Press, London.

Kent, J.T. 1975, *Lectures on Homœopathic Materia Medica*, 3rd impression, Sett Dey & Co., Calcutta.

Kent, J.T. 1995, *Lectures on Homœopathic Philosophy*, B. Jain, New Delhi.

Kleijnen, J., Knipschild, P. and ter Riet, G. 1991, 'Clinical trials of homœopathy' *British Medical Journal* 302: 316–23.

Linde, K., Clausius, N., Ramirez, G., Melchart, D., Eitel, F. and Hedges, L. 1997, 'Are the clinical effects of homœopathy placebo effects? A meta analysis of placebo controlled trials' *The Lancet* 350: 834–43.

Linde, K. and Melchart, D. 1988, 'Randomised controlled trials of individualised homœopathy: a state-of-the-art review' *The Journal of Alternative & Complementary Medicine* 4(4): 371–88.

Moskowitz, R. 2002, 'Innovation and fundamentalism in homœopathy' *American Journal of Homœopathy* 95(2).

Paracelsus, T. 1973, *The Prophecies of Paracelsus; Occult Symbols and Magic Figures with Esoteric Explanations*, by Theophrastus Paracelsus of Hohenheim, and *The life and Teachings of Paracelsus*, by Franz Hartmann. Introduction by Paul M. Allen, Blauvelt, New York.

Reilly, D., Taylor, M.A., Beattie, N.G., Campbell, J.H., McSharry, C., Aitchison, T.C., Carter, R. and Stevenson, R. 1994, 'Is evidence for homœopathy reproducible?' *The Lancet* 344: 1601–6.

Sankaran, R. 1992, *The Spirit of Homœopathy*, Homœopathic Medical Publishers, Bombay.

Schmidt, J.J. 1994, 'History and relevance of the 6th edition of the Organon of Medicine (1842)' *The British Homœopathic Journal* 83: 1, 46.

Scholten, J. 1993, *Homœopathy and Minerals*, Stichting Alonnissos, the Netherlands.

Scholten, J. 1997, *Homœopathy and the Elements*, Stichting Alonnissos, the Netherlands.

Schwartz, G. and Russek, L. 1998, 'The plausibility of homœopathy: the systemic memory mechanism' *Integrative Medicine* 1(2): 53–9.

Steiner, R. 1985, *The Origins of Natural Science*, Anthroposophic Press, New York.

Vannier, L. 1955, *Homœopathy: Human Medicine*, Homœopathic Publishing Co., Bombay.

Vermeulen, F. 2002, *Prisma The Arcana of Materia Medica Illuminated*, Emryss, the Netherlands.

Vithoulkas, G. 1989, *The Science of Homœopathy*, Grove Press, New York.

Whitmont, E. 1980, *Psyche and Substance*: Essays on Homœopathy in the light of Jungian Psychology, North Atlantic Books, US.

Winston, J. 1999, *The Faces of Homœopathy*, Great Auk Publishing, New Zealand.

Winston, J. 2001, *The Heritage of Homœopathic Literature*, Great Auk Publishing, New Zealand.

Chapter 12 Massage therapy

Beard, G. 1952, 'A history of massage technic' *The Physical Therapy Review* 32(12): 613–24.

Beck, M. 1988, *The Theory and Practice of Therapeutic Massage*, Milady Publishing Co., New York.

Cafarelli, E. and Flint, F. 1993, 'The role of massage in preparation for and recovery from exercise—an overview' *Physiotherapy in Sport* 16(1): 17–20.

Callaway, K.E. 2002, 'History of Massage', in C.C. Tuchtan, V.M. Tuchtan, D.P. Stelfox, C.P. Valkenburg and D.K. Moran (eds) *Principles and Philosophies of Massage*, Australian College of Natural Medicine, Melbourne.

Calvert, R.N. 2002, *The History of Massage: An Illustrated Survey from Around the World*, Healing Arts Press, Rochester.

Cassar, M. 1999, *Handbook of Massage Therapy: A Complete Guide for the Student and Professional Massage Therapist*, Butterworth Heinemann, Oxford.

Clews, W. 1988, *The Role of Massage in Sports Medicine—2nd Elite Coaches Seminar*, Australian Institute of Sport, Canberra.

Davis, G.C., Cortez, C. and Rubin, B.R. 1990, 'Pain management in the older adult with rheumatoid arthritis or osteoarthritis' *Arthritis Care and Research* 3(3): 127–31.

De Domenico, G. and Wood, E.C. 1997, *Beard's Massage*, 4th edn, W.B. Saunders Co., Philadelphia.

Diego, M.A., Field, T., Hernandez-Reif, M., Shaw, K., Friedman, L. and Ironson, G. 2001, 'HIV adolescents show improved immune function following massage therapy' *International Journal of Neuroscience* 106: 35–45.

Elton, D. 1995, 'Injury and pain', in M. Zuluaga, C. Briggs, J. Carlisle, V. McDonald, J. McMeeken, W. Nickson, P. Oddy and D. Wilson. (eds) *Sports Physiotherapy—Applied Science and Practice*, Churchill Livingstone, Australia.

Ernst, E., Matrai, A., Magyarosy, I., Liebermeister, R., Eck, M. and Breu, M. 1987, 'Massages cause changes in blood fluidity' *Physiotherapy* 73(1): 43–5.

Ferrell-Torry, A.T. and Glick, O.J. 1993, 'The use of therapeutic massage as a nursing intervention to modify anxiety and the perception of cancer pain' *Cancer Nursing* 16(2): 93–101.

Field, T., Delage, J. and Hernandez-Reif, M. 2003, 'Movement and massage therapy reduce fibromyalgia pain' *Journal of Bodywork and Movement Therapies* January: 49–52.

Field, T., Grizzle, N., Scafidi, F. and Schanberg, S. 1996, 'Massage and relaxation therapies' effects on depressed adolescent mothers' *Adolescence* 31(124): 903–11.

Field, T., Hernandez-Reif, M., Seligman, S., Krasnegor, J. and Sunshine, W. 1997, 'Juvenile rheumatoid arthritis: benefits from massage therapy' *Journal of Pediatric Psychology* 22(5): 607–17.

Field, T., Morrow, C., Valdeon, C., Larson, S., Kuhn, C. and Schanberg, S. 1993, 'Massage reduces anxiety in children and adolescent psychiatric patients' *International Journal of Alternative and Complementary Medicine* July: 22–7.

Fraser, J. and Kerr, J. 1993, 'Psychophysiological effects of back massage on elderly institutionalized patients' *Journal of Advanced Nursing* 18: 238–45.

Fritz, S. 2000, *Mosby's Fundamentals of Therapeutic Massage*, 2nd edn, Mosby, Missouri.

Harmer, P.A. 1991, 'The effect of pre-performance massage on stride frequency in sprinters' *Athletic Training* 26(1): 55–9.

Hernandez-Reif, M., Field, T., Krasnegor, J., Theakston, H., Hossain, Z. and Burman, I. 2000, 'High blood pressure and associated symptoms were reduced by massage therapy' *Journal of Bodywork and Movement Therapies* 4(1): 31–8.

Kamenetz, H.L. 1980, 'History of massage', in J.B. Rogoff (ed.) *Manipulation, Traction and Massage*, 2nd edn, Williams & Wilkins, Baltimore.

Kellogg, J.H. 1895, 'The art of massage', <www.meridianinstitute.com/eamt/files/kellogg/ch.1.html>, 20 February 2003.

Maanum, A. 1985, *The Complete Book of Swedish massage*, Winston Press, Minneapolis.

Matuszewski, W. 1985, 'Rehabilitative regeneration in sports' *Science Periodical on Research and Technology in Sport* January: 1–5.

Melzack, R. and Wall, P.D. 1965, 'Pain mechanisms: a new theory' *Science* 150: 971.

Mennell, J.B. *c.* 1917, *Massage: Its Principles and Practice*, J. & A. Churchill, London.

Nixon, M., Teschendorff, J., Finney, J. and Karnilowicz, W. 1997, 'Expanding the nursing repertoire—the effect of massage on post operative pain' *Australian Journal of Advanced Nursing* 14(3): 21–6.

Ortolani, A. 1978, 'Massage & injuries' *American Swimming Coaches Association World Clinic Year Book*, 17–21.

Pyves, G. 2001, 'No-hands massage: squaring the circle of practitioner damage' *Journal of Bodywork and Movement Therapies* July: 173–80.

Rich, G.J. 2002, *Massage Therapy: The Evidence for Practice*, Mosby, London.

Salvo, S.G. 1999, *Massage Therapy: Principles and Practice*, W.B. Saunders, Philadelphia.

Smith, L.L., Keating, M.N., Holbert, D., Spratt, D.J., McCammon, M.R., Smith, S.S. and Israel, R.G. 1994, 'The effects of athletic massage on delayed onset muscle soreness, creatine kinase, and neutrophil count: a preliminary report' *Journal of Orthopaedic and Sports Physical Therapy* 19(2): 93–9.

Stelfox, D.P. 2002, 'Philosophy, principles and definitions', in C.C. Tuchtan, V.M. Tuchtan, D.P. Stelfox, C.P. Valkenburg and D.K Moran (eds) *Principles and Philosophies of Massage*, Australian College of Natural Medicine, Melbourne.

Tappan, F.M. and Benjamin, P.J. 1998, *Tappan's Handbook of Healing Massage Techniques: Classic, Holistic, and Emerging Methods*, 3rd edn, Appleton & Lange, Connecticut.

Trevelyan, J. 1993, 'Massage' *Nursing Times* 89(19): 45–7.

Tuchtan, C.C. and Tuchtan, V.M. 2002, 'Endangerment sites and indications for the use of therapuetic massage', in C.C. Tuchtan, V.M. Tuchtan, D.P. Stelfox, C.P. Valkenburg and D.K. Moran (eds) *Principles and Philosophies of Massage*, Australian College of Natural Medicine, Melbourne.

Veith, I. 1949 (translator), *Huang Ti: Nei Ching Su Wen (The Yellow Emperor's Classic Internal Medicine)* Lippincott Williams & Wilkins, Baltimore.

Weinberg, R., Jackson, A. and Kolodny, K. 1988, 'The relationship of massage and exercise to mood enhancement' *The Sport Psychologist* 2: 202–11.

Weinrich, S.P. and Weinrich, M.C. 1990, 'The effect of massage on pain in cancer patients' *Applied Nursing Research* 3(4): 140–5.

Yamazaki, Z., Idezuki, Y., Nemoto, T. and Togawa, T. 1988, 'Clinical experiences using pneumatic massage therapy for edematous limbs over the last 10 years' *Angiology—The Journal of Vascular Diseases* February: 154–63.

Chapter 13 Nutrition

Atkins, R. 1992, *Atkin's New Diet Revolution*, M. Evans, New York.

Australian Adverse Drug Reactions 2002 (ADRAC) Bulletin. MIMS. <www.mims.com.au>, November 2002.

Ballantine, R. 1978, *Diet and Nutrition—A Holistic Approach*, The Himalayan Institute, Pennsylvania.

Bland, J. (ed.) 1999, *Clinical Nutrition: A Functional Approach*, Institute of Functional Medicine, Washington.

Brand-Miller, J. *et al.* 1998, *The G.I. Factor*, 3rd edn, Hodder, Sydney.

Bridgman, K. 2000, *We Are What We Eat*, Vols 4–6, Starflower Pty Ltd, Sydney.

Briggs, D. and Wahlquist, M. 1983, *Food Facts*, Penguin, Melbourne.

Brothwell, D. and Brothwell, P. 1998, *Food In Antiquity—A Survey of the Diet of Early Peoples*, Johns Hopkins University Press, Baltimore.

Buist, R. 1984, 'Drug–nutrient interactions—an overview' *International Clinical Nutrition Review* 4(3): 114–21.

D'Adamo, P. 1998, *Eat Right 4 Your Type*, Century, London.

Eaton, S. and Konner, M. 1985, 'Paleolithic nutrition: a consideration of its nature and current implications' *New England Journal of Medicine* 312: 283–9.

Eaton, S. *et al.* 1988, 'Stone agers in the fast lane: chronic degenerative diseases in evolutionary perspective' *American Journal of Medicine* 84: 739–49.

Horrobin, D. 2001, *The Madness of Adam and Eve—How Schizophrenia shaped Humanity*, Bantam Books, London.

Kushi, M. 1985, *The Macrobiotic Way*, Avery Pub., New Jersey.

Pitchford, P. 1993, *Healing with Whole Food—Oriental Traditions and Modern Nutrition*, Atlantic Books, California.

Pritikin, N. 1979, *The Pritikin Program of Diet and Exercise*, Bantam, New York.

Sears, B. and Lawren, W. 1995, *The Zone—A Dietary Road Map*, HarperCollins, New York.

Shephard, S. 2000, *Pickled, Potted and Canned—The Story of Food Preserving*, Headline, London.

Shils, M. *et al.* 1994, *Modern Nutrition in Health and Disease*, Vols 1 and 2, Lea and Febiger, Pennsylvania.

Spencer, C. (ed.) 1993, *The Faber Book of Food*, Faber & Faber, London.

Truswell, A.S. (ed.) 1990, *Recommended Nutrient Intakes Australian Papers*, Australian Professional Publications, Sydney.

Wahlqvist, M. 1981, *Food and Nutrition in Australia*, Nelson, Melbourne.

Wardlaw, G. and Insel, P. 1990, *Perspectives in Nutrition*, Times/Mirror/Mosby Publishing, St Louis.

Chapter 14 Osteopathy

AACOM 1997, Glossary of osteopathic terminology, in R.C. Ward (ed.) *Foundations for Osteopathic Medicine*, Williams & Wilkins, Baltimore.

ACC 1997, *New Zealand Acute Low Back Pain Guide*, Accident Rehabilitation and Compensation Insurance Corporation of New Zealand and the National Health Committee, Wellington, New Zealand.

Achterberg, J. 1996, 'What is medicine?' *Alternative Therapies* 2: 58–61.

AHCPR 1994, *Management Guidelines for Acute Low Back Pain*, Agency for Health Care Policy and Research, US Department of Health and Human Services, Rockville, MD.

Andersson, G.B., Lucente, T., Davis, A.M., Kappler, R.E., Lipton, J.A. and Leurgans, S. 1999, 'A comparison of osteopathic spinal manipulation with standard care for patients with low back pain [see comments]' *New England Journal of Medicine* 341: 1426–31.

Bogduk, N. 1997, *Clinical Anatomy of the Lumbar Spine and Sacrum*, Churchill Livingstone, New York.

Brodeur, R. 1995, 'The audible release associated with joint manipulation' *Journal of Manipulative and Physiological Therapeutics* 18: 155–64.

Burton, A.K. 1981, 'Back pain in osteopathic practice' *Rheumatology and Rehabilitation* 20: 239–46.

Cameron, M. 1998, 'A comparison of osteopathic history, education and practice in Australia and the United States of America' *Australasian Osteopathic Medicine Review* 2: 6–12.

Cameron, M. 2002, *Worldwide Source Book of Osteopathy*, Melanie Cameron, Melbourne.

DiGiovanna, E.L. and Schiowitz, S. 1997, *An Osteopathic Approach to Diagnosis and Treatment*, Lippincott Williams & Wilkins, Baltimore.

Engel, G.L. 1977, 'The need for a new medical model: a challenge for biomedicine' *Science* 137: 129–36.

Evans, D.W. 2002, 'Mechanisms and effects of spinal high-velocity, low-amplitude thrust manipulation: previous theories' *Journal of Manipulative and Physiological Therapeutics* 25: 251–62.

Frank, J.D. 1973, *Persuasion and Healing*, Johns Hopkins University Press, Baltimore.

Fryer, G. 2000, 'Muscle energy concepts: a need for change' *Journal of Osteopathic Medicine* 3: 54–9.

Gerteis, M., Edgman-Levitan, S. and Daley, J. (eds) 1993, *Understanding and Promoting Patient-Centred Care: Through Patient's Eyes*, Jossey-Bass, San Francisco.

Gevitz, N. 1991, *The D.O.'s: Osteopathic Medicine in America*, Johns Hopkins University Press, Baltimore.

Gibbons, P. and Tehan, P. 2000, *Manipulation of the Spine, Thorax and Pelvis: An Osteopathic Perspective*, Churchill Livingstone, Edinburgh.

Greenman, P.E. 1995, *Principles of Manual Medicine*, Lippincott Williams & Wilkins, Baltimore.

GSAC 1994, *Report on Back Pain*, Clinical Standards Advisory Group, HMSO, London.

Hagi, J. 1999, Thesis, 'The transition from student to osteopath', School of Health Sciences, Victoria University, Melbourne.

Hartman, S.E. and Norton, J.M. 2002, 'Interexaminer reliability and cranial osteopathy' *The Scientific Review of Alternative Medicine* 6: 23–34.

Hawkins, P. and O'Neill, A. 1990, *Osteopathy in Australia*, Phillip Institute of Technology Press, Melbourne.

Hoving, J.L., Koes, B.W., de Vet, H.C., van der Windt, D.A., Assendelft, W.J., van Mameren, H., Deville, W.L., Pool, J.J., Scholten, R.J. and Bouter, L.M. 2002, 'Manual therapy, physical therapy, or continued care by a general practitioner for patients with neck pain. A randomized, controlled trial' *Annals of International Medicine* 136: 713–22.

Kendall, N.A.S., Linton, S.J. and Main, C.J. 1997, *Guide to Assessing Psychosocial Yellow Flags in Acute Low Back Pain: Risk Factors for Long Term Disability and Work Loss*, Accident and Rehabilitation and Compensation Insurance Corporation of New Zealand and the National Health Committee, Wellington, New Zealand.

Koes, B.W., Assendelft, W.J., van Der Heijen, G.J.M.G. and Bouter, L.M. 1996, 'Spinal manipulation for low back pain. An updated systematic review of randomised clinical trials' *Spine* 21: 2860–71.

Koes, B.W., Assendelft, W.J., van Der Heijen, G.J.M.G., Bouter, L.M. and Knipschild, P.J. 1991, 'Spinal manipulation and mobilisation for back and neck pain: a blinded review' *British Medical Journal* 303: 1298–303.

Kuchera, M.L. and Kuchera, W. 1994, *Osteopathic Principles in Practice*, Greyden Press, Colombo, Ohio.

Linton, S.J. 1998, 'The socioeconomic impact of chronic back pain: is anyone benefiting?' *Pain* 75: 163–8.

MAA 2001, *Guidelines for the Management of Whiplash-Associated Disorders*, Motor Accidents Authority, NSW.

McIlwraith, B. 2003, 'A survey of 1200 patients in osteopathic practice in the United Kingdom' *Journal of Osteopathic Medicine* 6: 7–12.

Martin, P. 1997, *The Sickening Mind. Brain, Behaviour, Immunity and Disease*, Flamingo, London.

Moran, R.W. and Gibbons, P. 2001, 'Intraexaminer and interexaminer reliability for palpation of the cranial rhythmic impulse at the head and sacrum' *Journal of Manipulative and Physiological Therapeutics* 24: 183–90.

NHMRC 1998, *Acute Pain Management*, National Health and Medical Research Council, Canberra.

Palmer, R. 2000, 'FIMM update' *Australasian Musculoskeletal Medicine* 5: 48.

Peterson, B.A. 1997, 'Major events in osteopathic history', in R.C. Ward (ed.) *Foundations for Osteopathic Medicine*, Williams & Wilkins, Baltimore.

Pringle, M. and Tyreman, S. 1993, 'Study of 500 patients attending an osteopathic practice' *British Journal of General Practice* 43: 15–18.

RCGP 1996, *Clinical Guidelines for the Management of Acute Low Back Pain*, Royal College of General Practitioners, London.

Rosen, M. 1994, *The Clinical Standards Advisory Group Report on Back Pain*, HMSO, London.

Seffinger, M.A. 1997, 'Osteopathic philosophy', in R.C. Ward (ed.) *Foundations for Osteopathic Medicine*, Williams & Wilkins, Baltimore.

Stoddard, A. 1969, *Manual of Osteopathic Practice*, Hutchinson, London.

Surkitt, D., Gibbons, P. and McLaughlin, P. 2000, 'High velocity low amplitude manipulation of the atlanto-axial joint: effect on atlanto-axial and cervical spine rotation asymmetry in asymptomatic subjects' *Journal of Osteopathic Medicine* 3: 13–19.

Truhlar, R.E. *Doctor A.T. Still in the Living*, Robert E. Truhlar, D.O., Chagrin Falls, Ohio.

Waddell, G. 1998, *The Back Pain Revolution*, Churchill Livingstone, Edinburgh.

Ward, R.C. (ed.) 2003, *Foundations for Osteopathic Medicine*, 2nd edn, Lippincott Williams & Wilkins, Baltimore.

WHO 1992, *ICD-10. International Classification of Diseases and Related Health Problems*, World Health Organization, Geneva.

Willard, F.H., Mokler, J.M. and Morgane, P.J. 1997, 'Neuroendocrine-immune system and homœostasis', in R.C. Ward (ed.) *Foundations for Osteopathic Medicine*, Williams & Wilkins, Baltimore.

Wright, A. 2000, 'Hypoalgesia post-manipulative therapy: a review of a potential neuro-physiological mechanism' *Journal of Manipulative Therapy* 1: 11–16.

Chapter 15 Yoga and meditation

Aagaard, P., Simonsen, E.B., Andersen, J.L., Magnusson, S.P., Bojsen-Miller, F. and Dyhre Poulsen, P. 2000, 'Antagonist muscle co-activation during isokinetic knee extension' *Scandinavian Journal of Medical Science and Sports* Apr 10(2): 58–67.

Aftanas, L.I. and Golocheikine, S.A. 2001, 'Human anterior and frontal midline theta and lower alpha reflect emotionally positive state and internalized attention: high-resolution EEG investigation of meditation' *Neuroscience letters* 310(1): 57–60.

Alexander, C.N., Langer, E.J., Newman, R.I., Chandler, H.M. and Davies, J.L. 1989, 'Transcendental meditation, mindfulness, and longevity: an experimental study with the elderly' *Journal of Personality and Social Psychology* 57(6): 950–64.

Alter, M.J. 1996, *Science of Flexibility*, Human Kinetics, South Australia.

Arambula, P., Peper, E., Kawakami, M. and Gibney, K.H. 2001, 'The physiological correlates of Kundalini Yoga meditation: a study of a yoga master' *Applied Psychophysiology and Biofeedback* 26(2): 147–53.

Atwood, J.D. and Maltin, L. 1991, 'Putting eastern philosophies into western psychotherapies' *American Journal of Psychotherapy* XLV: 368–82.

Backon, J., Matamoros, N., Ramirez, M., Sanchez, R.M., Ferrer, J., Brown, A. and Ticho, U. 1990, 'A functional vagotomy induced by unilateral forced right nostril breathing decreases intraocular pressure in open and closed angle glaucoma' *The British Journal of Ophthalmology* 74(10): 607–9.

Badawi, K., Wallace, R.K., Orme-Johnson, D. and Rouzere, A.M. 1984, 'Electrophysiologic characteristics of respiratory suspension periods occurring during the practice of the Transcendental Meditation Program' *Psychosomatic Medicine* 46(3): 267–76.

Balasubramanian, B. and Pansare, M.S. 1991, 'Effect of yoga on aerobic and anaerobic power of muscles' *Indian Journal of Physiology and Pharmacology* 35(4): 281–2.

Barbeau, H., Marchand-Pauvert, V., Meunier, S., Nicolas, G. and Pierrot-Deseilligny, E. 2000, 'Posture-related changes in heteronymous recurrent inhibition from quadriceps to ankle muscles in humans' *Experimental Brain Research*, 130(3): 345–61.

Barnes, V.A., Treiber, F.A. and Davis, H. 2001, 'Impact of transcendental meditation on cardiovascular function at rest and during acute stress in adolescents with high normal blood pressure' *Journal of Psychosomatic Research* 51(4): 597–605.

Barnes, V.A., Treiber, F.A., Turner, J.R., Davis, H. and Strong, W.B. 1999, 'Acute effects of transcendental meditation on hemodynamic functioning in middle-aged adults' *Psychosomatic Medicine* 61(4): 525–31.

Bazak, I. 1990, 'Clinical use of the Valsalva manoeuvre' *Harefuah* 323–5.

Benca, R.M., Obermeyer, W.H., Larson, C.L., Yun, B., Dolski, I., Kleist, K.D., Weber, S.M. and Davidson, R.J. 1999, 'EEG alpha power and alpha power asymmetry in sleep and wakefulness' *Psychophysiology* 36(4): 430–6.

Benson, H., Malhotra, M.S., Goldman, R.F., Jacobs, G.D. and Hopkins, P.J. 1990, 'Three case reports of the metabolic and electroencephalographic changes during advanced Buddhist meditation techniques' *Behavioral Medicine* 16(2): 90–5.

Bernardi, L., Passino, C., Wilmerding, V., Dallam, G.M., Parker, D.L., Robergs, R.A. and Appenzeller, O. 2001a, 'Breathing patterns and cardiovascular autonomic modulation during hypoxia induced by simulated altitude' *Journal of Hypertension* 19(5): 947–58.

Bernardi, L., Sleight, P., Bandinelli, G., Cencetti, S., Fattorini, L., Wdowczyc-Szulc, J. and Lagi, A. 2001b, 'Effect of rosary prayer and yoga mantras on autonomic cardiovascular rhythms: comparative study' *British Medical Journal* 323(7327): 1446–9.

Bharucha, A.E., Camilleri, M., Ford, M.J., O'Connor, M.K., Hanson, R.B. and Thomforde, G.M. 1996, 'Hyperventilation alters colonic motor and sensory function: effects and mechanisms in humans' *Gastroenterology* 111(2): 368–77.

Brown, D., Forte, M. and Dysart, M. 1984, 'Visual sensitivity and mindfulness meditation' *Perceptual and Motor Skills* 58(3): 775–84.

Cantero, J.L., Atienza, M., Salas, R.M. and Gomez, C. 1999, 'Alpha power modulation during periods with rapid oculomotor activity in human REM sleep' *Neuroreport* 10(9): 1817–20.

Chohan, I.S., Nayar, H.S., Thomas, P. and Geetha, N.S. 1984, 'Influence of yoga on blood coagulation' *Thrombosis and Haemostasis* 51(2): 196–7.

Cholewicki, J., Panjabi, M.M. and Khachatryan, A. 1997, 'Stabilizing function of trunk flexor-extensor muscles around a neutral spine posture' *Spine* 22(19) 2207–12.

Corby, J.C., Roth, W.T., Zarcone, V.P. Jr and Kopell, B.S. 1978, 'Psychophysiological correlates of the practice of Tantric Yoga meditation' *Archives of General Psychiatry* 35(5): 571–7.

Craven, J.L. 1989, 'Meditation and psychotherapy' *Canadian Journal of Psychiatry* 34: 648–53.

Dash, M. and Telles, S. 2001, 'Improvement in hand grip strength in normal volunteers and rheumatoid arthritis patients following yoga training' *Indian Journal of Physiology and Pharmacology* 45(3): 355–60.

Dembner, A. 2003, 'Om . . . Om . . . oh my aching back'. Increases in the number of yoga-related injuries', reprinted from the *Boston Globe* in *The Sydney Morning Herald*, 14 January: 8.

Desikachar, T.K.V. 1998, *Health Healing and Beyond*, Krishnamacharya Yoga Mandiram.

Desikachar, T.K.V. 2000, *Yoga-yajnavalkya Samhita*, Krishnamacharya Yoga Mandiram.

Dillbeck, M.C. 1977, 'The effect of the Transcendental Meditation technique on anxiety level' *Journal of Clinical Psychology* 33(4): 1076–8.

Dillbeck, M.C. and Bronson, E.C. 1981, 'Short-term longitudinal effects of the transcendental meditation technique on EEG power and coherence' *International Journal of Neuroscience* 14(3–4): 147–51.

Dillbeck, M.C. and Orme-Johnson, D.W. 1987, 'Psychological differences between transcendental meditation and rest' *American Psychology* 42: 879–81.

Dillbeck, M.C. and Vesely, S.A. 1986, 'Participation in the transcendental meditation program and frontal EEG coherence during concept learning' *International Journal of Neuroscience* 29(1–2): 45–55.

Dua, J.K and Swinden, M.L. 1992, 'Effectiveness of negative-thoughts-reduction, meditation and placebo training treatment in reducing anger' *Scandinavian Journal of Psychology* 33(2): 135–46.

Elias, A.N. and Wilson, A.F. 1995, 'Serum hormonal concentrations following transcendental meditation: potential role of gamma aminobutyric acid' *Medical Hypotheses* 44: 287–91.

Eppley, K.R., Abrams, A.I. and Shear, J. 1989, 'Differential effects of relaxation techniques on trait anxiety: a meta-analysis' *Journal of Clinical Psychology* 45(6): 957–74.

Fairey, A.S., Courneya, K.S., Field, C.J. and Mackey, J.R. 2002, 'Physical exercise and immune system function in cancer survivors: a comprehensive review and future directions' *Cancer* 94(2): 539–51.

Farrow, J.T. and Hebert, J.R. 1982, 'Breath suspension during the transcendental meditation technique' *Psychosomatic Medicine* 44(2): 133–53.

Feuerstein, G. 1996, *The Shambala Guide to Yoga*, Shambala Publications, Boston.

Fink, J.B. 2002, 'Positioning versus postural drainage' *Respiratory Care* 47(7): 769–77.

Gallois, P. 1984, 'Modifications neurophysiologiques et respiratoires lors de la pratique des techniques de relaxation [Neurophysiologic and respiratory changes during the practice of relaxation techniques]' *L'Encephale* 10(3): 139–44.

Gardner, A.W., Katzel, L.I., Sorkin, J.D., Bradham, D.D., Hochberg, M.C., Flinn, W.R. and Goldberg, A.P. 2001, 'Exercise rehabilitation improves functional outcomes and peripheral circulation in patients with intermittent claudication: a randomized controlled trial' *Journal of the American Geriatrics Society* 49(6): 755–62.

Garfinkel, M.S., Schumacher, H.R. Jr, Husain, A., Levy, M. and Reshetar, R.A. 1994, 'Evaluation of a yoga based regimen for treatment of osteoarthritis of the hands' *The Journal of Rheumatology* 21(12): 2341–3.

Garfinkel, M.S., Singhal, A., Katz, W.A., Allan, D.A., Reshetar, R. and Schumacher, H.R. 1998, 'Yoga-based intervention for carpal tunnel syndrome: a randomized trial' *Journal of the American Medical Association* 280(18): 1601–3.

Ghosh, S. 1999, *The Original Yoga: As expounded in Sivasamhita, Gherandasamhita and Patanjala Yogasutra*, Munshiram Manoharlal Publishers Pvt. Ltd, New Delhi.

Gioia, G., Lin, B., Katz, R., DiMarino, A.J., Ogilby, J.D., Cassel, D., DePace, N.L., Heo, J. and Iskandrian, A.S. 1995, 'Use of a tantalum-178 generator and a multiwire gamma camera to study the effect of the Mueller maneuver on left ventricular performance: comparison to hemodynamics and single photon emission computed tomography perfusion patterns' *American Heart Journal* 130(5): 1062–7.

Glasscock, N.F., Turville, K.L., Joines, S.B. and Mirka, G.A. 1999, 'The effect of personality type on muscle coactivation during elbow flexion' *Human Factors* 1: 51–60.

Goswami, S.S. 1980, *Layayoga: An Advanced Method of Concentration*, Routledge & Kegan Paul, London.

Harte, J.L., Eifert, G.H. and Smith, R. 1995, 'The effects of running and meditation on beta-endorphin, corticotrophin-releasing hormone and cortisol in plasma and on mood' *Biological Psychology* 40(3): 251–65.

Herbert, R.D. and Gabriel, M. 2002, 'Effects of stretching before and after exercising on muscle soreness and risk of injury: systematic review' *British Medical Journal* 325: 7362–468.

Herzog, H., Lele, V.R., Kuwert, T., Langen, K.J., Kops, E.R. and Feinendegen, L.E. 1990, 'Changed pattern of regional glucose metabolism during yoga meditative relaxation' *Neuropsychobiology* 23(4): 182–7, 91.

Hewitt, J. 1983, *The Yoga of Breathing Posture and Meditation*, Random House, London.

Hillman, D.R. and Finucane, K.E. 1987, 'A model of the respiratory pump' *Journal of Applied Physiology* 63(3): 951–61.

Hudetz, J.A., Hudetz, A.G. and Klayman, J. 2000, 'Relationship between relaxation by guided imagery and performance of working memory' *Psychological Reports* 86(1): 15–20.

Iyengar, B.K.S. 1988, *The Tree of Yoga*, Shambala Publications, Massachusetts.

Iyengar, B.K.S. 1993, *Light on the Yoga Sutras of Patanjali*, Aquarian Press, London.

Iyengar, B.K.S. 2001, *Yoga: The Path to Holistic Health*, Dorling Kindersley Limited, London.

Jella, S.A. and Shannahoff-Khalsa, D.S. 1993, 'The effects of unilateral forced nostril breathing on cognitive performance' *The International Journal of Neuroscience* 73(1–2): 61–8.

Jevning, R., Anand, R., Biedebach, M. and Fernando, G. 1996, 'Effects on regional cerebral blood flow of transcendental meditation' *Physiology and Behavior* 59(3): 399–402.

Jevning, R., Wallace, R.K. and Beidebach, M. 1992, 'The physiology of meditation: a review. A wakeful hypometabolic integrated response' *Neuroscience and Biobehavioral Reviews* 16(3): 415–24.

Jin, P. 1992, 'Efficacy of Tai Chi, brisk walking, meditation, and reading in reducing mental and emotional stress' *Journal of Psychosomatic Research* 36(4): 361–70.

Junker, A. and Dworkis, S. 1986, 'Investigation of brain wave activity during yoga postures and meditation', PhD thesis, Dayton, Ohio. Results of a research project at Wright Patterson Air Force Base also incorporated into Andrew Junker's PhD thesis. For more information see <www.extensionyoga.com/7Principles.htm>.

Kamei, T., Toriumi, Y., Kimura, H., Ohno, S., Kumano, H. and Kimura, K. 2000, 'Decrease in serum cortisol during yoga exercise is correlated with alpha wave activation' *Perceptual and Motor Skills* 90(3), Pt 1: 1027–32.

Kannus, P., Alosa, D., Cook, L., Johnson, R.J., Renstrom, P., Pope, M., Beynnon, B., Yasuda, K., Nichols, C. and Kaplan, M. 1992, 'Effect of one-legged exercise on the strength, power & endurance of the contralateral leg. A randomized, controlled study using isometric & concentric isokinetic training' *European Journal of Applied Physiology* 64: 117–26.

Kesterson, J. and Clinch, N.F. 1989, 'Metabolic rate, respiratory exchange ratio, and apneas during meditation' *American Journal of Physiology* 256(3), Pt 2: R632–8.

Kocher, H.C. 1976, 'Effects of savasana on the extent of knee-jerk' *Yoga Mimamsa* XVIII(3–4): 40–7. (Quarterly journal of the Kaivalyadhama Yoga Research Institution, Lonavala, India.)

Kominars, K.D. 1997, 'A study of visualization and addiction treatment' *Journal of Substance Abuse Treatment* 14(3): 213–23.

Kroner-Herwig, B., Hebing, G., van Rijn-Kalkmann, U., Frenzel, A., Schilkowsky, G. and Esser, G. 1995, 'The management of chronic tinnitus—comparison of a cognitive-behavioural group training with yoga' *Journal of Psychosomatic Research* 39(2): 153–65.

Kubota, Y., Sato, W., Toichi, M., Murai, T., Okada, T., Hayashi, A. and Sengoku, A. 2001, 'Frontal midline theta rhythm is correlated with cardiac autonomic activities during the performance of an attention demanding meditation procedure' *Brain Research. Cognitive Brain Research* 11(2): 281–7.

Kutz, I., Burysenko, J.K. and Benson, H. 1985a, 'Meditation and psychotherapy: a rationale for the integration of dynamic psychotherapy, the relaxation response and mindfulness meditation' *American Journal of Psychiatry* 142: 1–8.

Kutz, I., Leserman, J., Dorrington, C., Morrison, C.H., Borysenko, J. and Benson, H. 1985b, 'Meditation as an adjunct to psychotherapy, an outcome study' *Psychotherapy Psychosomatics* 43: 209–18.

Kuvalayananda, S. 1925, 'X ray experiments on uddiyana and nauli in relation to the colon contents' *Yoga Mimamsa* I(1–4): 15–254. (Quarterly journal of the Kaivalyadhama Yoga Research Institution, Lonavala, India.)

Lazar, S.W., Bush, G., Gollub, R.L., Fricchione, G.L., Khalsa, G. and Benson, H. 2000, 'Functional brain mapping of the relaxation response and meditation' *Neuroreport* 11(7): 1581–5.

Liu, G.L., Cui, R.Q., Li, G.Z. and Huang, C.M. 1990, 'Changes in brainstem and cortical auditory potentials during Qi-Gong meditation' *The American Journal of Chinese Medicine* 18(3–4): 95–103.

Lowe, G., Bland, R., Greenman, J., Kirkpatrick, N. and Lowe, G. 2001, 'Progressive muscle relaxation and secretory immunoglobulin A' *Psychological Reports* 88(3), Pt 1: 912–14.

MacLean, C.R., Walton, K.G., Wenneberg, S.R., Levitsky, D.K., Mandarino, J.P., Waziri, R., Hillis, S.L. and Schneider, R.H. 1997, 'Effects of the Transcendental Meditation program on adaptive mechanisms: changes in hormone levels and responses to stress after 4 months of practice' *Psychoneuroendocrinology* 22(4): 277–95.

Madanmohan, Thombre, D.P., Balakumar, B., Nambinarayanan, T.K., Thakur, S., Krishnamurthy, N. and Chandrabose, A. 1992, 'An effect of yoga training on reaction time, respiratory endurance and muscle strength' *Indian Journal of Physiology and Pharmacology* 36(4): 229–33.

Malathi, A. and Damodaran, A. 1999, 'Stress due to exams in medical students—role of yoga' *Indian Journal of Physiology and Pharmacology* 43(2): 218–24.

Manchanda, S.C., Narang, R., Reddy, K.S., Sachdeva, U., Prabhakaran, D., Dharmanand, S., Rajani, M. and Bijlani, R. 2000, 'Retardation of coronary atherosclerosis with yoga lifestyle intervention' *The Journal of the Association of Physicians of India* 48(7): 687–94.

Manjunath, N.K. and Telles, S. 2001, 'Improved performance in the Tower of London test following yoga' *Indian Journal of Physiology and Pharmacology* 45(3): 351–4.

Miyamura, M., Nishimura, K., Ishida, K., Katayama, K., Shimaoka, M. and Hiruta, S. 2002, 'Is man able to breathe once a minute for an hour?: the effect of yoga respiration on blood gases' *Japanese Journal of Physiology* 52(3): 313–16.

Mohan, A.G. 2000, *Yoga-yajnavalkya*, Ganesh & Co., Madras.

Mohan, S.M. 1996, 'Svara (nostril dominance) and bilateral volar GSR' *Indian Journal of Physiology and Pharmacology* 40(1): 58–64.

Monteiro Pedro, V., Vitti, M., Bérzin, F. and Bevilaqua Grosso, D. 1999, 'The effect of free isotonic and maximal isometric contraction exercises of the hip adduction on vastus medialis oblique muscle: an electromyographic study' *Electromyographic Clinical Neurophysiology* 39(7): 435–40.

Moorthy, A.M. 1982, 'Effect of selected yoga asanas and physical exercises on flexibility' *Yoga Review* II(3): 161–6.

Motoyama, H. 1993, *A Study of Yoga from Eastern & Western Medical Viewpoints—Control of Body & Mind through the Activation of Prana (Ki)*, Human Science Press, Japan.

Nagarathna, R. and Nagendra, H.R. 1985, 'Yoga for bronchial asthma: a controlled study' *British Medical Journal* 291: 1077–9.

Narayan, R., Kamat, A., Khanolkar, M., Kamat, S., Desai, S.R. and Dhume, R.A. 1990, 'Quantitative evaluation of muscle relaxation induced by kundalini yoga with the help of E.M.G. integrator' *Indian Journal of Physiology and Pharmacology* 34(4): 279–81.

Naveen, K.V., Nagarathna, R., Nagendra, H.R. and Telles, S. 1997, 'Yoga breathing through a particular nostril increases spatial memory scores without lateralized effects' *Psychological Reports* 81(2): 555–61.

O'Brien, M. 2001, 'Exercise and osteoporosis' *Irish Journal of Medical Science* 170(1): 58–62.

Orsted, H.L., Radke, L. and Gorst, R. 2001, 'The impact of musculoskeletal changes on the dynamics of the calf muscle pump' *Ostomy Wound Management* 47(10): 18–24.

Panjwani, U., Gupta, H.L., Singh, S.H., Selvamurthy, W. and Rai, U.C. 1995, 'Effect of Sahaja yoga practice on stress management in patients of epilepsy' *Indian Journal of Physiology and Pharmacology* 39(2): 111–16.

Pansare, M.S., Kulkarni, A.N. and Pendse, U.B. 1989, 'Effect of yogic training on serum LDH levels' *The Journal of Sports Medicine and Physical Fitness* 29(2): 177–8.

Parrino, L., Smerieri, A. and Terzano, M.G. 2001, 'Combined influence of cyclic arousability and EEG syncrony on generalized interictal discharges within the sleep cycle' *Epilepsy Research* 44(1): 7–18.

Patel, C. and North, W.R. 1975, 'Randomised controlled trial of yoga and bio-feedback in management of hypertension' *The Lancet* 93–5.

Pedersen, B.K. and Toft, A.D. 2000, 'Effects of exercise on lymphocytes and cytokines' *British Journal of Sports Medicine* 34(4): 246–51.

Peng, C.K., Mietus, J.E., Liu, Y., Khalsa, G., Douglas, P.S., Benson, H. and Goldberger, A.L. 1999, 'Exaggerated heart rate oscillations during two meditation techniques' *International Journal of Cardiology* 70(2): 101–7.

Pranavananda, Y. 1992, *Pure Yoga*, Motilal Banarsidass Publishers Pvt Ltd, New Delhi.

Proske, U., Wise, A.K. and Gregory, J.E. 2000, 'The role of muscle receptors in the detection of movements' *Progress in Neurobiology* 60(1): 85–96.

Raghuraj, P., Nagarathna, R., Nagendra, H.R. and Telles, S. 1997, 'Pranayama increases grip strength without lateralized effects' *Indian Journal of Physiology and Pharmacology* 41(2): 129–33.

Raghuraj, P. and Telles, S. 1997, 'Muscle power, dexterity skill and visual perception in community home girls trained in yoga or sports and in regular school girls' *Indian Journal of Physiology and Pharmacology* 41(4): 409–15.

Raju, P.S., Kumar, K.A., Reddy, S.S., Madhavi, S., Gnanakumari, K., Bhaskaracharyulu, C., Reddy, M.V., Annapurna, N., Reddy, M.E., Girijakumari, D. 1986, 'Effect of yoga on exercise tolerance in normal healthy volunteers' *Indian Journal of Physiology and Pharmacology* 30(2): 121–32.

Raju, P.S., Madhavi, S., Prasad, K.V., Reddy, M.V., Reddy, M.E., Sahay, B.K. and Murthy, K.J. 1994, 'Comparison of effects of yoga & physical exercise in athletes' *Indian Journal of Medical Research* 100: 81–6.

Ray, U.S., Mukhopadhyaya, S., Purkayastha, S.S., Asnani, V., Tomer, O.S., Prashad, R., Thakur, L. and Selvamurthy, W. 2001, 'Effect of yogic exercises on physical and mental health of young fellowship course trainees' *Indian Journal of Physiology and Pharmacology* 45(1): 37–53.

Rood, Y.R., Bogaards, M., Goulmy, E. and Houwelingen, H.C. 1993, 'The effects of stress and relaxation on the *in vitro* immune response in man: a meta-analytic study' *Journal of Behavioral Medicine* 16(2): 163–81.

Scheler, M.F. 1992, 'Effects of optimism on psychological and physical wellbeing: theoretical and empirical update' *Cognitive Therapy and Research* 16: 201–28.

Schell, F.J., Allolio, B. and Schonecke, O.W. 1994, 'Physiological and psychological effects of Hatha-Yoga exercise in healthy women' *International Journal of Psychosomatics* 41(1–4): 46–52.

Schiff, B.B. and Rump, S.A. 1995, 'Asymmetrical hemispheric activation and emotion: the effects of unilateral forced nostril breathing' *Brain Cognition* 29(3): 217–31.

Sei, H. and Morita, Y. 1996, 'Acceleration of EEG theta wave precedes the phasic surge of arterial pressure during REM sleep in the rat' *Neuroreport* 7(18): 3059–62.

Selvamurthy, W., Sridharan, K., Ray, U.S., Tiwary, R.S., Hegde, K.S., Radhakrishan, U. and Sinha, K.C. 1998, 'A new physiological approach to control essential hypertension' *Indian Journal of Physiology and Pharmacology* 42(2): 205–13.

Shaffer, H.J., LaSalvia, T.A. and Stein, J.P. 1997, 'Comparing Hatha yoga with dynamic group psychotherapy for enhancing methadone maintenance treatment: a randomized clinical trial' *Alternative Therapies in Health and Medicine* 3(4): 57–66.

Shah, C.S. 2001, 'The Tantras and the concept of Kundalini Shakti', at <www.boloji.com/hinduism/kundalini.htm>.

Shannahoff-Khalsa, D.S. and Kennedy, B. 1993, 'The effects of unilateral forced nostril breathing on the heart' *The International Journal of Neuroscience* 73(1–2): 47–60.

Shapiro, D.H. 1992, 'Adverse effects of meditation: a preliminary investigation of long-term meditators' *International Journal of Psychosomatics* 39(1–4): 62–7.

Sim, M.K. and Tsol, W.F. 1992, 'The effects of centrally acting drugs on the EEG correlates of meditation' *Biofeedback Self-Regulation* 17(3): 215–20.

Singh, V., Wisniewski, A., Britton, J. and Tattersfield, A. 1990, 'Effect of yoga breathing exercises (pranayama) on airway reactivity in subjects with asthma' *The Lancet* 335: 1381–3.

Solberg, E.E., Ingjer, F., Holen, A., Sundgot-Borgen, J., Nilsson, S. and Holme, I. 2000, 'Stress reactivity to and recovery from a standardised exercise bout: a study of 31 runners practising relaxation techniques' *British Journal of Sports Medicine* 34(4): 268–72.

Stancak, A. Jr, Pfeffer, D., Hrudova, L., Sovka, P. and Dostalek, C. 1993, 'Electro-encephalographic correlates of paced breathing' *Neuroreport* 4(6): 723–6.

Stancak, A. Jr and Kuna, M. 1994, 'EEG changes during forced alternate nostril breathing' *International Journal of Psychophysiology* 18(1): 75–9.

Stanescu, D.C., Nemery, B., Veriter, C. and Marechal, C. 1981, 'Pattern of breathing and ventilatory response to CO_2 in subjects practising hatha-yoga' *Journal of Applied Physiology* 51: 1625–9.

Stigsby, B., Rodenberg, J.C. and Moth, H.B. 1981, 'Electroencephalographic findings during mantra meditation (transcendental meditation). A controlled, quantitative study of experienced meditators' *Electroencephalography and Clinical Neurophysiology* 51(4): 434–42.

Sudsuang, R., Chentanez, V. and Veluvan, K. 1991, 'Effect of Buddhist meditation on serum cortisol and total protein levels, blood pressure, pulse rate, lung volume and reaction time' *Physiology and Behavior* 50(3): 543–8.

Telles, S., Hanumanthaiah, B., Nagarathna, R. and Nagendra, H.R. 1993, 'Improvement in static motor performance following yogic training of school children' *Perceptual and Motor Skills* 76(3), Pt 2: 1264–6.

Telles, S., Hanumanthaiah, B.H., Nagarathna, R. and Nagendra, H.R. 1994a, 'Plasticity of motor control systems demonstrated by yoga training' *Indian Journal of Physiology and Pharmacology* 38(2): 143–4.

Telles, S., Nagarathna, R. and Nagendra, H.R. 1994b, 'Breathing through a particular nostril can alter metabolism and autonomic activities' *Indian Journal of Physiology and Pharmacology* 38(2): 133–7.

Telles, S., Nagarathna, R. and Nagendra, H.R. 1995, 'Autonomic changes during "OM" meditation' *Indian Journal of Physiology and Pharmacology* 39(4): 418–20.

Telles, S., Nagarathna, R. and Nagendra, H.R. 1996, 'Physiological measures of right nostril breathing' *Journal of Alternative and Complementary Medicine* (New York) 2(4): 479–84.

Teramoto, S., Sugai, M., Saito, E., Matsuse, T., Eto, M., Toba, K. and Ouchi, Y. 1997, 'Hyperventilation syndrome in a very old woman' *Nippon Ronen Igakkai Zasshi* March: 226–9.

Tooley, G.A., Armstrong, S.M., Norman, T.R. and Sali, A. 2000, 'Acute increases in night-time plasma melatonin levels following a period of meditation' *Biological Psychology* 53(1): 69–78.

Travis, F., 2001, 'Autonomic and EEG patterns distinguish transcending from other experiences during Transcendental Meditation practice' *International Journal of Psychophysiology* 42(1): 1–9.

Travis, F.T. and Orme-Johnson, D.W. 1989, 'Field model of consciousness: EEG coherence changes as indicators of field effects' *International Journal of Neuroscience* 49: 203–11.

Travis, F. and Pearson, C. 2000, 'Pure consciousness: distinct phenomenological and physiological correlates of "consciousness itself"' *The International Journal of Neuroscience* 100(1–4): 77–89.

Travis, F. and Wallace, R.K. 1997, 'Autonomic patterns during respiratory suspensions: possible markers of Transcendental Consciousness' *Psychophysiology* 34(1): 39–46.

Vempati, R.P. and Telles, S. 2002, 'Yoga-based guided relaxation reduces sympathetic activity judged from baseline levels' *Psychological Reports* 90(2): 487–94.

Vishnu-Devananda, S. 1987, *Hatha Yoga Pradipika of Swatmarama: The Classic Guide for the Advanced Practice of Hatha Yoga*, with 1897 commentary of Brahmananda and 1987 commentary of Vishnu-Devandana, OM Lotus Publishing Company, New York.

Wallace, R.K., Dillbeck, M., Jacobe, E. and Harrington, B. 1982, 'The effects of the transcendental meditation and TM-Sidhi program on the aging process' *International Journal of Neuroscience* 16(1): 53–8.

Weber, S. 1996, 'The effects of relaxation exercises on anxiety levels in psychiatric inpatients' *Journal of Holistic Nursing* 14(3): 196–205.

Wenneberg, S.R., Schneider, R.H., Walton, K.G., Maclean, C.R., Levitsky, D.K., Salerno, J.W., Wallace, R.K., Mandarino, J.V., Rainforth, M.V. and Waziri, R. 1997, 'A controlled study of the effects of the Transcendental Meditation program on cardiovascular reactivity and ambulatory blood pressure' *The International Journal of Neuroscience* 89(1–2): 15–28.

Werntz, D.A., Bickford, R.G. and Shannahoff-Khalsa, D. 1987, 'Selective hemispheric stimulation by unilateral forced nostril breathing' *Human Neurobiology* 6(3): 165–71.

Wilson, A.F., Jevning, R. and Gulch, S. 1987, 'Marked reduction of forearm carbon dioxide production during states of decreased metabolism' *Physiology and Behavior* 41: 347–52.

Wolkove, N., Kreisman, H., Darragh, D., Cohen, C. and Frank, H. 1984, 'Effect of transcendental meditation on breathing and respiratory control' *Journal of Applied Physiology: Respiratory, Environmental and Exercise Physiology* 56(3): 607–12.

Wood, C. 1993, 'Mood change and perceptions of vitality: a comparison of the effects of relaxation, visualization and yoga' *Journal of the Royal Society of Medicine* 86(5): 254–8.

Yan, Q. and Sun, Y. 1996, 'Quantitative research for improving respiratory muscle contraction by breathing exercise' *Chinese Medical Journal* 109(10): 771–5.

Yeshe, L. 1999, *Make Your Mind an Ocean: Aspects of Buddhist Psychology*, Lama Yeshe Wisdom Archive, Boston.

Zeier, H., 1984, 'Arousal reduction with biofeedback-supported respiratory meditation' *Biofeedback Self-Regulation* 9(4): 497–508.

Conclusion Challenges facing integrated medicine

Bensoussan, A. and Myers, S.P. 1996, *Towards a Safer Choice: The Practice of Traditional Chinese Medicine in Australia*, University of Western Sydney, Sydney.

Bensoussan, A., Myers, S.P. and Carlton, A.L. 2000, 'Risks presented by the practice of Chinese herbal medicine: an Australian study' *Archives of Family Medicine* 9(10): 1071–8.

BMA Scientific Division 1993, *Complementary Medicine. New Approaches to Good Practice*, Oxford University Press, Oxford.

Chalmers, I., Enkin, M. and Keirse, M.J.N.C. (eds) 1989, *Effective Care in Pregnancy and Childbirth*, Oxford University Press, Oxford.

Delbridge, A. and Bernard, J.R.L. (eds) 1998, *Macquarie Dictionary*, Macquarie Library Pty Ltd, Sydney.

Fulder, S. 1996, *The Handbook of Alternative and Complementary Medicine*, Oxford University Press, Oxford.

Linde, K. and Mulrow, C.D. 2001, 'St John's Wort for depression (Cochrane Review)', in *The Cochrane Library*, Issue 2, Update Software, Oxford.

Sackett, D.L., Rosenburg, W.M.C., Grey, J.A.M., Haynes, R.B. and Richardson, W.S. 1996, 'Evidence-based medicine: what it is and what it isn't' *British Medical Journal* 312(7023): 71–2.

St George, D. 2001, 'Integrated medicine. Integrated medicine means doctors will be in charge' *British Medical Journal* 322(7300): 1484.

Wilk, C.A. 1996, *Medicine, Monopolies and Malice*, Avery Publishing Group, New York.

Wilson, K. and Mills, E.J. 2002, 'Introducing evidence-based complementary and alternative medicine: answering the challenge' *The Journal of Alternative and Complementary Medicine* 8(2): 103–5.

INDEX

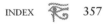

Havering College Sixth Form Library

6537254

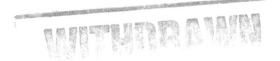

Resource Centre 01277 220808

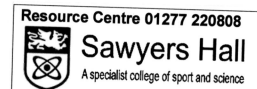

Sawyers Hall

A specialist college of sport and science